Obstetrical Anesthesia

Editors

MAY C.M. PIAN-SMITH
REBECCA D. MINEHART

ANESTHESIOLOGY CLINICS

www.anesthesiology.theclinics.com

Consulting Editor
LEE A. FLEISHER

December 2021 • Volume 39 • Number 4

ELSEVIER

1600 John F. Kennedy Boulevard • Suite 1800 • Philadelphia, Pennsylvania, 19103-2899

http://www.theclinics.com

ANESTHESIOLOGY CLINICS Volume 39, Number 4
December 2021 ISSN 1932-2275, ISBN-13: 978-0-323-84942-5

Editor: Joanna Collett
Developmental Editor: Arlene Campos

Anesthesiology Clinics (ISSN 1932-2275) is published quarterly by Elsevier Inc., 360 Park Avenue South, New York, NY 10010-1710. Months of issue are March, June, September, and December. Periodicals postage paid at New York, NY and at additional mailing offices. Subscription prices are $100.00 per year (US student/resident), $368.00 per year (US individuals), $455.00 per year (Canadian individuals), $957.00 per year (US institutions), $1000.00 per year (Canadian institutions), $100.00 per year (Canadian student/resident), $225.00 per year (foreign student/resident), $488.00 per year (foreign individuals), and $1000.00 per year (foreign institutions). To receive student and resident rate, orders must be accompanied by name of affiliated institution, date of term, and the *signature* of program/residency coordinator on institutions letterhead. Orders will be billed at individual rate until proof of status is received. Foreign air speed delivery is included in all *Clinics'* subscription prices. All prices are subject to change without notice. POSTMASTER: Send address changes to *Anesthesiology Clinics,* Elsevier Health Sciences Division, Subscription Customer Service, 3251 Riverport Lane, Maryland Heights, MO 63043. Customer Service (orders, claims, online, change of address): Elsevier Health Sciences Division, Subscription Customer Service, 3251 Riverport Lane, Maryland Heights, MO 63043. **Tel:1-800-654-2452 (U.S. and Canada); 314-447-8871 (outside U.S. and Canada). Fax: 314-447-8029. E-mail: journalscustomerservice-usa@elsevier.com (for print support); journalsonlinesupport-usa@elsevier.com (for online support).**

Reprints. For copies of 100 or more of articles in this publication, please contact the Commercial Reprints Department, Elsevier Inc., 360 Park Avenue South, New York, NY 10010-1710. Tel.: 212-633-3874; Fax: 212-633-3820; E-mail: reprints@elsevier.com.

Anesthesiology Clinics, is also published in Spanish by McGraw-Hill Inter-americana Editores S. A., P.O. Box 5-237, 06500 Mexico D. F., Mexico.

Anesthesiology Clinics, is covered in *MEDLINE/PubMed (Index Medicus), Current Contents/Clinical Medicine, Excerpta Medica, ISI/BIOMED*, and *Chemical Abstracts*.

Contributors

CONSULTING EDITOR

LEE A. FLEISHER, MD
Professor and Former Chair of Anesthesiology and Critical Care, Professor of Medicine, Perelman School of Medicine, University of Pennsylvania, Philadelphia, Pennsylvania, USA

EDITORS

MAY C.M. PIAN-SMITH, MD, MS
Division Chief, Quality and Safety, Associate Professor, Department of Anesthesia, Critical Care and Pain Medicine, Massachusetts General Hospital, Harvard Medical School, Boston, Massachusetts, USA

REBECCA D. MINEHART, MD, MSHPEd
Interim Division Chief of Obstetric Anesthesia, Program Director, Obstetric Anesthesia Fellowship, Assistant Professor of Anesthesia, Department of Anesthesia, Critical Care and Pain Medicine, Massachusetts General Hospital, Harvard Medical School, Boston, Massachusetts, USA

AUTHORS

GILLIAN ABIR, MBChB, FRCA
Clinical Professor, Department of Anesthesiology, Perioperative and Pain Medicine, Center for Academic Medicine, Stanford University School of Medicine, Palo Alto, California, USA

JEANETTE R. BAUCHAT, MD, MS
Associate Professor of Anesthesiology, Vanderbilt University Medical Center, Nashville, Tennessee, USA

JENNIFER M. BANAYAN, MD
Associate Professor, Department of Anesthesiology, Northwestern University, Northwestern McGaw Medical Center, Northwestern University Feinberg School of Medicine, Chicago, Illinois, USA

ERICA COFFIN, MD
Director, Obstetric Anesthesia, Department of Anesthesiology, West Penn Hospital/Allegheny Health Network, Pittsburgh, Pennsylvania, USA

JENNIFER E. DOMINGUEZ, MD, MHS
Associate Professor of Anesthesiology, Duke University Medical Center, Durham, North Carolina, USA

ROBERT A. DYER, MBChB (UCT), FCA (SA), PhD
Department of Anaesthesia and Perioperative Medicine, University of Cape Town, D23
Department of Anaesthesia and Perioperative Medicine, Groote Schuur Hospital, Cape Town, South Africa

NICOLE L. FERNANDES, MBChB (UCT), MMed (UCT), FCA (SA)
Department of Anaesthesia and Perioperative Medicine, University of Cape Town, D23
Department of Anaesthesia and Perioperative Medicine, Groote Schuur Hospital, Cape Town, South Africa

JACQUELINE M. GALVAN, MD
Associate Professor, Department of Anesthesiology, University of Illinois at Chicago, Chicago, Illinois, USA

REBECCA S. HIMMELWRIGHT, MD
Duke University Medical Center, Durham, North Carolina, USA

DANIEL KATZ, MD
Associate Professor of Anesthesiology, Perioperative and Pain Medicine, Associate Professor of Obstetrics, Gynecology and Reproductive Science, Vice Chair of Education, Department of Anesthesiology, Perioperative and Pain Medicine, Mount Sinai Hospital, New York, New York, USA

KLAUS KJAER, MD, MBA
Professor of Clinical Anesthesiology, Weill Cornell Medical College, New York, New York, USA

SARAH KROH, MD
Fellow, Obstetric Anesthesiology, UPMC Magee Women's Hospital, University of Pittsburgh Medical School, Pittsburgh, Pennsylvania, USA

ELIZABETH LUEBBERT, DO
PGY3 Anesthesiology Resident, Department of Anesthesiology, Perioperative and Pain Medicine, Mount Sinai Morningside and West Hospitals, New York, New York, USA

BRYAN MAHONEY, MD
Associate Professor, Department of Anesthesiology, Perioperative and Pain Medicine, Mount Sinai Morningside and West Hospitals, New York, New York, USA

DAVID G. MANN, MD, DBe
Associate Professor, Department of Pediatric Anesthesiology, Perioperative, and Pain Medicine, Chief, Clinical Ethics, Texas Children's Hospital, Baylor College of Medicine, Houston, Texas, USA

LESLIE J. MATTHEWS, MD, PharmD
Obstetric Anesthesiology Fellow, Department of Anesthesiology, The Ohio State University, Pediatric Anesthesiologist, Department of Anesthesiology and Pain Medicine, Nationwide Children's Hospital, Columbus, Ohio, USA

ALICIA MENCHACA, MD
Abigail Wexner Research Institute, Center for Regenerative Medicine, Nationwide Children's Hospital, Columbus, Ohio, USA

REBECCA D. MINEHART, MD, MSHPEd
Interim Division Chief of Obstetric Anesthesia, Program Director, Obstetric Anesthesia Fellowship, Assistant Professor, Department of Anesthesia, Critical Care and Pain Medicine, Massachusetts General Hospital, Harvard Medical School, Boston, Massachusetts, USA

EMILY E. NAOUM, MD
Instructor in Anesthesia, Department of Anesthesia, Critical Care and Pain Medicine, Massachusetts General Hospital, Boston, Massachusetts, USA

KAITLYN E. NEUMANN, MD, MEd
Instructor, Department of Anesthesiology, Northwestern University, Northwestern McGaw Medical Center, Northwestern University Feinberg School of Medicine, Chicago, Illinois, USA

HEATHER C. NIXON, MD
Associate Professor, Department of Anesthesiology, University of Illinois at Chicago, Chicago, Illinois, USA

OLUTOYIN A. OLUTOYE, MD, MSc
Department of Anesthesiology, Perioperative and Pain Medicine, Texas Children's Hospital, Baylor College of Medicine, Houston, Texas, USA

KATHERINE M. SELIGMAN, MD, FRCPC, D.ABA
Clinical Assistant Professor, Department of Anesthesiology, Pharmacology and Therapeutics, University of British Columbia, Vancouver, British Columbia, Canada

LAURA L. SORABELLA, MD
Assistant Professor of Anesthesiology, Vanderbilt University Medical Center, Nashville, Tennessee, USA

DAVID L. STAHL, MD
Associate Clinical Professor, Department of Anesthesiology, The Ohio State University, Columbus, Ohio, USA

CANDACE STYLE, MD, MS
Abigail Wexner Research Institute, Center for Regenerative Medicine, Nationwide Children's Hospital, Columbus, Ohio, USA

CAITLIN D. SUTTON, MD
Assistant Professor, Department of Pediatric Anesthesiology, Perioperative, and Pain Medicine, Chief, Division of Maternal-Fetal Anesthesia, Texas Children's Hospital, Baylor College of Medicine, Houston, Texas, USA

DOMINIQUE VAN DYK, MBChB (UCT), FCA (SA)
Department of Anaesthesia and Perioperative Medicine, University of Cape Town, D23 Department of Anaesthesia and Perioperative Medicine, Groote Schuur Hospital, Cape Town, South Africa

TRACEY M. VOGEL, MD
Obstetric Anesthesiologist, Perinatal Trauma-Informed Care Specialist, Department of Anesthesiology, West Penn Hospital/Allegheny Health Network, Pittsburgh, Pennsylvania, USA

ELISA C. WALSH, MD
Instructor in Anesthesia, Department of Anesthesia, Critical Care and Pain Medicine, Massachusetts General Hospital, Boston, Massachusetts, USA

JONATHAN H. WATERS, MD
Professor, Anesthesiology and Perioperative Medicine, Chief of Anesthesiology, UPMC Magee-Womens Hospital, Medical Director, Patient Blood Management Program, Pittsburgh, Pennsylvania, USA

Contents

> Obstetric hemorrhage is a leading cause of morbidity and mortality. Prevention includes identifying patients with risk factors and actively managing the third stage of labor. The anesthesiologist should be ready to manage hemorrhage with general strategies as well as strategies tailored to the specific cause of hemorrhage. Both neuraxial anesthesia and general anesthesia are appropriate in different situations. Treatments proven to be effective include increasing the oxytocin infusion, administering tranexamic acid early, guiding transfusion with point-of-care tests, and using cell salvage. Utilization of protocols and checklists within systems that encourage effective communication between teams should be implemented.

> Quality assurance (QA) is the maintenance of a desired level of quality, whereas quality improvement (QI) is the continuous process of creating systems to make things better. Implementation science promotes the systematic uptake of best practices. Bundles are a structured list of best practices whereas toolkits provide the necessary details, rationale, and implementation materials, such as sample policies and protocols. Metrics that can guide care on the labor and delivery (L&D) floor may be related to team structure (obstetric, multidisciplinary, anesthetic), processes (patient monitoring, team effects), and outcomes (postpartum hemorrhage, venous thromboembolism). Multiple anesthetic quality metrics have been proposed, including the mode of anesthesia for cesarean delivery.

> Utilization of emergency resources in obstetrics can help to optimize health care providers' care to pregnant and postpartum patients. There is a vast array of resources with various accessibility modalities that can be used before, during, and/or after an obstetric emergency. These resources can also be included as teaching material to increase knowledge and awareness with the aim to reduce maternal morbidity and mortality and improve patient outcomes.

Simulation has played a critical role in medicine for decades as a pedagogical and assessment tool. The labor and delivery unit provides an ideal setting for the use of simulation technology. Prior reviews of this topic have focused on simulation for individual and team training and assessment. The COVID-19 pandemic has provided an opportunity for educators and leaders in obstetric anesthesiology to rapidly train health care providers and develop new protocols for patient care with simulation. This review surveys new developments in simulation for obstetric anesthesiology with an emphasis on simulation use during the COVID-19 pandemic.

Maternal morbidity and mortality are rising due in part to the rising prevalence of chronic illness, socioeconomic and racial disparities, and advanced maternal age. Prevention of maternal adverse outcomes requires prompt escalation of care to facilities with appropriate capabilities including intensive care services. The development of obstetrical-specific risk assessment tools and protocolized care for the most common causes of maternal intensive care unit (ICU) admission has helped to reduce preventable complications. However, significant work remains to address barriers to the escalation of maternal care and minimize delays in appropriate management.

Postpartum respiratory depression is a complex, multifactorial issue that encompasses a patient's baseline preexisting conditions, certain pregnancy-specific conditions or complications, as well as the iatrogenic element of various medications given in the peripartum period. In this review, we discuss many of these factors including obesity, sleep-disordered breathing, chronic lung disease, neuromuscular disorders, opioids, preeclampsia, peripartum cardiomyopathy, postpartum hemorrhage, amniotic fluid embolism, sepsis, acute respiratory distress syndrome (ARDS), and medications such as analgesics, sedatives, anesthetics, and magnesium. Current recommendations for screening, treatment, and prevention are also discussed.

The authors provide a review of recent advances in the understanding of pathophysiology and perioperative management of preeclampsia and eclampsia, from the perspective of the anesthesiologist. This review includes aspects of assessment of severity of disease, hemodynamic monitoring, peripartum anesthesia care, and postpartum management. The perioperative management of patients with eclampsia is also discussed.

Jacqueline M. Galvan and Heather C. Nixon

Pharmacologic thromboprophylaxis from venous thromboembolism (VTE) and thrombocytopenia in pregnancy results in conditions that may preclude the use of neuraxial anesthesia due to a perceived risk of spinal/epidural hematoma. Spinal epidural hematoma is a recognized complication in patients who are hypocoagulable and may lead patients to undergo general anesthesia for delivery or other procedures, which carries numerous complications in obstetric care. A robust understanding of maternal physiologic changes in coagulation status, review of consensus statements, and safety bundles may help to maximize the use of neuraxial anesthesia in obstetric patients who might otherwise be denied these anesthetic techniques.

Laura L. Sorabella and Jeanette R. Bauchat

This review summarizes the importance of enhanced recovery after surgery (ERAS) implementation for cesarean deliveries (CDs) and explores ERAS elements shared with the non-obstetric surgical population. The Society for Obstetric Anesthesia and Perinatology (SOAP) consensus statement on ERAS for CD is used as a template for the discussion. Suggested areas for research to improve our understanding of ERAS in the obstetric population are delineated. Strategies and examples of anesthesia-specific protocol elements are included.

David L. Stahl and Leslie J. Matthews

Parturients with substance use disorder require expertise to manage the complexity of intoxication, withdrawal, and chronic use as well as ensure adequate analgesia throughout labor. Opioid use disorder in pregnancy has increased more than 4-fold in the past decade, with a 50-fold geographic variability that now dwarfs other substance use in this population. Understanding not only the medical but also the public health and criminal justice implications of substance use disorder is essential to providing optimal care to this at-risk population.

Tracey M. Vogel and Erica Coffin

The integration of trauma-informed care practices into the care of obstetric patients requires an understanding of psychological trauma, its impact on this population, and how trauma-informed care can be adapted to improve outcomes for those patients with a previous history of trauma or for those that experience peripartum trauma. System-based changes to policies, protocols, and practices are needed to achieve sustainable change. Maternal morbidity and mortality that result from trauma-related and other mental health conditions in the peripartum period are significant. Innovative approaches to the prevention of negative birth experiences and retraumatization during labor and delivery are needed.

ANESTHESIOLOGY CLINICS

SERIES OF RELATED INTEREST

Advances in Anesthesia
Critical Care Clinics

THE CLINICS ARE AVAILABLE ONLINE!
Access your subscription at:
www.theclinics.com

ANESTHESIOLOGY CLINICS

FORTHCOMING ISSUES

March 2022
Enhanced Recovery after Surgery and Perioperative Medicine
Michael Scott, Anton Krige, and Michael Grocott, Editors

September 2022
Total Well-being
Alison J Brainard and Lyndsay M. Hoy, Editors

RECENT ISSUES

September 2021
Perioperative Monitoring
Gabriella Iohom and Girish P. Joshi, Editors

June 2021
Anesthesiologists in Times of Disaster
Jesse Raiten and Lee A. Fleisher, Editors

March 2021
Neuroanesthesia
Jeffrey R. Kirsch and Cynthia A. Lien, Editors

SERIES OF RELATED INTEREST

Advances in Anesthesia
Critical Care Clinics

THE CLINICS ARE AVAILABLE ONLINE!
Access your subscription at:
www.theclinics.com

Foreword

Care of the Obstetric Patient: Mitigating Risk

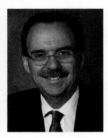

Lee A. Fleisher, MD
Consulting Editor

Maternal morbidity and mortality have been increasing over the last several decades, and anesthesiologists need to be engaged in working with their obstetric colleagues in mitigating risk. In addition, there are wide disparities in complications when stratified by race and ethnicity. Most of us trained in obstetric anesthesia care during our residency and may not be aware of these trends or our ability to intervene. In this issue of *Anesthesiology Clinics*, the editors have assembled a series of articles that highlight the anesthesiologist's role in addressing peripartum complications and high-risk individuals. They have also included articles on ERAS (enhanced recovery after surgery) and ethics. It will allow us to assume shared accountability for peripartum care.

In order to commission an issue on obstetric anesthesia care, I have turned to colleagues at Massachusetts General Hospital (MGH). May Pian-Smith is Associate Professor of Anesthesia at Harvard Medical School and Division Chief for Quality and Safety in the Department of Anesthesia, Critical Care, and Pain Medicine at MGH. Her research has been focused on improving the health care of women. She has pursued fellowship training in Medical Education and Patient Safety and lectures on fostering trust. Rebecca Minehart is Assistant Professor of Anaesthesia at Harvard Medical School and Program Director for Obstetric Anesthesia Fellowship at MGH. She has received grant funding for research in education from the Foundation for Anesthesia Education and Research as well as the Executive Committee on Teaching and Education at MGH. In addition, she is a member of the ASA's Interactive Computer-Based Education Editorial Board, and the Chair of the Society

Anesthesiology Clin 39 (2021) xiii–xiv
https://doi.org/10.1016/j.anclin.2021.10.001
1932-2275/21/© 2021 Published by Elsevier Inc.

for Obstetric Anesthesia and Perinatology Fellowship Program Directors' Committee. Together, they have edited an important issue.

Lee A. Fleisher, MD
Perelman School of Medicine at
University of Pennsylvania
3400 Spruce Street, Dulles 680
Philadelphia, PA 19104, USA

E-mail address:
Lee.Fleisher@pennmedicine.upenn.edu

Preface

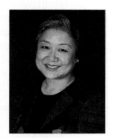 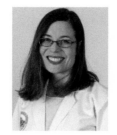

May C.M. Pian-Smith, MD, MS   Rebecca D. Minehart, MD, MSHPEd
Editors

It has been our privilege to bring together this collection of articles on key issues in obstetrical anesthesiology. The last issue of *Anesthesiology Clinics* devoted to obstetrical anesthesia was published in 2017. So much has changed in the intervening years, reflecting the increasingly significant impact that skilled and informed anesthetists can have on improving maternal care. As our pregnant patients are becoming more medically complex, our management of obstetrical anesthesia has also become more tailored, nuanced, and impactful. We are appreciating ways we can influence the difference between good obstetrical anesthesia care and excellent obstetrical anesthesia care.

One tangible acknowledgment of the value of excellent obstetrical care was the establishment in 2018 of the Society of Obstetric Anesthesia and Perinatology Centers of Excellence. This competitive designation is awarded to institutions and programs that have implemented programming and invested in resources to offer the highest possible quality of obstetrical anesthesia care, nationally and internationally.

The articles in this issue were chosen to reflect topics whereby anesthesiologists contribute to truly exceptional obstetrical care. Together, they offer some historic perspective and are important updates from known experts. Most importantly, they are meant to inspire our readers to think about ways we anesthesiologists can be innovative clinicians, and effective leaders in collaborative teams, system improvements, and collective learning.

We would like to thank Dr Lee Fleisher for entrusting us with editing this issue, and to our publishing partners, Arlene Campos and Joanna Collette, who demonstrated enormous patience throughout this process. It was a true pleasure to work with them on this endeavor.

Finally, we need to thank our individual authors, for whom this issue became a labor of love during the unprecedented professional and personal challenges of the COVID-19 pandemic. Anesthesiologists across the world rose to the occasion, flexing and pivoting to meet rapidly evolving clinical needs. For obstetrical anesthesiologists, the patients kept coming; there was never an option to cancel "elective" cases. We are so grateful to our authors for making this *Anesthesiology Clinics* project a priority. Their

Anesthesiology Clin 39 (2021) xv–xvi
https://doi.org/10.1016/j.anclin.2021.09.001
anesthesiology.theclinics.com
1932-2275/21/© 2021 Elsevier Inc. All rights reserved.

dedication is truly a gift to fellow clinicians who strive to bring their absolute best to the care of every obstetrical patient, every day, everywhere.

May C.M. Pian-Smith, MD, MS
Department of Anesthesia, Critical Care &
Pain Medicine
Massachusetts General Hospital
Harvard Medical School
55 Fruit Street, GRJ 440
Boston, MA 02114, USA

Rebecca D. Minehart, MD, MSHPEd
Department of Anesthesia, Critical Care &
Pain Medicine
Massachusetts General Hospital
Harvard Medical School
55 Fruit Street, GRJ 440
Boston, MA 02114, USA

E-mail addresses:
MPIANSMITH@mgh.harvard.edu (M.C.M. Pian-Smith)
RMINEHART@mgh.harvard.edu (R.D. Minehart)

Obstetrical Hemorrhage

Sarah Kroh, MD[a,*], Jonathan H. Waters, MD[b]

KEYWORDS

- Postpartum hemorrhage • Obstetric hemorrhage • Obstetric emergency
- Obstetric anesthesia • Maternal morbidity • Uterine atony • Transfusion • Cell saver

KEY POINTS

- Many patients who experience postpartum hemorrhage, defined as blood loss of greater than 1000 mL accompanied by symptoms, show no risk factors beforehand, and early diagnosis of hemorrhage is challenging.
- Uterine atony is the most common cause of hemorrhage, and the anesthesiologist should understand active management of the third stage of labor for prevention.
- Both neuraxial anesthesia and general anesthesia are appropriate during ongoing hemorrhage, and the decision of which to use will be made based on the situation.
- There is evidence that up-titration of oxytocin infusions, administration of tranexamic acid, guided transfusion strategies, and cell salvage are effective in obstetric hemorrhage.
- It is beneficial to have system-level protocols and readiness in place to help communication and coordination between the different teams involved in responding to hemorrhage. The California Maternal Quality Care Collaborative offers guidance on "best practices" to standardize and improve coordinated care.

HISTORY

In prior centuries, although pregnancy was viewed as a joy, it was also seen as a threat to a woman's life. Obstetric hemorrhage, currently defined as blood loss greater than 1000 mL per the American College of Obstetricians and Gynecologists (ACOG), played a great role in this.[1] In the early to mid-1900s, several crucial advances were made that drastically decreased maternal deaths related to hemorrhage.[2] In the 1930s, the British physician Chassar Moir pioneered using ergometrine, an ergot alkaloid and precursor to the currently used methylergonovine, as the first uterotonic.[3] With the advent of widespread antibiotic use in the 1940s, maternal hemorrhage related to sepsis plummeted.[2] Later in the 1950s, an American chemist Vincent du Vigneaud received a Nobel Prize for his work in synthesizing oxytocin.[4] In this same period, a citrate solution that permitted storage of blood for several days after

[a] Obstetric Anesthesiology, UPMC Magee Women's Hospital, University of Pittsburgh Medical School, 300 Halket Street, Pittsburgh, PA 15213, USA; [b] Anesthesiology & Perioperative Medicine, UPMC Magee-Womens Hospital, Patient Blood Management Program, 300 Halket Street, Pittsburgh, PA 15213, USA
* Corresponding author.
E-mail address: SarahJaneKroh@gmail.com

Anesthesiology Clin 39 (2021) 597–611
https://doi.org/10.1016/j.anclin.2021.08.009   **anesthesiology.theclinics.com**
1932-2275/21/© 2021 Elsevier Inc. All rights reserved.

collection was developed. Blood banks began to be formed in hospitals, and The American Red Cross began organized systems of blood donation. By the 1960s, deaths from maternal hemorrhage were at an all-time low.[2] Despite great progress, obstetric hemorrhage is the most significant cause of maternal mortality worldwide.[5] Although hemorrhage accounts for a larger portion of maternal deaths in the developing world, it remains a problem in developed nations.[6,7] Morbidity and mortality from hemorrhage have been increasing in the United States since the 1990s, primarily because of increasing rates of atony.[8,9] This increase has been significant across all demographics.[10]

Contributors to this trend are multifactorial and include increases in placenta accreta spectrum (PAS) related to increased cesarean section (CS) rates and changing demographics of women giving birth, with a higher percentage being obese and of advanced maternal age.[11,12] Implicit bias likely contributes, as a disproportionate amount of harm falls on black women even when controlling for comorbidities and mode of delivery.[10] Work to mitigate the recent increase in hemorrhage morbidity and mortality is needed; however, it is important to recognize that treatment and prognosis are still overall improved from previous historical levels because of blood transfusion, blood salvage, antibiotics, tranexamic acid (TXA), and advancing obstetric methods to stop ongoing blood loss (**Fig. 1**).

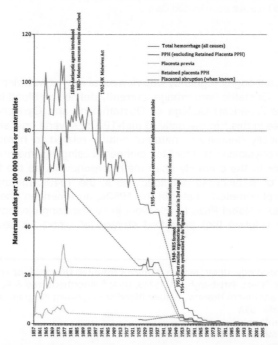

Fig. 1. Maternal deaths from obstetrical hemorrhage between 1857-2005. NHS, National Health Service. (*From* Kerr RS, Weeks AD. Lessons from 150 years of UK maternal hemorrhage deaths. Acta Obstet Gynecol Scand 2015;94:664-668. Reprinted with permission.)

RISK FACTORS AND PREVENTION

Obstetric hemorrhage has a high preventability index, and clinicians have the ability to interrupt the progression when it occurs.[13] Before delivery, it is helpful to identify patients at risk for hemorrhage, although 33% of patients with hemorrhage have no risk factors before delivery.[14] Risk factors for hemorrhage and related morbidity include prior uterine surgery, high parity, multiple gestation, uterine anomalies, history of previous obstetric hemorrhage, placental abnormalities, such as previa and PAS, known coagulopathy, prolonged labor, and laboratory values, such as low initial hemoglobin (Hgb) and platelet count. Obesity, which is increasing in prevalence, is a known risk factor for postpartum hemorrhage (PPH).[15] A recent meta-analysis showed that hypertension, diabetes, and ethnicity also correlated with PPH.[16]

Active management of the third stage of labor is recommended to prevent PPH.[1,17,18] The main role for the anesthesiologist will be oxytocin administration. Oxytocin is administered by the obstetrics team following vaginal birth but is commonly given by the anesthesiologist following CS. A typical dose is 10 units and is administered via an intramuscular (IM) injection or a diluted infusion.[17] Although both IM and intravenous (IV) administration are effective, a randomized controlled trial of more than 4000 women in Egypt demonstrated IV administration to be more effective.[19] Patients previously exposed to oxytocin during their labor require higher doses to prevent hemorrhage.[20] In the commonly used infusion of 30 units per 500 mL, the ED90 for women not previously exposed to oxytocin is 300 mL/h (0.3 IU/min) until atony resolves, whereas the ED90 for women exposed to oxytocin during labor is 700 mL/h (0.7 IU/min).[21] Unfortunately, the addition of a second uterotonic, such as prostaglandins or methylergonovine, has not proven more effective than oxytocin alone for the prevention of hemorrhage.[22] Oxytocin protocols differ by hospital, but a commonly used infusion is 0.33 IU/min for 30 minutes after delivery, which corresponds to 333 mL/h[23] This dose is lower than the ED90 for women exposed to oxytocin before delivery but has the potential to be titrated up. The lower dose attenuates the risk of adverse effects, such as hypotension and tachycardia. Coadministration of phenylephrine can be considered to help mitigate the hemodynamic effects.[24] There is also a risk of hyponatremia because oxytocin is structurally similar to vasopressin; this risk is increased when oxytocin is given at the same time as a large volume of IV fluids.[25]

Carbetocin is a longer-acting alternative to oxytocin that was recently shown in a randomized double-blinded noninferiority trial to be effective for managing the third stage of labor.[26] There are cost concerns with carbetocin, and it is not currently used in the United States.

TXA has also been studied as a potential medication for prevention of PPH in vaginal deliveries; in one study, it did not result in a lower rate of hemorrhage, although there was less need for additional uterotonics and lower rates of provider-assessed PPH in the TXA group.[27] A similar study looking at whether TXA would prevent PPH in women undergoing CS did reveal a significantly lower incidence of visually estimated blood loss (EBL) greater than 1000 mL, but it was not supported by a corresponding decrease in gravimetrically determined EBL.[28] More evidence is needed before recommending prophylactic TXA.

A study of women receiving neuraxial anesthesia compared immediate versus delayed (often called "laboring down") pushing after full cervical dilation and found that the immediate pushing group had lower rates of PPH.[29] Laboring down is not standard practice, although it continues to be used in certain situations.

DIAGNOSIS

The first step in preventing the morbidity and mortality associated with obstetric hemorrhage is early diagnosis. Pregnant women have more physiologic reserve than other surgical patients because of increased blood volume and being generally younger and healthier. Thus, there is frequently significant blood loss (~15%) before a patient begins to show changes in vital signs and clinical symptoms.[30] Because of the high blood flow to the uterus at term (700 mL/min), hemorrhage can be precipitous and severe. The current definition of hemorrhage per ACOG is a blood loss of 1000 mL accompanied by symptoms.[1] Because blood volume is normally increased by 1250 mL in pregnancy,[31] a blood loss of a liter can be well tolerated while still significant. (For reference, the average woman has just more than 5000 mL of blood volume before pregnancy.) Timely diagnosis can be hampered by occult bleeding. The postpartum uterus can hold up to 1000 mL of blood that may not be immediately apparent. The most dangerous obstetric hemorrhage for the mother is acute hemorrhage within 24 hours of delivery. Causes of early PPH can be categorized within the "4 Ts": "Tone, Trauma, Tissue, Thrombin" (see the tailored anesthetic management section later). In contrast, the fetus is most at risk during antepartum hemorrhage that occurs before delivery. Causes of antepartum hemorrhage include abruption, placenta previa, vasa previa, and uterine rupture. Patients should be counseled that delayed hemorrhage can occur between 24 hours' and 12 weeks' postpartum. Appropriate follow-up is needed for obstetric reasons and because coagulation factors begin to decrease toward prepregnancy levels.[32,33]

A challenge with diagnosis is that simple visual estimates of blood loss are often inaccurate.[34] A prospective cohort study of 150 patients demonstrated that when visually determined EBL was compared with EBL determined via weighing techniques, visual estimates underestimated true blood loss by around 30%.[35] Accuracy of EBL can be enhanced by using devices that weigh surgical lap pads and special drapes that collect blood to be used for quantitative measurement during both vaginal and cesarean birth. Although ACOG suggests more evidence is required to demonstrate effectiveness, they do recommend using gravimetric methods of calculating blood loss when feasible.[36] Cumulative blood loss that occurs antepartum, intrapartum, and postpartum must be considered.

BASICS OF ANESTHETIC MANAGEMENT

In all obstetric hemorrhage, the anesthesiologist should not discount the basics. Additional large-bore IV access should be obtained; laboratory values like Hgb should be closely monitored (a point-of-care fashion is ideal), and volume resuscitation should be started. The international, randomized controlled WOMAN trial demonstrated that TXA, if given within 3 hours of birth, decreases the risk of mortality regardless of the underlying cause of hemorrhage.[37] TXA is given as a 1-g dose over 10 minutes. The severity of hemorrhage varies greatly, and further escalation of care at the discretion of the anesthesiologist is warranted. Prompt initiation of a proper transfusion strategy should not be delayed if indicated and is discussed later in the transfusion management section. If hemodynamic changes become deleterious, invasive monitors, such as an arterial line, should be considered. Central line placement may be advantageous, particularly large-bore catheters of 6 to 8.5F for rapid infusion. Although vasopressors are ideally administered via central lines, they can be administered safely through peripheral IVs, especially at lower drug concentrations. The largest concern in infusing vasopressors through a peripheral line is extravasation, causing tissue necrosis, but this is rare with infusions of less than 4 hours' duration.[38]

Coordinated efforts are needed for successful cardiocerebral resuscitation, and the initiation of ACLS (advanced cardiac life support) protocols is a leadership opportunity for anesthesiologists.[39]

Of note, neuraxial anesthesia is an option during ongoing hemorrhage of any cause, even during hysterectomy for placenta accreta.[40] It has been used successfully for both planned and emergent hysterectomies. Neuraxial anesthesia has been used for placenta previa with suspected PAS with a success rate approaching 80%.[41] An epidural or combined spinal epidural allows for longer duration of surgical anesthesia. Still, the decision to use neuraxial anesthesia has challenges: It is often the responsibility of the anesthesiologist to manage the patient's experience during an acute crisis, including mitigating the harm of psychological trauma when keeping the patient's support person in the room may be impractical. As severity of hemorrhage increases, general anesthesia becomes preferred. Conversion to general anesthesia should not be delayed when patient instability threatens airway protection or is associated with large fluid shifts, or if general anesthesia would better facilitate obtaining needed vascular access. Just as with other patients, induction of general anesthesia in a hemodynamically unstable obstetric patient can precipitate cardiovascular collapse and even death.[42,43] As with nonobstetric patients, an existing neuraxial block (with its attendant anesthetic and sympathectomy effects) may affect drug choices for the induction and maintenance of general anesthesia.

TAILORED ANESTHETIC MANAGEMENT

Successful treatment of obstetric hemorrhage depends on identifying and addressing the cause. This will require good communication with the obstetricians who are most likely to be making the diagnosis. A popular mnemonic incorporates 4 of the most common causes of hemorrhage that all begin with T: tone, trauma, tissue, and thrombin (**Table 1**).[33] In theory, the anesthesiologist should tailor treatment to the underlying cause of hemorrhage, as is outlined in later discussion, and in practice, strategies to cover all causes of obstetric hemorrhage are often initiated simultaneously. In

Table 1
Risk factors and frequency of maternal hemorrhage by etiology

Cause	Details	Frequency	Risk Factors
Tone	Uterus fails to contract adequately for hemostasis	Most common	General anesthesia, prolonged exposure to oxytocin, uterine anomalies, infection, high parity, multiple gestation
Trauma	Lacerations to the reproductive tract (cervical, vaginal, iatrogenic)	Common	Operative delivery, shoulder dystocia, instrumented delivery, prime delivery
Tissue	Retained placenta or products of conception, placenta accreta spectrum	Less common	Previous uterine surgery or procedures, placental abnormalities, such as previa or accreta
Thrombin	Defects of coagulation	Least common	Preeclampsia, disseminated intravascular coagulation, amniotic fluid embolism, inherited coagulopathy, medical anticoagulation

all instances, timely and informative 2-way communication allows the team to be updated as clinical conditions evolve and for interventions to be adapted accordingly.

Tone

If uterine tone is the primary cause of hemorrhage, the oxytocin infusion should be titrated up. A stepwise increase to 0.6 IU/min and then to 0.9 IU/min if atony continues during CS is one example.[20] The rate of oxytocin infusion should be decreased once atony resolves. There is no benefit to infusing oxytocin at higher rates, and a previous strategy of running oxytocin wide open is increasingly questioned in the obstetric anesthesiology community. Rather, if increasing oxytocin is unsuccessful, other uterotonics, which work via different mechanisms, should be considered. Methylergonovine is typically given as a 0.2-mg IM injection. It has a duration of 2 to 4 hours and produces tetanic contractions. Inadvertent IV administration can cause serious complications, such as hypertensive emergency and myocardial ischemia. Prostaglandin F2 alpha, known as carboprost, is another drug given by IM injection, and the most common dose is 250 µg. It has a propensity to induce bronchospasm and pulmonary shunting and thus should be avoided in asthmatics. Although prostaglandin E1 or misoprostol is another uterotonic to consider, it is not effective in women already receiving high-dose oxytocin infusion.[44]

Trauma

Anesthesiologists will use different strategies depending on the location and severity of bleeding from the reproductive tract. For small lacerations to the vagina or cervix, augmenting preexisting epidural analgesia facilitates comfort while the obstetrician performs repair. The epidural frequently needs to be redosed before the repair, and shorter-acting local anesthetics, such as 5 to 10 cc 1% to 2% lidocaine with epinephrine, or 3% chloroprocaine can benefit the patient while minimizing the prolongation of anesthetic recovery. More serious injuries, such as laceration of uterine arteries and retroperitoneal hematomas, require escalation of care as described earlier in the basic anesthetic management section.

Tissue

If tissue is the problem, it may not be immediately evident to the anesthesiologist, and communication with the obstetrics team can help elucidate appropriate plans. For retained placenta or uterine inversion, nitroglycerin helps facilitate removal of placenta and replacement of the uterus, respectively. Reported doses range from 50 to 500 µg.[45] The amount given can be titrated to effect, as nitroglycerin has a short onset and duration of action.[46] Sublingual formulations are also effective. A significant drop in blood pressure with nitroglycerin should be anticipated, and small boluses of vasopressors to counteract the drop should be available. Other modalities of uterine relaxation include volatile anesthetics, terbutaline, and magnesium sulfate.[47] If PAS is diagnosed, the anesthesiologist should anticipate massive blood loss and need for care escalation. Predelivery diagnosis of PAS via ultrasound or MRI is imperfect; thus, it is important to be ready to manage an unexpected accreta at any time.

Thrombin

If the bleeding issue is a coagulopathy ("thrombin"), the possibilities include underlying preeclampsia, HELLP syndrome, inborn errors of coagulation, antiplatelet or anticoagulant medications, and disseminated intravascular coagulation. Treatment will depend on the underlying cause. If the cause is due to a medication, the anesthesiologist should investigate whether a reversal agent is available. In cases of coagulopathy, it is useful to obtain viscoelastic testing, and coagulation laboratory tests, including a fibrinogen level to guide management and transfusion strategies. Fibrinogen levels normally increase in pregnancy to more than 300 mg/dL; thus, it is concerning if fibrinogen drops to less than 150 mg/dL during vaginal delivery or 200 mg/dL during cesarean delivery.[48]

TRANSFUSION MANAGEMENT

In anticipation of the potential need for blood transfusion, all obstetric patients should be screened for antibodies.[49] In patients with no antibodies and low to medium risk of hemorrhage, crossmatch is not necessarily required. Ideally, Hgb is optimized before delivery. Anemic patients require oral or IV iron supplementation during pregnancy, although this does not have a role in the acute setting. Risk factors for transfusion include general anesthesia, operative delivery, chorioamnionitis, fetal demise, preterm labor, and prolonged labor.[50] Transfusion of obstetric patients is not uncommon and occurs in 0.5% to 3% of patients with PPH.[11]

Ideal transfusion strategies are moving away from the traditional 1:1:1 ratios of packed red blood cells (PRBC):plasma:platelets and more toward "guided transfusion" strategies. The evidence for ratio-based transfusion comes mostly from trauma literature, and there is no evidence that demonstrates it is effective in obstetrics. There is no clear survival benefit to this copious transfusion strategy,[51] and there is evidence that guided transfusion strategies lead to less morbidity.[52] A study comparing a guided transfusion strategy based on laboratory tests drawn every 2 hours with a ratio-based transfusion strategy showed decreased survival in the latter.[53]

Using viscoelastic testing to guide transfusion has shown great promise and can decrease blood transfusion.[54] Systems of viscoelastic testing include thromboelastography (TEG), a rotational thromboelastometry, and Sonoclot.[55] A practical and basic way to remember normal values of TEG is the rule of 6: R time should be around 6 minutes; alpha angle should be around 60°; maximum amplitude (MA) should be around 60 mm; and lysis at 30 minutes should be around 6%. (This mnemonic is a generalization and does not replace referencing the normal values for each type of viscoelastic testing). When R time is increased, consider fresh frozen plasma; when alpha angle is decreased, consider cryoprecipitate. When MA is decreased, consider platelets, and when lysis is increased, consider antifibrinolytics. A study looking at plasma infusion within the first 60 minutes of PPH refractory to initial measures did not show improved outcomes compared with later plasma administration.[56] This supports the thinking that in certain situations it is not dangerous to wait for laboratory results before transfusion.

Ongoing investigations are exploring whether fibrinogen concentrate is beneficial. Fibrinogen level is one of the only markers shown to actively predict severity of PPH.[57] In the trauma literature, there is a clear association between decreased fibrinogen concentration and death.[58] Fibrinogen concentrate is shown to rapidly correct hypofibrinogenemia in obstetric patients.[59] Unfortunately, fibrinogen concentrate is very costly, and cryoprecipitate may be a more cost-effective method of fibrinogen replacement. However, in certain geographic areas, notably Europe, the use of cryoprecipitate is rare. There is currently inadequate evidence to recommend fibrinogen concentrate outside of congenital hypofibrinogenemia or afibrinogenemia.[60] This may change in the future.

Monitoring laboratory values can also be used to guide transfusion of red blood cells. This can be done with point-of-care testing, such as arterial blood gas, or other rapid tests, such as Hemocue (manufactured by Danaher Corporation). Because there is a lag time in laboratory testing, transfusion of red blood cells (either allogenic or autologous) can be considered at Hgb ≤8 g/dL if bleeding is ongoing or Hgb <7 g/dL if bleeding is controlled. Patients are often able to tolerate lower levels of Hgb than we realize, and there are case reports of patients surviving major surgeries with levels as low as 2 g/dL.[61] Despite this, transfusion should never be delayed in cases of significant blood loss and hemodynamic instability. Lactate level is another marker of inadequate resuscitation and can be measured from a point-of-care arterial blood gas sample. Although guided transfusion strategies are ideal, they are not without challenges because their utility requires rapid test value turnaround time. Although Hemocue offers a Hgb measurement immediately, there are some concerns about accuracy,[62] possibly when capillary blood is used instead of traditionally drawn blood. Hospitals face difficulties in implementing guided transfusion strategies when there is limited access to, and sustained maintenance of, the technologies required.

Allogenic blood transfusion carries a higher risk than autologous blood transfusion. Historically, cell salvage was thought to be unadvisable in obstetrics because of concern for contamination with amniotic fluid and possible iatrogenic amniotic fluid embolism. This has proven false. A 2000 study compared unwashed blood from the surgical field, washed and filtered blood (cell salvage), and maternal blood drawn from a central line. The washed and filtered blood showed significant removal of bacteria and components of amniotic fluid, including squamous cells and lamellar bodies, and there were no discernible differences in these parameters when comparing the washed and filtered blood with maternal blood.[63] Cell salvage resulted in significant although not complete removal of bacteria from frankly contaminated blood, and additional filtering could be afforded with an additional leukocyte depletion filter.[64]

When cell salvage is used during CS, there are 2 separate suction systems. An autotransfusion suction tubing is connected to a cell salvage machine and is used both before and after amniotomy, whereas a traditional wall suction is used to remove as much amniotic fluid as possible following rupture of membranes.[65] A prospective randomized controlled trial of intraoperative cell salvage in obstetrics showed a decreased need for allogeneic transfusion, lower incidence of infection, lower risk of cardiovascular events, and shorter hospital stay.[66] Cell salvage is cost-effective and can even reduce overall costs.[67] Even when hemorrhage is unanticipated and cell salvage was not used at the onset of bleeding, the laparotomy sponges can be rinsed to collect the blood for salvage.[68] It is not limited to CSs and can be used for hemorrhage after vaginal deliveries as well.[69]

Massive transfusion is needed in the most severe cases of hemorrhage, notably when 4 or more units of PRBC are needed within 4 hours of bleeding, when greater than 10 units of products are given in 24 hours, or when there is greater than 1500 mL of blood loss with hemodynamic decompensation.[49] In these cases, a massive transfusion protocol should be initiated, and additional help should be called for. Success depends on excellent teamwork, and close collaboration with operating room and blood bank personnel. In most instances, anesthesiologists play a central role to lead and coordinate these efforts.

SYSTEMS-BASED MANAGEMENT

One of the most significant barriers to effective treatment of obstetric hemorrhage (and thus one of the most significant areas with opportunities for impact) occurs at the systems level. Many teams, including anesthesiology, obstetrics, nursing, technical support, blood bank, and other stakeholders, must all communicate effectively and collaborate in order to address a time-sensitive and high-acuity problem. It is

Obstetric Hemorrhage Emergency Management Plan: Table Chart Format
version 2.0

	Assessments	Meds/Procedures	Blood Bank
Stage 0	**Every woman in labor/giving birth**		
Stage 0 focuses on risk assessment and active management of the third stage.	• Assess every woman for **risk factors** for hemorrhage • Measure **cumulative quantitative blood loss** on every birth	**Active Management 3rd Stage:** • **Oxytocin** IV infusion or 10u IM • **Fundal Massage-** vigorous, 15 seconds min.	• If **Medium Risk**: T & Scr • If **High Risk**: T&C 2 U • If **Positive Antibody Screen** (prenatal or current, exclude low level anti-D from RhoGam):T&C 2 U
Stage 1	**Blood loss: > 500ml vaginal or >1000 ml Cesarean, or VS changes (by >15% or HR ≥110, BP ≤85/45, O2 sat <95%)**		
Stage 1 is short: activate hemorrhage protocol, initiate preparations and give Methergine IM.	• Activate OB Hemorrhage Protocol and Checklist • Notify Charge nurse, OB/CNM, Anesthesia • VS, O2 Sat q5' • Record **cumulative** blood loss q5-15' • **Weigh** bloody materials • Careful inspection with good exposure of vaginal walls, cervix, uterine cavity, placenta	• **IV Access:** at least 18gauge • Increase IV fluid (LR) and **Oxytocin** rate, and repeat **fundal massage** • **Methergine** 0.2mg IM (if not hypertensive) May repeat if good response to first dose, BUT otherwise **move on** to 2nd level uterotonic drug (see below) • Empty bladder: straight cath or place foley with urimeter	• **T&C 2 Units PRBCs** (if not already done)
Stage 2	**Continued bleeding with total blood loss under 1500ml**		
Stage 2 is focused on sequentially advancing through medications and procedures, mobilizing help and Blood Bank support, and keeping ahead with volume and blood products.	**OB back to bedside** (if not already there) • **Extra help:** 2nd OB, Rapid Response Team (per hospital), assign roles • VS & cumulative blood loss q 5-10 min • Weigh bloody materials • **Complete evaluation** of vaginal wall, cervix, placenta, uterine cavity • Send additional labs, including DIC panel • If in Postpartum: Move to L&D/OR • Evaluate for special cases: -Uterine Inversion -Amn. Fluid Embolism	**2nd Level Uterotonic Drugs:** • **Hemabate** 250 mcg IM or • **Misoprostol** 800 mcg SL **2nd IV Access** (at least 18gauge) Bimanual massage **Vaginal Birth:** (typical order) • Move to OR • Repair any tears • D&C: r/o retained placenta • Place intrauterine balloon • Selective Embolization (Interventional Radiology) **Cesarean Birth:** (still intra-op) (typical order) • Inspect broad lig, posterior uterus and retained placenta • B-Lynch Suture • Place intrauterine balloon	• Notify Blood Bank of **OB Hemorrhage** • **Bring 2 Units PRBCs to bedside, transfuse per clinical signs – do not wait for lab values** • Use blood warmer for transfusion • Consider thawing 2 FFP (takes 35+min), use if transfusing > 2u PRBCs • Determine availability of additional RBCs and other Coag products
Stage 3	**Total blood loss over 1500ml, or >2 units PRBCs given or VS unstable or suspicion of DIC**		
Stage 3 is focused on the Massive Transfusion protocol and invasive surgical approaches for control of bleeding.	• **Mobilize team** -Advanced GYN surgeon -2nd Anesthesia Provider -OR staff -Adult Intensivist • **Repeat labs** including coags and ABG's • Central line • Social Worker/ family support	• **Activate Massive Hemorrhage Protocol** • Laparotomy: -B-Lynch Suture -Uterine Artery Ligation -Hysterectomy • Patient support -Fluid warmer -Upper body warming device -Sequential compression stockings	**Transfuse Aggressively** Massive Hemorrhage Pack • Near 1:1 PRBC:FFP • 1 PLT apheresis pack per 4-6 units PRBCs **Unresponsive Coagulopathy:** After 8-10 units PRBCs and full coagulation factor replacement: may consult re rFactor VIIa risk/benefit

Fig. 2. Improving health care response to obstetric hemorrhage version 2.0. A California quality improvement toolkit. cath, catheter; Coag., coagulant; FFP, fresh frozen plasma; in-traop, intraoperative; labs, laboratory tests; Meds, medications; O2 sat, oxygen saturation;

an unreasonable expectation that even highly skilled clinicians can align perfectly in the heat of the moment, and thus, standardized "best practice" systems must be organized and put in place before hemorrhage occurs.

The California Maternal Quality Care Collaborative (CMQCC) convened a task force to address obstetric hemorrhage, and their recommendations were published in 2015. To date, this is the most comprehensive resource (version 2 is now available) on the management of obstetric hemorrhage. Specifically, they advocate for having systems in place for readiness, recognition, response, and reporting as well as avoidance of delay and denial.[14] Readiness includes establishing easy access to needed supplies, identifying response teams, and establishing transfusion protocols. An excellent example of a management plan developed by the CMQCC is shown in **Fig. 2**. Recognition includes predelivery assessment of risk factors and accurate measurement of cumulative blood loss. Response includes a standardized and stage-based (escalating) management plan, including a checklist. Finally, reporting involves debriefing and review of hemorrhagic events so providers can share hindsight perspectives and improvements can be made. The CMQCC paper and a corresponding power point are both available for free online and serve as excellent references for any anesthesia provider.

All providers involved in managing PPH require nontechnical skills (NTS), such as communication and teamwork. A small randomized trial showed that providers randomized to receive NTS training went on to receive higher scores when these skills were evaluated in a high-fidelity simulation scenario.[70] Another study showed that although team training was appreciated, in practice, it failed to decrease Adverse Outcome Index-5 in a cluster randomized trial.[71] Despite mixed evidence, team training and simulation are unlikely to cause harm, and shared experiential learning can promote team familiarity with personnel and protocols.

OBSTETRIC MANAGEMENT

Targeted obstetric management of hemorrhage depends on the cause. Understanding the tactics obstetricians use allows anesthesiologists to anticipate the next steps and be more effective partners. Atony is the most common cause of hemorrhage, and uterine contraction is necessary to control the bleeding that occurs once the placenta separates from the uterus.[22] The first step to control atony is bimanual massage of the uterus: after vaginal delivery, uterine compression is performed by placing one hand in the vagina and pushing against the uterus while the other hand compresses the fundus from above through the abdominal wall. During CS, both hands can simultaneously massage the anterior and posterior s surface of the uterus. Massage is of benefit for fundal atony but is unlikely to help lower uterine segment atony. Other strategies include intrauterine devices, such as balloons, to tamponade blood loss (an example is the Bakri balloon), or gentle vacuum pressure to induce contraction (an example is the Jada system).[72,73] Compression B-Lynch sutures can be placed around the exterior of the uterus if there is a laparotomy.[74] Traumatic injury to the reproductive tract can be controlled with surgical repair or intravascular arterial embolization. Sometimes

---

OB, obstetrics; OB/CNM, obstetrician/certified nurse-midwife; PLT, platelet. (Lyndon A, Lagrew D, Shields L, Main E, Cape V. Improving Health Care Response to Obstetric Hemorrhage. (California Maternal Quality Care Collaborative Toolkit to Transform Maternity Care) Developed under contract #11-10006 with the California Department of Public Health; Maternal, Child and Adolescent Health Division; Published by the California Maternal Quality Care Collaborative, 3/17/15.)

this requires return to the operating room or transfer to interventional radiology. Retained placenta can be removed manually or with forceps.[1] The gold-standard treatment for morbidly adherent placenta, placenta accreta, is peripartum hysterectomy; however, conservative management is sometimes attempted in patients with a strong desire to preserve fertility.[75] These conservative attempts to manage accreta have a high failure rate and morbidity.[76] Regardless of underlying cause of hemorrhage, there are certain more extreme measures that can be taken when the hemorrhage cannot be adequately controlled. These include emergent hysterectomy and uterine artery embolization, which have absolute and high risks of future infertility, respectively.[77] Risk factors for requiring hysterectomy include increased maternal age and CS.[78] Other options when hemorrhage is life threatening include surgical clamping of the aorta and resuscitative endovascular occlusion of the aorta. Significant risks include aortic injury and peripheral ischemia.[79]

SUMMARY

Obstetric hemorrhage continues to be a leading cause of maternal morbidity and mortality worldwide. Many advances have been made in the understanding of the use of uterotonics to manage bleeding, nuanced transfusion strategies, and the safety and efficacy of cell-saver techniques. Ultimately, the ability to anticipate and respond to these emergencies depends on coordinated efforts of interdisciplinary and interprofessional teams, and moving the needle on this threat to maternal well-being will depend on the dissemination of standardized and sustainable "best practices."

CLINICS CARE POINTS

- There should be a high index of suspicion for obstetric hemorrhage because classic risk factors are not always present; there may be occult bleeding, and even visible bleeding is usually underestimated.
- Basic strategies for resuscitation are in many ways similar to those for nonobstetric patients.
- The classic 1:1:1 ratio of transfused packed red blood cells:plasma:platelets is based on the trauma literature and is no longer considered best practices for obstetric hemorrhage; ideally, transfusion strategies are more nuanced and guided by point-of-care testing.
- CMQCC.org offers the most comprehensive and updated reference on management of obstetric hemorrhage, including recommendations and checklists for improving readiness, recognition, response, and reporting.

DISCLOSURE

S. Kroh: No financial disclosures. J.H. Waters: Strategic Advisory Committee: Haemonetics (manufacturer of TEG and Cell Saver). Consultant for LivaNova (manufacturer of Cell Saver).

REFERENCES

1. Practice Bulletin No. 183: postpartum hemorrhage. Obstet Gynecol 2017;130: e168–86.
2. Kerr RS, Weeks AD. Lessons from 150 years of UK maternal hemorrhage deaths. Acta Obstet Gynecol Scand 2015;94:664–8.

3. Dudley HW, Moir C. The substance responsible for the traditional clinical effect of ergot. BMJ 1935;1:520–3.

4. Vigneaud VD, Ressler C, Swan CJM, et al. The synthesis of an octapeptide amide with the hormonal activity of oxytocin. J Am Chem Soc 1953;75:4879–80.

5. Kassebaum NJ, Bertozzi-Villa A, et al. Global, regional and national levels and causes of maternal mortality during 1990-2013: a systematic analysis for the Global Burden of Disease Study 2013. Lancet 2014;384:980–1004.

6. Say L, Chou D, et al. Global causes of maternal death: a WHO systematic analysis. Lancet Glob Health 2014;2:e323–33.

7. Picetti R, Miller L, et al. The WOMAN trial: clinical and contextual factors surrounding the deaths of 483 women following post-partum haemorrhage in developing nations. BMC Pregnancy Childbirth 2020;20(1):409.

8. Knight M, Callaghan WM, et al. Trends in postpartum hemorrhage in high resource countries: a review and recommendations from the International Postpartum Hemorrhage Collaborative Group. BMC Pregnancy Childbirth 2009;9:7.

9. Callaghan WM, Kuklina EV, et al. Trends in postpartum hemorrhage: United States, 1994-2006. Am J Obstet Gynecol 2010;202:353.e1–6.

10. Leonard SA, Main EK, Scott KA, et al. Racial and ethnic disparities in severe maternal morbidity prevalence and trends. Ann Epidemiol 2019;33:30–6.

11. Bateman BT, Berman MF, et al. The epidemiology of postpartum hemorrhage in a large nationwide sample of deliveries. Anes Analg 2010;110:1368–73.

12. Butwick AJ, Abreo A, et al. Effect of maternal body mass index on postpartum hemorrhage. Anesthesiology 2018;128:774–83.

13. Berg CJ, Harper MA, et al. Preventability of pregnancy-related deaths: results of a statewide review. Obset Gynecol 2005;106(6):1228–34.

14. Lyndon A, Lagrew D, Shields L et al. Improving health care response to obstetric hemorrhage version 2.0. California Maternal Quality Care Collaborative Toolkit to Transform Maternity Care (CMQCC). Developed under contract #11-10006 with the California Department of Public Health; Maternal, Child and Adolescent Health Division; published by the California Maternal Quality Care Collaborative 3/17/15

15. Dalbye R, Gunnes N, et al. Maternal body mass index and risk of obstetric, maternal and neonatal outcomes: a cohort study of nulliparous women with spontaneous onset of labor. Acta Obstet Gynecol Scand 2021;100(3):521–30.

16. Ende HB, Lozada MJ, Chestnut DH, et al. Risk factors for atonic postpartum hemorrhage: a systematic review and meta-analysis. Obstet Gynecol 2021;137(2): 305–23.

17. World Health Organization. WHO recommendations for the prevention and treatment of postpartum haemorrhage. Geneva: WHO; 2012.

18. Westoff G, Cotter AM, et al. Prophylactic oxytocin for the third state of labour to prevent postpartum haemorrhage. Cochrane Database Syst Rev 2013;(10):CD001808.

19. Charles D, Anger H, et al. Intramuscular injection, intravenous infusion, and intravenous bolus of oxytocin in the third stage of labor for prevention of postpartum hemorrhage: a three-arm randomized control trial. BMC Childbirth 2019;19(1):38.

20. Foley A, Gunter A, Nunes KJ, et al. Patients undergoing cesarean delivery after exposure to oxytocin during labor require higher postpartum oxytocin doses. Anesth Analg 2018;126(3):920–4.

21. Lavoie A, McCarthy RJ. The ED90 of prophylactic oxytocin infusion after delivery of the placenta during cesarean delivery in laboring compared with nonlaboring

women: an up-down sequential allocation dose-response study. Anes Analg 2015;121:159–64.

22. Mousa HA, Blum J, et al. Treatment for primary postpartum haemorrhage. Cochrane Database Syst Rev 2014;(2):CD003249.

23. Dagraca J, Malladi V, Nunes K, et al. Outcomes after institution of a new oxytocin infusion protocol during the third stage of labor and immediate postpartum period. J Obstet Anesth 2013;22:194–9.

24. Dyer RA, Reed AR, et al. Hemodynamic effects of ephedrine, phenylephrine and the coadministration of phenylephrine with oxytocin during spinal anesthesia for elective cesarean delivery. Anesthesiology 2009;111:753–65.

25. Bergum D, Lonnee H, et al. Oxytocin infusion: acute hyponatremia, seizures and coma. Acta Anaesthesiol Scand 2009;53:826–7.

26. Widmer M, Piaggio G, et al. Heat-stable carbetocin versus oxytocin to prevent hemorrhage after vaginal birth. N Engl J Med 2018;379(8):743–52.

27. Sentilhes L, Winer N, Azria E, et al. Tranexamic acid for the prevention of blood loss after vaginal delivery. N Eng J Med 2018;379(8):731–42.

28. Sentilhes L, Senat M, et al. Tranexamic acid for the prevention of blood loss after cesarean delivery. N Engl J Med 2021;384(17):1623–34.

29. Cahill A, Srinivas SK, et al. Effect of immediate vs delayed pushing on rates of spontaneous vaginal delivery among nulliparous women receiving neuraxial analgesia: a randomized clinical trial. JAMA 2018;320(14):1444–54.

30. Pacagnella RC, Souza JP, et al. Factors associated with postpartum hemorrhage with vaginal birth. Obstet Gynecol 1991;77:69–76.

31. Hytten F. Blood volume changes in normal pregnancy. Clin Haematol 1985;14(3):601–12.

32. Alexander J, Thomas P, et al. Treatments for secondary postpartum haemorrhage. Cochrane Database Syst Rev 2002;(1):CD002867.

33. Likis FE, Sathe NA, Morgans AK, et al. Management of postpartum hemorrhage. Rockville (MD): Agency for Healthcare Research and Quality (US); 2015.

34. Dildy GA, Pain AR, et al. Estimating blood loss: can teaching significantly improve visual estimation? Obstet Gynecol 2004;104:601–6.

35. Al Kadri HM, Al Anazi BK. Visual estimation versus gravimetric measurement of postpartum blood loss: a prospective cohort study. Arch Gynecol Obstet 2011;283:1207–13.

36. American College of Obstetricians and Gynecologists. Committee Opinion No 794. Quantitative blood loss in obstetric hemorrhage. obstet Gynecol 2019;134(6):e150–6.

37. Effect of early tranexamic acid administration on mortality, hysterectomy and other morbidities in women with post-partum haemorrhage (WOMAN): an international, randomized, double-blind, placebo-controlled trial. WOMAN Trial Collaborators. Lancet 2017;389:2105–16.

38. Loubani OM, Green RS. A systematic review of extravasation and local tissue injury. J Crit Care 2015;30(3). 653.e9-653.e6.53E17.

39. Ewy GA. Cardiocerebral and cardiopulmonary resuscitation - 2017 update. Acute Med Surg 2017;4(3):227–34.

40. Chestnut DH, Dewan DM, et al. Anesthetic management for obstetric hysterectomy: a multi-institutional study. Anesthesiology 1989;70:607–10.

41. Markley JC, Farber MK, et al. Neuraxial anesthesia during cesarean delivery for placenta previa with suspected MAP: a retrospective analysis. Anes Analg 2018;131:930–8.

42. Bonnet MP, Deneux-Tharaux C, et al. Critical care and transfusion management in maternal deaths from postpartum haemorrhage. Eur J Obstet Gynecol Reprod Biol 2011;158:183–8.
43. Anderson JM, Etches D. Prevention and management of postpartum hemorrhage. Am Fam Physician 2007;75:875–82.
44. Widmer M, Blum J, et al. Misoprostol as an adjunct to standard uterotonics for treatment of postpartum-hemorrhage: a multicenter, double-blind randomized trial. Lancet 2010;375:1808–13.
45. Desimone CA, Norris MC, et al. Intravenous nitroglycerin aids manual extraction of retained placenta. Anesthesiology 1990;73:787.
46. Chandraharan E, Arulkumaran S. Acute tocolysis. Obstet Gynecol 2005;17:151–6.
47. Dufour P, Vinatier D, et al. The use of intravenous nitroglycerin for cervico-uterine relaxation: a review of the literature. Arch Gynecol Obstet 1997;261:1–7.
48. Kobayashi T, Terao T, et al. Congenital afibrinogenmia: prenatal and peripartum management" Japanese. J Thromb Hemost 2001;12:57–65.
49. Waters JH, Bonnet MP. When and how should I transfuse during obstetric hemorrhage? Int J Obstet Anesth 2021;46:102973.
50. Pressly MA, Parker RS, Waters JH, et al. Improvements and limitations in developing multivariate models of hemorrhage and transfusion risk for the obstetric population. Transfusion 2021;61(2):423–34.
51. Mesar T, Larentzakis A, Dzik W, et al. Association between ration of fresh frozen plasma to red blood cells during massive transfusion and survival among patients without traumatic injury. JAMA Surg 2017;152:574–80.
52. Snegovskikh D, Souza D, Walton Z, et al. Point-of-care viscoelastic testing improves the outcome of pregnancies complicated by severe postpartum hemorrhage. J Clin Anesth 2018;44:50–6.
53. Nascimento B, Callum J, Tien H, et al. Effect of a fixed ratio (1:1:1) transfusion protocol versus laboratory-results-guided transfusion with severe trauma: a randomized feasibility trial. CMAJ 2013;185:E583–9.
54. Dias JD, Sauaia A. Thromboelastography-guided therapy improves patient blood management and certain clinical outcomes in elective cardiac and liver surgery and emergency resuscitation: a systematic review and analysis. J Thromb Haemost 2019;17:984–94.
55. Shen L, Tabaie S, Ivascu N. Viscoelastic testing inside and beyond the operating room. J Thorac Dis 2017;9(4):S299–308.
56. Henriquez DD, Caram C, et al. Association of timing of plasma transfusion with adverse maternal outcomes in women with persistent postpartum hemorrhage. JAMA Netw Open 2019;2(11):e1915628.
57. Charbit B, Mandelbrot L, Samain E, et al. The decrease in fibrinogen is an early predictor of the severity of postpartum hemorrhage. J Thromb Haemost 2007;5(2):266–73.
58. Bouzat P, Ageron FX, Charbit J, et al. Modelling the association between fibrinogen concentration on admission and mortality in patients with massive transfusion after severe trauma: an analysis of a large regional database. Scand J Trauma Resusc Emerg Med 2018;26:55.
59. Matsunaga S, Takai Y, Seki H. Fibrinogen for the management of critical obstetric hemorrhage. J Obstet Gynaecol Res 2019;45(1):13–21.
60. Zaidi A, Kohli R, Daru J, et al. Early use of fibrinogen replacement therapy in postpartum hemorrhage – a systematic review. Transfus Med Rev 2020;35:101.

61. Kariya T, Nobuku I, Kitamura T, et al. Recovery from extreme hemodilution (hemoglobin level of 0.6 g/dL) in cadaveric liver transplantation. A A Case Rep 2015; 4(10):132–6.
62. Butwick A, Hilton G, Carvalho B. Non-invasive haemoglobin measurement in patients undergoing elective Cesarean section. Br J Anaest 2012;108:271–7.
63. Waters JH, Biscotti C, Potter PS. Amniotic fluid removal during cell salvage in the cesarean section patient. Anesthesiology 2000;92:1531–6.
64. Waters JH, Tuohy MJ, Hobson DF. Bacterial reduction by cell salvage washing and leukocyte depletion filtration. Anesthesiology 2003;99:652–5.
65. Waters JH, Beck S, Yazer M. How do I perform cell salvage in obstetrics? Transfusion 2019;59(7):2199–202.
66. Liu Y, Li X, Che X, et al. Intraoperative cell salvage for obstetrics: a prospective randomized controlled clinical trial. BMC Pregnancy Childbirth 2020;20(1):452.
67. Frank SM, Sikorski RA, Konig G, et al. Clinical utility of autologous salvaged blood: a review. J Gastrointest Surg 2020;24:464–72.
68. Waters JH. Patient blood management in obstetrics. Int Anesthesiol Clin 2014; 52(3):85–100.
69. Lim G, Kotsis E, Zorn JM, et al. Cell salvage for postpartum haemorrhage during vaginal delivery: a case series. Blood Transfus 2018;16(6):498–501.
70. Michelet D, Barre J, et al. Benefits of screen-based postpartum hemorrhage simulation on nontechnical skills training: a randomized simulation study. Simul Healthc 2018;14(6):391–7.
71. Romijn A, Ravelli A, et al. Effect of a cluster randomized team training intervention on adverse perinatal and maternal outcomes: a stepped wedge study. BJOG 2019;126(7):907–14.
72. Patacchiola F, D'Alfonso A, et al. Intrauterine balloon tamponade as management of postpartum haemorrhage related to low-lying placenta. Clin Exp Obstet Gynecol 2012;39:498–9.
73. D'Alton M, Rood KM, et al. Intrauterine vacuum-induced hemorrhage-control device for rapid treatment of postpartum hemorrhage. Obstet Gynecol 2020;136(5): 882–91.
74. B-Lynch C, Coker A, et al. The B-Lynch surgical technique for the control of massive postpartum haemorrhage: an alternative to hysterectomy? Five cases reported. Br J Obstet Gynaecol 1997;104:372–5.
75. American College of Obstetricians and Gynecologists. Committee Opinion No 529: placenta Accreta. Reaffirmed 2017. Obstet Gynecol 2012;120:207–11.
76. Pather S, Strockyj S, et al. Maternal outcome after conservative management of placenta percreta at cesarean section: a report of three cases and a review of the literature. Aust N Z J Obstet Gynaecol 2014;54:84–7.
77. Zwart JJ, Dijk PD, et al. Peripartum hysterectomy and arterial embolization for major obstetric hemorrhage: a 2-year nationwide cohort study in the Netherlands. Am J Obstet Gynecol 2010;202:150e1–7.
78. Huque S, Roberts I, et al. Risk factors for peripartum hysterectomy among women with postpartum haemorrhage: analysis of data from the WOMAN trial. BMC Pregnancy Childbirth 2018;18(1):186.
79. Riazanova OV, Reva VA, et al. Open versus endovascular REBOA control of blood loss during cesarean delivery in placenta accreta spectrum: a single-center retrospective case control study. Eur J Obstet Gynecol Reprod Biol 2021;258:23–8.

Quality Assurance and Quality Improvement in the Labor and Delivery Setting

Klaus Kjaer, MD, MBA

KEYWORDS

- Obstetric • Anesthesia • Quality • Improvement

KEY POINTS

- Quality assurance (QA) is the maintenance of a desired level of quality, a way to make sure that agreed-upon standards are met. It is the first step toward quality improvement (QI), which is the continuous process of creating systems to make things better.
- Designing a quality and patient safety project should involve one of the 6 desirable outcomes of care systems defined by the Institute of Medicine—that care should be safe, effective, efficient, personalized, timely, and equitable.
- Project management involves asking these questions: What is a need on the labor and delivery (L&D) floor that is not currently being met? What is in scope? What resources do you need for your project? What are the deliverables of the project? What is your timeline?
- Implementation of the proposed solution requires a tactical approach, drawing from both art and science. There is an art to persuading participants to engage in a project. Implementation science promotes the systematic uptake of best practices.
- Metrics that can guide care on the L&D floor may be related to team structure (obstetric, multidisciplinary, anesthetic), processes (patient monitoring, team effects), and outcomes (postpartum hemorrhage, venous thromboembolism).

DEFINITIONS

Quality assurance (QA) is the maintenance of a desired level of quality, a way to make sure that agreed-upon standards are met. It is the first step toward quality improvement (QI), which is the continuous process of creating systems to make things better. QA and QI are both important and reinforce each other. So how do we approach QA and QI on the labor and delivery (L&D) floor? Putting the right processes in place, and making sure they are executed reliably, are both important drivers of achieving the best possible outcomes. Obstetric anesthesiologists, as key players on the L&D clinical care team, are well positioned to do both.

Weill Cornell Medical College, 525 East 68th Street, New York, NY 10065, USA
E-mail address: Klk9001@med.cornell.edu

Anesthesiology Clin 39 (2021) 613–630
https://doi.org/10.1016/j.anclin.2021.08.010   anesthesiology.theclinics.com
1932-2275/21/© 2021 Elsevier Inc. All rights reserved.

BACKGROUND

As with any change management work, it is useful to consider the business case when launching a quality and patient safety project, as this may affect the availability of resources. On the revenue side, achieving quality metrics may be tied to facility accreditation status and reimbursement for physician services. On the cost side, a reduced frequency of patient safety events may lower costs related to the management of complications, medical malpractice, and reputational risk.[1] Note that the key to promoting patient safety is building a culture of safety, which, in turn, requires psychological safety. Psychological safety is a shared belief held by members of a team that the team is safe for interpersonal risk taking.[2]

GOALS

Designing a quality and patient safety project to improve patient care on the L&D floor requires identifying an area of unmet need. That need should ideally map to one of the 6 desirable outcomes of care systems defined by the Institute of Medicine—that care should be safe, effective, efficient, personalized, timely, and equitable.[3] This means that there will be many opportunities. How do you choose whereby to apply your time and energy? A good place to start is to ask 3 questions (**Box 1**).

Project Management

One way to consider these questions is to organize them in project management terms

Step 1: What is a need on the L&D floor that is, not currently being met? This involves defining the problem in detail, determining whether the solution to the problem is strategically aligned with all stakeholders on the L&D floor, clarifying how the solution adds value, and thinking about the business case to secure resources.

Step 2: What is in scope? Where will you focus your attention? For example, will your project involve only scheduled cesarean deliveries? What are the specific goals of the project, and what metrics will indicate that these goals have been reached? Also, if successful, are you going to be able to scale that success up to more patients and/or more settings? Finally, what is out of scope? What are you specifically not taking on to make the project focused enough that it is doable with your time and resources?

Step 3: What resources do you need for your project? Is there existing infrastructure you can use, such as automated reports generated by the electronic health record? Who needs to be on your team? Do you have a budget? If you are asking for people's time to participate in the project, who pays for that time? And who will sponsor your project at the executive leadership level and help you secure both formal and informal approval from participants?

Step 4: What are the deliverables of the project? What specific activities are involved with the implementation of the project?[4,5] What data will you collect, and at what intervals? What are the sources of that data, and how will you collect it? Finally, how will you summarize the data in reports? What will be the format and frequency of these reports? What will be your distribution channel, and who will need to see them?

Box 1
Questions to get started

What do you want to improve?

How do you want to improve it?

How will you know you are successful?

Step 5: What is your timeline? By what dates do you plan to have ready the various deliverables to which you have committed?

Strategically Selecting the Problem

It's not just about finding the right solution to a problem—it's also about finding the right problem to solve. If you will be looking at a project to reduce error frequency, think about the types of errors most frequently made. These include diagnostic, treatment, preventive, and communication errors.[6] Once a problem has been chosen, be clear about how you want to approach it. As stated by Toby Cosgrove, "The first step in any strategic transformation is to clarify the goal. What, exactly, do leaders want physicians to engage with?"[7]

There are many ways to structure the solution, including the Six Sigma methodology developed by Motorola, the Lean methodology developed by Toyota, and the Model for Improvement developed by the Institute for Healthcare Improvement. In all of these methodologies, an important tool is the control chart, which tracks a metric over time and indicates whether that metric stays within predefined upper and lower acceptable limits (**Fig. 1**).

Tracking with control charts is foundational to both quality assurance and quality improvement (QA/QI), as it allows for the systematic detection of deviation from goals and real-time evaluation of solutions put into place to correct the deviation. As famously stated by Peter Drucker, "If you can't measure it, you can't improve it." That is, you can't know whether or not you are successful unless success is clearly defined and tracked. It is important to know that once the measurement is initiated and participants in a process are aware that their work is being observed, they may change their behavior even without any other interventions. This is known as the Hawthorne effect. If improvements are based on the Hawthorne Effect and measurement is stopped, then those improvements may be short-lived.

Protocols and checklists are another important foundation of all the methodologies. The reliability of a process, and the likelihood of consistently achieving a desired outcome, is profoundly affected by checklists.[8]

APPROACH FOR IMPLEMENTING CHANGE

Implementation of the proposed solution requires a tactical approach, drawing from both art and science. There is an art to persuading participants to engage in a project.

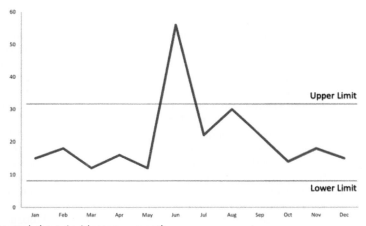

Fig. 1. Control chart, incidents per month.

Implementation science promotes the systematic uptake of best practices. Think about the culture, incentives, metrics, and making the case for why team members should engage.

Culture

To think about a persuasive pitch for engagement, it is important to assess the local culture. This involves understanding the local set of expectations around job performance, barriers to implementing new workflows, and perceptions of shared purpose.

Incentives

Understanding the incentive structure involves how participants in a project are rewarded. Are they rewarded for the productivity, efficiency, or quality of their work? Who on the care team will incur costs as the project moves forward (eg, providers having to perform extra steps in patient care), and who will benefit (eg, other providers may need to perform fewer steps in patient care)? It is useful to think about identifying the least expensive team of providers and staff who can perform the services to be delivered at the required level of proficiency.

Metrics

Choosing metrics that will reflect the successful achievement of project goals requires careful thought. Goals that are specific, measurable, assignable, realistic, and time-related (SMART goals) make this process easier. Quality metrics fall into 3 categories, assigned by whether they measure structures, processes, or outcomes. Outcome measures are usually most closely related to what we care about but can be difficult to capture, mostly because outcomes may be related to multiple independent factors. As a result, we frequently use structure and process measures. When choosing quality metrics, we also anticipate unintended consequences, such as the diversion of resources away from high-importance activities to activities that support a focus on the metrics. The unfortunate effect of some quality measures is just to create an effort to produce data. Obtaining the data should involve as little manual work as possible; automated data collection is faster, less error-prone, less resource-intensive, and more sustainable. Economy of metrics is important as well. They should be used selectively and efficiently, keeping in mind that there will always be some things that are important but cannot be measured.

Making the Case

Making the case for the project to get genuine buy-in and engagement from the team is essential and needs to be conducted continually. This is about helping providers and staff sees the alignment of the chosen metrics with a purpose and the organization's strategic framework through learning conversations and targeted education. It requires relentless follow-up, which can be conducted by providing frequent insight into the data gathered to date. Reactions, or stages of engagement, may unfold much like the Kubler-Ross stages of grief (**Table 1**).[9]

It is important to choose the messenger carefully, as to how well people respond may depend less on the message and more on their relationship with the messenger. Difficult conversations may be needed if teams react emotionally to changing long-standing workflows.[10] Continued attention is needed over time. As noted by Michael Shabot, "When we change a process to eliminate a source of error or a problem, it isn't like a project that runs for 3 months. We change our work standard to avoid problems indefinitely. We talk about it at every board meeting and every medical staff meeting."[11]

Table 1
Stages of engagement (from[9])

Kübler-Ross	Shannon Sims, MD, PhD
Denial	There's not a problem
Anger	Data are completely wrong
Bargaining	Need different metrics
Depression	Our patients are sicker
Acceptance	OK, maybe we can do better

APPLICATION OF QUALITY AND SAFETY PRINCIPLES TO LABOR AND DELIVERY CARE

Authors in the quality and patient safety literature in obstetric anesthesia have carefully chosen problems to address by asking some of the following questions. Do you want to make a change at scale or local change? Do you want to work on efficiency or maternal health outcomes? Which of the elements of the "quadruple aim" will you focus on—patient experience, patient health, cost of care, or care team well-being?[12,13] Will you focus on structure, process, or outcome measures?[14] A common starting place is to identify an unmet need, then stratify the relevant data and look for variation to rein in the outliers.[15–17] There are many opportunities for obstetric anesthesiologists to be impactful along the continuum of care from prepartum to postpartum.[18,19] Let's look at some examples.

Impacting Obstetric Care

There are many proposed indicators to monitor the quality of obstetric care using maternal near-miss cases and maternal deaths.[20] An example is emergency hysterectomy.[21] Access to consistent and high-quality data to track these indicators can be a challenge and a barrier. When a pregnancy question was added to the 2003 revision of the US standard death certificate to improve ascertainment of maternal mortality, reported maternal mortality rates increased. In response to new and better data, collaborative developed evidence-based toolkits to address 2 of the most common, preventable contributors to maternal death—obstetric hemorrhage and preeclampsia.[22] Hospital-based administrative databases that make up the Nationwide Inpatient Sample are primarily used for billing, and hence are subject to errors of omission and commission by medical coders as well as changes over time in coding practices. Although the identification of severe complications is based on an algorithm that uses ICD-9-CM codes and several data-driven criteria such as in-hospital mortality transfers from or to another health care facility, and length of hospital stay, the severity of these conditions can be difficult to assess. This highlights the difficulty of obtaining high-quality data.[23]

Creanga stratified contributors to pregnancy-related deaths and found not only racial disparities but also an increasing contribution of chronic disease, suggesting a change in the risk profile of the birthing population over time. These data can be useful in constructing metrics to drive improvement.[24]

Glance found that women undergoing a cesarean delivery at a low-performing hospital were nearly five times more likely to experience a major complication (20.93%) than women undergoing a cesarean delivery at a high-performing hospital (4.37%). At low-performing hospitals, 22.55% of patients delivering vaginally experienced major complications than 10.42% of similar patients delivering vaginally at high-performing hospitals.[25]

Howell noted that risk-standardized severe maternal morbidity rates among New York City hospitals ranged from 0.8 to 5.7 per 100 deliveries, and concluded that more research is needed to understand the attributes of high-performing centers.[26] In a study by Goffman, race remained significant while controlling for other significant factors and markers of socioeconomic status. The authors noted that some risk factors can be modified through medical care, education, or social support systems, but that racial disparity is unexplained by traditional risk factors.[27]

Markow noted that the average time required for national guidelines to be adopted into widespread practice is 17 years and made several recommendations to shorten the time for change and achieve success at scale. In addition to timely and transparent data, recommendations include toolkits with best practices as guidance, bringing together hands-on collaboratives to develop capacity, and establishing a coalition of partners. Data collection and analysis should be rapid-cycle and low-burden, and safety bundles and toolkits must be individualized to local resources. Bundles are a structured list of best practices that should be addressed for all facilities. Toolkits provide the necessary details, rationale, and implementation materials, such as sample policies and protocols. The nulliparous term singleton vertex (NTSV) cesarean rate was selected as a quality metric by the National Quality Forum, The Joint Commission, Centers for Medicare & Medicaid Services, and Leapfrog Group, among others. There was significant variation, with a range in 2015 from 11% to 77% (**Fig. 2**), which was an important incentive for engagement.[28]

The California Maternal Quality Care Collaborative (CMQCC) was formed in 2006 as a public–private partnership at Stanford. A review found that 60% to 75% of maternal deaths were preventable. Their first task was reducing early elective deliveries, followed by reducing the NTSV cesarean rate. The CMQCC data site, which tracks more than 50 maternal/infant performance measures and houses additional data quality tools, became a key resource. A web-based user interface allows hospitals to access their data using data visualization strategies to promote multiple peer comparisons, benchmark in multiple ways, and track progress over time. It was noted that not all L&D units have the QI experience or leadership skills needed to drive the work.[28]

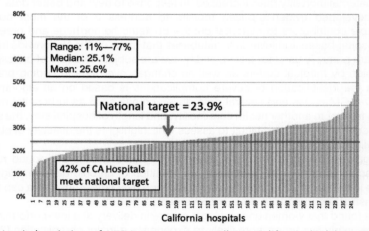

Fig. 2. Hospital variation of NTSV cesarean rates. All 248 California (CA) hospitals, 2015. (*From* Markow C, Main EK. Creating Change at Scale: Quality Improvement Strategies used by the California Maternal Quality Care Collaborative. Obstet Gynecol Clin North Am. 2019;46(2):317-328. *Reprinted with permission from* the American College of Obstetricians and Gynecologists and the Foreign Policy Research Institute.)

Impacting Multidisciplinary Care

Projects may also be focused on local unit efficiency measures rather than broader population health outcomes. This is an important way of developing QA/QI capability and can have many desirable downstream effects. Vago used Toyota Lean principles to improve care delivery on an L&D unit: During a monthly rapid improvement event (RIE) that focused on patient recoveries and transfers, the group found that it took an average of 1 hour to have patient epidurals discontinued by an anesthesiologist. They discovered that with training, a registered nurse (RN) could discontinue the epidural instead of waiting for the anesthesiologist.[29]

As part of that same effort, Bell found that with a focus on streamlining operations, on-time case initiation for labor induction and cesarean birth improved, length of stay in obstetric triage decreased, postanesthesia recovery care was reorganized to be completed within the expected 2-h standard time frame, and emergency transfers to the main hospital operating room and intensive care units were standardized and enhanced for efficiency and safety. Patients scheduled for labor inductions who were called in on time increased from 47% to 98%, cesarean deliveries that started on time increased from 52% to 74%, and PACU recovery times that were less than 2 hours increased from 29% to 50%. The authors note that RIEs are valuable because they engage frontline clinicians with direct knowledge of the work as participants to develop strategies for success and that respect for the coworker is what creates the foundation for continuous improvement.[30]

After delivery, the transition to home is an important step in the care of new mothers. Fleischman and colleagues focused on improving discharge preparation, which was measured by an increase in the Hospital Consumer Assessment of Hospital Providers and Systems (HCAHPS) discharge domain question scores, particularly, "During your hospital stay, did doctors, nurses, or other hospital staff talk to you about whether you would have the help you need when you left the hospital?" HCAHPS ratings on the discharge domain increased from the 34th percentile to the 96th percentile.[31]

The prescribing of unnecessary opioid, which often happens as part of the discharge process, is an important metric in the setting of the prescription opioid epidemic. A shared decision-making approach to opioid prescribing after cesarean delivery was associated with approximately a 50% decrease in the number of opioids prescribed postoperatively.[32] In a larger follow-up study by the same group, the mean number of oxycodone tablets patients took decreased from 33 to 21, representing a 35% decrease.[33]

Sometimes multiple systems interventions can make it difficult to trace improvement in care back to a specific factor. One L&D Unit reduced its cesarean delivery rate after the implementation of several different quality initiatives. These included consultant review, L&D team training, electronic intrapartum medical records, chain of communication protocol, dedicated gynecology attending, limitation of misoprostol to nonviable fetus, standardized oxytocin protocol, premixed and safety color-coded magnesium sulfate and oxytocin solutions, electronic templates for shoulder dystocia and operative deliveries, early identification of potential obstetric professional liability cases, obstetric patient safety nurse, electronic L&D whiteboard to simplify sign out, physician assistants added to L&D staff, electronic fetal monitoring interpretation certification, electronic antepartum medical records, routine thromboprophylaxis for all cesarean deliveries, obstetric emergency drills, recruitment of laborist, oxytocin initiation checklist, postpartum hemorrhage (PPH) kit, internet-based reading assignment and testing, and elimination of scheduled labor induction before 39 weeks gestation without medical indications.[34]

Impacting Anesthetic Care

What metrics are specific to obstetric anesthesia? Bamber did a Delphi survey of providers and patients from 220 maternity units in the United Kingdom to identify metrics related to obstetric anesthesia service provision, service quality, and outcomes. A list of 31 indicators was narrowed down to 5: percent of patients with wet tap, use of antenatal consult guidelines, dedicated elective Cesarean section schedule and staff, point-of-care hemoglobin testing, and percent of patients with analgesia within 45 minutes of request.[35]

Wikner has attributed the difficulty of agreeing on quality metrics in obstetric anesthesia to the fact that anesthesia is characterized by a low incidence of direct complications, a shared responsibility for many outcomes, and a patient population who are frequently unable to witness the care they are receiving.[36]

Pritchard noted that, based on a response to a survey of lead obstetric anesthesiologists with 98/191 respondents, only 54% of centers routinely analyzed their data, and the most common approach was reactive rather than proactive analysis. Routinely data collected for obstetric anesthesia include those listed later in discussion. Many of these were considered by Bamber 2020 but did not land in their top 5 (**Table 2**).[37]

Lucas, in the 2020 Messages for Improving Anesthetic Care report for Mother and Babies: Reducing Risk through Audits and Confidential Enquiries (MBRRACE), identified recurring themes that point to opportunities, such as venous thromboembolism (VTE) prophylaxis, antenatal review, timely neuraxial block placement, PPH management, postop surveillance, timely provision of neuraxial analgesia, management of failed neuraxial anesthesia, and appropriate management of postdural puncture headache (PDPH), along with standardized handovers focusing on the sick, those at risk, follow-up, and active epidurals.[38]

McQuaid noted that health care providers in the obstetric unit should also recognize the unique training and skill set that anesthesiologists possess that allow them to manage a range of obstetrics crises, but that the challenge remains to translate performance into metrics.[39]

Pryde has suggested skillsets and toolkits for obstetric anesthesiologists, dividing these into antenatal, intrapartum, postpartum, and regionalization. An example under regionalization is the promotion of patient-safety science using team training and the deployment of checklists. Critical to the success of regional referral centers will be on-site, medically sophisticated clinicians fluent in maternal medicine, and capable of rapidly orchestrating interdisciplinary escalation of care. Obstetric anesthesiologists can have a major impact on the success of such a model (**Box 2**).[40]

Abir and Mhyre have pointed out that while anesthesia-related maternal mortality is exceptionally rare, airway management, high neuraxial blockade, and dural puncture remain significant safety hazards. They argue that to maximize the impact on maternal safety, anesthesiologists should lead interdisciplinary teams to implement system solutions directed at the leading causes of preventable maternal death, including sepsis, hemorrhage, VTE, and hypertensive disorders of pregnancy. Specific suggestions include monitoring strategies whereby maternal vital signs that show significant deviation should prompt careful consideration of differential diagnoses that include rare but serious complications, and participating in institutional, regional, and national reviews of maternal morbidity and mortality to generate lessons to improve safety. They also note that racial and ethnic disparities in maternal morbidity and mortality call for specific strategies to reduce them.[41]

Pardo has noted that a low rate of adverse outcomes in the overall population served by a hospital is not sufficient if, when stratified by race, a particular group is

Table 2
Proposed indicators vs collected data

Indicator	Proposed[a] Bamber et al,[35] 2020	Collected[b] Pritchard et al,[37] 2019
Mode of anesthesia for caesarean	—	58%
Conversion to GA	86%	—
Mode by the urgency level	88%	—
Complications of anesthesia	53%	—
Wet tap/headache/blood patch	92%	—
Headache	87%	—
Blood patch	98%	—
Patient satisfaction	—	47%
Pain relief within 45 min of insertion	87%	—
Effectiveness of postop analgesia	—	37%
Postnatal follow-up rate	80%	34%
Labor epidural resite rate	—	34%
Difficult intubation rate	91%	31%
Obstetric critical care admissions	—	31%
Labor epidural request response time	—	24%
Request response time within 30 min	47%	—

[a] Proportion of all participants in each Delphi Third phase who scored an indicator between 7 and 9 ('extremely important').
[b] Percentage of respondent hospitals.
Data from Refs.[35,37]

found to have rates above acceptable limits. The authors make a series of recommendations for performance improvement committees (**Box 3**).[42]

Tangel used stratification to show that black women were more likely than white women to receive general anesthesia for cesarean delivery. The authors also showed that black women were more likely to receive no analgesia for vaginal delivery.[43] White comments that Enhanced Recovery After Surgery (ERAS) programs can decrease disparities with an intent to deliver evidence-based perioperative care to all patients through a systematic approach. Standardized protocols can promote equality and reduce implicit bias.[44]

Essien has thoughtfully discussed postpartum transitions as an opportunity to decrease racial disparities, citing an urgent need for obstetricians and primary care providers to prevent adverse postpartum outcomes and improve the quality and safety of health care for women around the time of pregnancy.[45]

One way to hardwire structures and processes is to ask centers to follow a predefined set of standards. One such set of standards is offered the Society for Obstetric Anesthesia and Perinatology Center of Excellence (COE) designation. The criteria for COE designation cover various domains including personnel and staffing; equipment, protocols, and policies; simulation and team training; obstetric emergency management; cesarean delivery and labor analgesia care; recommendations and guidelines implementation; and QA and patient follow-up systems. The designation aims to recognize institutions that provide optimal care, improve standards nationally, and provide a broad surrogate quality metric for obstetric anesthesia care.[46]

Patient Monitoring

Wilkins conducted a survey showing that while postanesthesia competence checklists for perinatal nurses have been published, they do not seem to be widely adopted in obstetric PACUs.[47]

Box 2
Skillsets and toolkits[40]

Antenatal care

1. Collaboration in interdisciplinary medical high-risk antepartum clinic

2. Provision of antenatal anesthesiology consultation for medically and surgically complex maternal cases

3. Collaboration to create comprehensive interdisciplinary care plans including delivery plan, anesthetic plan, special monitoring considerations, and provisions for unanticipated or potential care complexities

Intrapartum care

1. Provision of 24/7 state-of-the-art and timely labor epidural analgesia and cesarean delivery anesthesia service (will require in-service training of nonspecialist anesthetists providing obstetric care)

2. Championing of interdisciplinary team training, with simulation and drills, for acute maternal crises (eg, local anesthetic systemic toxicity, maternal cardiac arrest, amniotic fluid embolism, high spinal, malignant hyperthermia)

3. Promotion of evidence-based care standardization including California Maternal Quality Care Collaboration or National Partnership for Maternal Safety bundles (eg, obstetric hemorrhage, severe hypertension, VTE prophylaxis, known and occult cardiac disease)

4. Optimization of maternal early warning system to assure the earliest detection of deteriorating maternal status in-hospital

5. Provision of expertise in recognition and advanced medical management of pregnancy-specific and pregnancy-aggravated conditions (eg, hypertensive disorders, hemorrhagic and septic shock, amniotic fluid embolism, VTE, and cardiac events)

6. Availability of on-site anesthesiologist to assist medical management of acute crises and initiation of critical care for maternity patients

Postpartum care

1. Transitioning to intensive care unit for postpartum critical care in cooperation with intensivists and maternal–fetal medicine

2. Leadership in protocol development to promote safe and appropriate use of prescription opioids

3. Championing of enhanced recovery after surgery protocols to optimize recovery, reduce the length of stay, and promote opioid sparing

Regionalization of maternal care

1. Promotion of regionalization of care, requiring obstetric anesthesia leadership at all levels III and IV hospitals

2. Support of regional and statewide high-quality interdisciplinary maternal mortality reviews

3. Study of the impact of regionalization, care bundles, and other practice improvement efforts

4. Promotion of a patient-safety science (eg, team training, deployment of well-conceived checklists)

5. Updating nonspecialist obstetric anesthesiology practicing colleagues about ongoing advances in obstetric anesthesia that often fail to become mainstream (eg, active management of labor epidural analgesia, appropriate use of vasoactive substances after neuraxial block for cesarean delivery, evidence-based fluid management protocols)

Box 3
Recommendations for performance improvement committees[42]

1. Integration of equity as a core principle for the entire department and as an overarching goal

2. Collaboration with expert(s) in equity-based research

3. Use of standardized tools to screen for social determinants of health and ensure appropriate linkages to community resources

4. Collection of disaggregated data on process and outcome measures, stratified by race, ethnicity, language, or any appropriate sociodemographic consideration based on the population served

5. Tracking of outcome measures that reflect sociodemographic barriers to care, such as missed visits or late initiation of prenatal care

6. Collaboration with departmental leadership to develop remediation plans

7. Possible inclusion of a patient-reported experience measure

Mhyre looked at 8 anesthesia-related and 7 anesthesia-contributing maternal deaths in Michigan between 1985 and 2003 and made 3 key findings. First, all anesthesia-related deaths from airway obstruction or hypoventilation took place during emergence and recovery, not during the induction of general anesthesia. Second, system errors played a role in most cases. Of concern, lapses in postoperative monitoring and inadequate supervision by an anesthesiologist seemed to contribute to more than half of the deaths. Third, obesity and African-American race were important risk factors for anesthesia-related maternal mortality.[48]

Early-warning systems have been recommended for nonobstetric patients to ensure timely recognition of patients who are developing an acute illness. A single-parameter risk assessment system favors simplicity and specificity over complexity and sensitivity (**Table 3**).[49] Maternal mortality reviews indicate that among women who died, a disproportionate number demonstrated frankly abnormal vital signs, suggesting that a single-parameter system should maximize specificity for patients who are developing critical illness. Multiparameter early-warning scoring systems rely on nurses to document, calculate, and interpret the scores, and are therefore more resource-intensive. An important component of early warning systems is clarifying who to notify, how to notify them, and when and how to activate the clinical chain of command to ensure an appropriate response.[49]

Shields used a maternal early-warning trigger tool designed to address 4 of the most common causes of maternal morbidity. Sepsis and hypertension were picked up in particular. Three components of this tool that made its use favorable were that the alarm frequency was relatively low, there was a reasonably good predictive value for patients who were ultimately admitted to the ICU, and it was tested in hospitals with delivery volumes varying between 860 and 3000.[50]

Team Effects

Another dynamic that results in variation and uneven outcomes is changes in staffing on different days of the week and times of the day. Pauls showed that hospital inpatients admitted during weekends may have a higher mortality rate compared with inpatients admitted during the weekdays.[51] Barnardo showed that difficult intubations in obstetrics are more likely to occur off-hours.[52]

Wagner showed that the presence of an obstetric fellowship-trained anesthesiologist may be a predictor of decreased rate of general anesthesia use in patients with

Table 3 Maternal early warning criteria	
Systolic BP (mm Hg)	<90 or >160
Diastolic BP (mm Hg)	>100
Heart rate (beats per min)	<50 or >120
Respiratory rate (breaths per min)	<10 or >30
Oxygen saturation on room air, at sea level	<95
Oliguria, mL/h for >2 h	<35
Maternal agitation, confusion, or unresponsiveness; Patient with preeclampsia reporting a nonremitting headache or shortness of breath	

Adapted from Ref.[49]

preexisting indwelling labor epidural catheters.[53] Campbell similarly showed that subspecialist obstetric anesthesiologists manage indwelling epidural catheters differently than generalist anesthesiologists and on average had a lower need for conversion of epidural to general anesthesia.[54] Riley found that factors associated with failure of the epidural block were an increased requirement for supplemental local anesthetic boluses during labor to provide adequate analgesia and that the attending anesthesiologist for the cesarean delivery was not a specialist in obstetric anesthesia.[55] Cobb found that treatment by an obstetric anesthesiologist was associated with lower odds of receiving general anesthesia for cesarean delivery, although this finding did not persist in a subgroup analysis restricted to evening and weekend deliveries.[56]

An important aspect of high-performance teamwork is learning from mistakes. Failure to debrief after critical events in anesthesia is associated with failures in communication during the event. If we don't learn from our critical events, we are likely to relive them.[57]

An emerging area for leveraging specialists in obstetric anesthesia is telemedicine. Telemedicine is a valuable tool by which evaluation, triaging, and multidisciplinary coordination can be provided for high-risk obstetric patients living in remote or rural communities without access to specialized, maternal care medical facilities. It has the potential to save cost, optimize transfer decisions, improve resource allocation, improve access, promote health provider education, increase patient satisfaction, increase range of care, and encourage community-based care (**Fig. 3**).[58] Only a limited number of studies have assessed the accuracy of preoperative anesthesia teleconsultation versus in-person consultation, and no study has examined patient outcomes. One telemedicine program was estimated to save patients in travel costs and lost wages per completed teleconsultation, and satisfaction was rated very highly among participants. Frequencies of cesarean sections, macrosomia, and fetal deaths were no different between telemedicine and in-person consultation groups; however, premature labor and neonatal intensive care unit use were noted to be lower in the telemedicine group. Overall, the program demonstrated that most telemedicine patients were able to be managed at their local hospital, with only 15% requiring transfer to a center with higher level of care. Obstetric anesthesia prelabor consultation should be an integral part of routine, high-risk, pregnancy medical care. However, due to a paucity of anesthesiologists trained in obstetric anesthesia with experience caring for high-risk parturients, access to care for many women in rural or remote areas is limited. Telemedicine has the potential to overcome this barrier.[58]

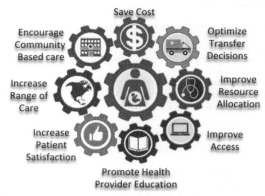

Fig. 3. Potential benefits of telemedicine in obstetric anesthesia.[58]

Postpartum Hemorrhage

PPH is included on most lists as an area of potential impact for obstetric anesthesiologists. It is most often caused by uterine atony resulting in transfusion, and often occurs in the absence of recognized risk factors.[59] Kacmar reported that despite the increasing emphasis on national QI in patient safety, there are no PPH protocols in at least 20% of US academic obstetric anesthesia units. Delivery case volume is the most important variable predicting the presence of a PPH protocol.[60] Reale found that among patients with PPH from 2010 to 2014, there was a decline in associated coagulopathy, acute respiratory failure, and maternal death, but an increase in sepsis and acute renal failure. Continued focus on PPH management is warranted.[61]

An example of a QI strategy for PPH is the better measurement of blood loss. Toledo hypothesized that adding calibrations to the vaginal delivery drapes would improve visual assessment of blood loss. Visual blood loss estimation with noncalibrated drapes underestimated blood loss, with worsening accuracy at larger volumes (16% error at 300 mL to 41% at 2000 mL). With calibrated drapes, the error was less than 15% at all volumes.[62]

An obstetric hemorrhage safety bundle was developed by the National Partnership for Maternal Safety and Council on Patient Safety in Women's Health Care. The multidisciplinary bundle consists of elements around (1) readiness, (2) recognition and prevention, (3) response, and (4) reporting and systems learning.[63] With a PPH protocol, Shields noted a significant shift toward resolution of maternal bleeding at an earlier stage, use of fewer blood products, and a 64% reduction in the rate of disseminated intravascular coagulation. In addition, there were significant improvements in staff and physician perceptions of patient safety.[64]

Venous Thromboembolism

Another toolkit developed by the National Partnership for Maternal Safety is the Consensus Bundle on VTE (**Box 4**).[65]

SOAP's Consensus Statement on the anesthetic management of pregnant and postpartum women receiving thromboprophylaxis or higher dose anticoagulants provides decision aids to help inform risk–benefit discussions with patients and facilitate shared decision making around anticoagulation and neuraxial anesthesia.[66]

DISCUSSION

QA/QI are ways to make sure that agreed-upon standards are met and to continuously improve systems to make things better. Multiple considerations go into designing

---

Box 4
Venous thromboembolism prevention maternal safety bundle[65]

Readiness
   Every unit should use a standardized thromboembolism risk assessment tool during:
   • Outpatient prenatal care
   • Antepartum hospitalization
   • Hospitalization after cesarean or vaginal birth
   • Postpartum period (up to 6 weeks after birth)

Recognition and prevention
   For every patient
   • Apply the standardized tool to all patients to assess VTE risk at time points designated under readiness
   • Apply the standardized tool to identify appropriate patients for thromboprophylaxis
   • Provide patient education
   • Provide all health care providers education regarding risk assessment tools and recommended thromboprophylaxis

Response
   Every unit should
   • Use standardized recommendations for mechanical thromboprophylaxis
   • Use standardized recommendations for dosing of prophylactic and therapeutic pharmacologic anticoagulation
   • Use standardized recommendations for appropriate timing of pharmacologic prophylaxis with neuraxial anesthesia

Reporting and systems learning
   Every unit should
   • Review all thromboembolism events for systems issues and compliance with protocols
   • Monitor process metrics and outcomes in a standardized fashion
   • Assess for complications of pharmacologic thromboprophylaxis

---

quality and patient safety project that will be successful, including carefully selecting the problem to be solved. Identifying variation in well-chosen metrics is an important way to find opportunities to improve quality, patient safety, and equity. Learning from the outliers is a valuable tool for improvement.[8] Using project management tools will increase the likelihood of achieving the desired goals. Making local change can pave the way for making change at scale. Additionally, QA/QI has to be approached from a perspective that considers provider burnout and well-being. Providers are overburdened with quality metrics, with one study estimating that providers spend $15.4B and 785 hours annually reporting quality metrics.[67]

Dyrbye showed that physicians identified on a brief screening tool as having increased risk of burnout were more likely to make medical errors.[68] Psychological safety and a culture of safety are foundational to identifying and addressing errors. Burnout is increased by disruptive behavior.[69] Convincing physicians that quality metrics are important and worthwhile often requires difficult conversations.[10]

Even while emphasizing measurement, we also have to recognize that providers do many things that cannot be measured. We do not want them to redirect their efforts away from those things as an unintended consequence of tracking selected metrics.[70]

SUMMARY

Safety and equity are both fundamental dimensions of health care quality. Sivashankar points out that "there is no such thing as high-quality, safe care that is, inequitable, and that there is a natural alignment between the framework we use to improve safety and the approach we can take to increase equity. Both frameworks encourage redesigning systems to make them more reliable and resilient. Both balance a systems focus with individual accountability. Both recognize the role of cognitive, often subconscious, biases in contributing to unintentional harm. Both highlight the importance of psychological safety to support difficult conversations. And both avoid excessive focus on individual or interpersonal blame." He argues that stratified data should be the norm in health care.[17]

Developing expertise in QA/QI is a major opportunity for obstetric anesthesiologists to impact care on the L&D floor to promote higher quality, safer, and more equitable care.

CLINICS CARE POINTS

- Skillsets and toolkits for obstetric anesthesiologists can be divided into antenatal, intrapartum, postpartum, and regionalization, and include the promotion of patient-safety science using team training and the deployment of checklists.

- Proposed quality metrics in obstetric anesthesia include mode of anesthesia for cesarean delivery, difficult intubation rate, wet tap rate, headache incidence after neuraxial anesthesia, blood patch rate, patient satisfaction, labor epidural request response time, labor epidural replacement rate, effectiveness of post-operative analgesia, and rate of obstetric critical care admissions.

- A single-parameter early-warning system based on abnormal vital signs can help with early identification of patients who are developing critical illness.

- Telemedicine is a valuable tool by which evaluation, triaging, and multidisciplinary coordination can be provided for high-risk obstetric patients living in remote or rural communities without access to specialized, maternal care medical facilities.

- Safety and equity are both fundamental dimensions of health care quality.

REFERENCES

1. Lynde GC. Working toward quality in obstetric anesthesia: a business approach. Curr Opin Anaesthesiol 2017;30(3):280–6.
2. Edmondson A. Psychological safety and learning behavior in work teams. Adm Sci Q 1999;44:350–83.
3. Institute of Medicine. Crossing the quality chasm: a new health system for the 21st century. Washington DC: National Academies Press (US); 2001.
4. Bauer MS, Damschroder L, Hagedorn H, et al. An introduction to implementation science for the non-specialist. BMC Psychol 2015;3(1):32.
5. Lane-Fall MB, Cobb BT, Cené CW, et al. Implementation science in perioperative care. Anesthesiol Clin 2018;36(1):1–15.
6. Institute of Medicine. In: Kohn LT, Corrigan JM, Donaldson MS, editors. To err is human: building a safer health system. Washington DC: National Academies Press (US); 2000.
7. Lee TH, Cosgrove T. Engaging doctors in the health care revolution. Harv Bus Rev 2014;92(6):104–11, 138.
8. Gawande A. The Bell Curve: What happens when patients find out how good their doctors really are? New York: The New Yorker; 2004.
9. Vizient. How integrated insights can transform care delivery. HIMSS20; 2020. Available at: https://himss20.mapyourshow.com. Accessed May 26, 2021.
10. Stone D, Patton B, Heen S. Difficult conversations: how to discuss what matters most. New York: Penguin Books; 2010.
11. The effects of CMS' star ratings: 5 things hospital leaders should know. Becker's Hospital Review; 2016.
12. Bodenheimer T, Sinsky C. From triple to quadruple aim: care of the patient requires care of the provider. Ann Fam Med 2014;12(6):573–6.

13. Sikka R, Morath JM, Leape L. The Quadruple Aim: care, health, cost and meaning in work. BMJ Qual Saf 2015;24(10):608–10.

14. Donabedian A. The quality of care. How can it be assessed? JAMA 1988;260(12): 1743–8.

15. Mhyre JM, Bateman BT, Leffert LR. Influence of patient comorbidities on the risk of near-miss maternal morbidity or mortality. Anesthesiology 2011;115(5):963–72.

16. Andreae MH, Maman SR, Behnam AJ. An electronic medical record-derived individualized performance metric to measure risk-adjusted adherence with perioperative prophylactic bundles for health care disparity research and implementation science. Appl Clin Inform 2020;11(3):497–514.

17. Sivashanker K, Gandhi TK. Advancing safety and equity together. N Engl J Med 2020;382(4):301–3.

18. Butwick A. What's new in obstetric anesthesia in 2011? Reducing maternal adverse outcomes and improving obstetric anesthesia quality of care. Anesth Analg 2012;115(5):1137–45.

19. Farquhar C, Sadler L, Masson V, et al. Beyond the numbers: classifying contributory factors and potentially avoidable maternal deaths in New Zealand, 2006-2009. Am J Obstet Gynecol 2011;205(4):331, e1–8.

20. Say L, Souza JP, Pattinson RC. Maternal near miss–towards a standard tool for monitoring quality of maternal health care. Best Pract Res Clin Obstet Gynaecol 2009;23(3):287–96.

21. Tunçalp O, Hindin MJ, Souza JP, et al. The prevalence of maternal near miss: a systematic review. BJOG 2012;119(6):653–61.

22. MacDorman MF, Declercq E, Cabral H, et al. Recent increases in the U.S. maternal mortality rate: disentangling trends from measurement issues. Obstet Gynecol 2016;128(3):447–55.

23. Callaghan WM, Creanga AA, Kuklina EV. Severe maternal morbidity among delivery and postpartum hospitalizations in the United States. Obstet Gynecol 2012; 120(5):1029–36.

24. Creanga AA, Berg CJ, Syverson C, et al. Pregnancy-related mortality in the United States, 2006-2010. Obstet Gynecol 2015;125(1):5–12.

25. Glance LG, Dick AW, Glantz JC, et al. Rates of major obstetrical complications vary almost fivefold among US hospitals. Health Aff (Millwood) 2014;33(8):1330–6.

26. Howell EA, Egorova NN, Balbierz A, et al. Site of delivery contribution to black-white severe maternal morbidity disparity. Am J Obstet Gynecol 2016;215(2):143–52.

27. Goffman D, Madden RC, Harrison EA, et al. Predictors of maternal mortality and near-miss maternal morbidity. J Perinatol 2007;27(10):597–601.

28. Markow C, Main EK. Creating change at scale: quality improvement strategies used by the California maternal quality care collaborative. Obstet Gynecol Clin North Am 2019;46(2):317–28.

29. Vago T, Bell A, Thompson H. Lean delivery. Qual Prog 2016;30.

30. Bell AM, Bohannon J, Porthouse L, et al. Process improvement to enhance quality in a large volume labor and birth unit. MCN Am J Matern Child Nurs 2016;41(6):340–8.

31. Fleischman E. Improving women's readiness for discharge postpartum. J Obstet Gynecol Neonatal Nurs 2015;44(1):S2.

32. Prabhu M, McQuaid-Hanson E, Hopp S, et al. A shared decision-making intervention to guide opioid prescribing after cesarean delivery. Obstet Gynecol 2017;130(1):42–6.

33. Prabhu M, Dubois H, James K, et al. Implementation of a quality improvement initiative to decrease opioid prescribing after cesarean delivery. Obstet Gynecol 2018;132(3):631–6.

34. Grunebaum A, Dudenhausen J, Chervenak FA, et al. Reduction of cesarean delivery rates after implementation of a comprehensive patient safety program. J Perinat Med 2013;41(1):51–5.
35. Bamber JH, Lucas DN, Plaat F, et al. The identification of key indicators to drive quality improvement in obstetric anaesthesia: results of the Obstetric Anaesthetists' Association/National Perinatal Epidemiology Unit collaborative Delphi project. Anaesthesia 2020;75(5):617–25.
36. Wikner M, Bamber J. Quality improvement in obstetric anaesthesia. Int J Obstet Anesth 2018;35:1–3.
37. Pritchard N, Lo Q, Wikner M, et al. Collecting data for quality improvement in obstetric anaesthesia. Int J Obstet Anesth 2019;39:142–3.
38. Lucas N, Bamber J. Messages for improving anaesthetic care. In: MBRRACE-UK: Saving lives, improving mothers' care 2020: lessons to inform maternity care from the UK and Ireland confidential Enquiries in maternal death and morbidity 2016-18. 2020. Available at: https://www.npeu.ox.ac.uk/mbrrace-uk/presentations. Accessed Mar 24, 2021.
39. McQuaid E, Leffert LR, Bateman BT. The role of the anesthesiologist in preventing severe maternal morbidity and mortality. Clin Obstet Gynecol 2018;61(2):372–86.
40. Pryde PG. Contemplating our maternity care crisis in the United States: reflections of an obstetrician anesthesiologist. Anesth Analg 2019;128(5):1036–41.
41. Abir G, Mhyre J. Maternal mortality and the role of the obstetric anesthesiologist. Best Pract Res Clin Anaesthesiol 2017;31(1):91–105.
42. Pardo C, Atallah F, Mincer S, et al. Reducing perinatal health disparities by placing equity at the heart of performance improvement. Obstet Gynecol 2021;137(3):481–5.
43. Tangel VE, Matthews KC, Abramovitz SE, et al. Racial and ethnic disparities in severe maternal morbidity and anesthetic techniques for obstetric deliveries: a multi-state analysis, 2007-2014. J Clin Anesth 2020;65:109821.
44. White RS, Matthews KC, Tangel V, et al. Enhanced recovery after surgery (ERAS) programs for cesarean delivery can potentially reduce healthcare and racial disparities. J Natl Med Assoc 2019;111(4):464–5.
45. Essien UR, Molina RL, Lasser KE. Strengthening the postpartum transition of care to address racial disparities in maternal health. J Natl Med Assoc 2019;111(4):349–51.
46. Carvalho B, Mhyre JM. Centers of excellence for anesthesia care of obstetric patients. Anesth Analg 2019;128(5):844–6.
47. Wilkins KK, Greenfield ML, Polley LS, et al. A survey of obstetric perianesthesia care unit standards. Anesth Analg 2009;108(6):1869–75.
48. Mhyre JM, Riesner MN, Polley LS, et al. A series of anesthesia-related maternal deaths in Michigan, 1985-2003. Anesthesiology 2007;106(6):1096–104.
49. Mhyre JM, D'Oria R, Hameed AB, et al. The maternal early warning criteria: a proposal from the national partnership for maternal safety. Obstet Gynecol 2014;124(4):782–6.
50. Shields LE, Wiesner S, Klein C, et al. Use of maternal early warning trigger tool reduces maternal morbidity. Am J Obstet Gynecol 2016;214(4):527.e1–6.
51. Pauls LA, Johnson-Paben R, McGready J, et al. The weekend effect in hospitalized patients: a meta-analysis. J Hosp Med 2017;12(9):760–6.
52. Barnardo PD, Jenkins JG. Failed tracheal intubation in obstetrics: a 6-year review in a UK region. Anaesthesia 2000;55(7):690–4.
53. Wagner JL, White RS, Mauer EA, et al. Impact of anesthesiologist's fellowship status on the risk of general anesthesia for unplanned cesarean delivery. Acta Anaesthesiol Scand 2019;63(6):769–74.
54. Campbell DC, Tran T. Conversion of epidural labour analgesia to epidural anesthesia for intrapartum Cesarean delivery. Can J Anaesth 2009;56(1):19–26.

55. Riley ET, Papasin J. Epidural catheter function during labor predicts anesthetic efficacy for subsequent cesarean delivery. Int J Obstet Anesth 2002; 11(2):81–4.
56. Cobb BT, Lane-Fall MB, Month RC, et al. Anesthesiologist specialization and use of general anesthesia for cesarean delivery. Anesthesiology 2019;130(2): 237–46.
57. Pian-Smith MCM, Cooper JB. If we don't learn from our critical events, we're likely to relive them: debriefing should be the norm. Anesthesiology 2019;130(6): 867–9.
58. Duarte SS, Nguyen TT, Koch C, et al. Remote obstetric anesthesia: leveraging telemedicine to improve fetal and maternal outcomes. Telemed J E Health 2020;26(8):967–72.
59. Bateman BT, Berman MF, Riley LE, et al. The epidemiology of postpartum hemorrhage in a large, nationwide sample of deliveries. Anesth Analg 2010;110(5): 1368–73.
60. Kacmar RM, Mhyre JM, Scavone BM, et al. The use of postpartum hemorrhage protocols in United States academic obstetric anesthesia units. Anesth Analg 2014;119(4):906–10.
61. Reale SC, Easter SR, Xu X, et al. Trends in postpartum hemorrhage in the United States from 2010 to 2014. Anesth Analg 2020;130(5):e119–22.
62. Toledo P, McCarthy RJ, Hewlett BJ, et al. The accuracy of blood loss estimation after simulated vaginal delivery. Anesth Analg 2007;105(6):1736–40, table of contents.
63. Main EK, Goffman D, Scavone BM, et al. National partnership for maternal safety: consensus bundle on obstetric hemorrhage. Obstet Gynecol 2015;126(1): 155–62.
64. Shields LE, Smalarz K, Reffigee L, et al. Comprehensive maternal hemorrhage protocols improve patient safety and reduce utilization of blood products. Am J Obstet Gynecol 2011;205(4):368, e1–8.
65. D'Alton ME, Friedman AM, Smiley RM, et al. National partnership for maternal safety: consensus bundle on venous thromboembolism. Anesth Analg 2016; 123(4):942–9.
66. Leffert LR, Dubois HM, Butwick AJ, et al. Neuraxial anesthesia in obstetric patients receiving thromboprophylaxis with unfractionated or low-molecular-weight heparin: a systematic review of spinal epidural hematoma. Anesth Analg 2017; 125(1):223–31.
67. Casalino LP, Gans D, Weber R, et al. US physician practices spend more than $15.4 billion annually to report quality measures. Health Aff (Millwood) 2016; 35(3):401–6.
68. Dyrbye LN, Satele D, Sloan J, et al. Utility of a brief screening tool to identify physicians in distress. J Gen Intern Med 2013;28(3):421–7.
69. Rehder KJ, Adair KC, Hadley A, et al. Associations between a new disruptive behaviors scale and teamwork, patient safety, work-life balance, burnout, and depression. Jt Comm J Qual Patient Saf 2020;46(1):18–26.
70. Shaywitz D. We are not a dashboard: contesting the Tyranny of metrics, measurement, and managerialism. New York: Forbes; 2018.

Emergency Resources in Obstetrics

Katherine M. Seligman, MD, FRCPC, D.ABA[a], Gillian Abir, MBChB, FRCA[b],*

KEYWORDS

- Cognitive aids • Emergency resources • Multidisciplinary
- Obstetrical anesthesiology

KEY POINTS

- Preparation for a response to an obstetric emergency includes the development of an appropriate response team, adequate supplies, and obstetrical-specific (or adaptable) management algorithms.
- Standardized communication tools and debriefing methods improve communication during critical events.
- Utilization of care tools, cognitive aids, and algorithms increases adherence to critical treatment steps during emergencies and should be used frequently.

INTRODUCTION

Preparation, anticipation, and early recognition of emergencies in obstetrics are paramount to improve patient outcomes. Maternal morbidity and mortality have been increasing in the United States (US), and is thought to be related to the increased medical comorbidity of this patient population.[1] Advanced planning and training for emergent situations allow efficient activation of emergency resources and appropriate escalation of care, and this requires a multidisciplinary team-based approach involving nursing, obstetricians, anesthesiologists, neonatologists, pharmacists, and other obstetric care team members.

Emergencies can be broadly classified into clinical emergencies, natural disasters, and man-made disasters (**Table 1**). This review will specifically identify and describe resources available for the preparation and management of clinical emergencies in obstetrics. Although obstetric emergencies are commonly sudden or unexpected,

[a] Department of Anesthesiology, Pharmacology & Therapeutics, University of British Columbia, 4500 Oak Street, Vancouver, BC V6H3N1, Canada; [b] Department of Anesthesiology, Perioperative and Pain Medicine, Center for Academic Medicine, Stanford University School of Medicine, MC 5663, 453 Quarry Road, Palo Alto, CA 94304, USA
* Corresponding author.
E-mail address: gabir@stanford.edu
Twitter: @gillyabir (G.A.)

Anesthesiology Clin 39 (2021) 631–647
https://doi.org/10.1016/j.anclin.2021.08.004
1932-2275/21/© 2021 Elsevier Inc. All rights reserved.
anesthesiology.theclinics.com

Table 1
Types of emergencies

Clinical Emergencies	Natural Disasters	Human-made Disasters
• Cardiac arrest	Geophysical	• Terrorist attacks
• Local anesthetic systemic toxicity	• Earthquake	• Biochemical weapons
• Anaphylaxis	• Landslide	• Nuclear weapons
• Difficult airway	• Tsunamis	• Radiation exposure
• Altered mental status	• Volcanic eruption	• Bombings
• High/total spinal	Hydrologic	• Cyber attacks
• Bronchospasm	• Avalanche	• Power outage
• Hypotension/hypertension	• Flooding	• War/civil disorder
• Malignant hyperthermia	• Limnic eruption	• Industrial accidents
OB Specific	Climatologic	• Transportation accidents
• Peripartum hemorrhage	• Extreme temperatures	• Complex humanitarian
• Amniotic fluid embolism	• Drought	disasters
• Abruption	• Wildfires	
• Uterine inversion	Meteorologic	
• Cord prolapse	• Cyclones	
• Eclampsia	• Storms	
• Stat cesarean delivery	Biologic	
• Shoulder dystocia	• Plague	
• Uterine rupture	• Pandemic/epidemics	

some can be anticipated, and they can all be prepared for. Obstetric emergencies can occur anywhere and at any time, as they are not only confined to labor and delivery (L&D) units. A culture of emergency preparedness, drills, debriefs, continuous process improvement, and access to emergency equipment and drugs promotes improvement in maternal and fetal outcomes.

DISCUSSION

Emergency resources in obstetrics are in abundance, and it is important that health care providers know how and where to access them, otherwise they may fail to reach the target audience. Resources range from institutional, to national, and international, and may be obstetrical-specific or adaptable for an obstetric patient. Resources are available on organizational and societal web sites, through online forums, podcasts, and webinars, and through platforms such as Twitter (Twitter, Inc., San Francisco, CA, US), WhatsApp (WhatsApp LLC., Menlo Park, CA, US), and Facebook groups (Facebook, Inc., Menlo Park, CA, US).[2]

Standardized Verbal Communication Tools

Suboptimal communication has been identified in root-cause analyses as a leading contributing factor in cases described in morbidity and mortality reports and closed claims reports.[3,4] In an anesthesiology closed claims report for massive hemorrhage for which obstetric cases accounted for 30% of the claims, one or more communication issues occurred in 60% of the claims and more than half of communication issues occurred between the anesthesiologist and surgeon.[3] Using standardized communication techniques helps with familiarity, and when team members utilize these techniques, awareness, and understanding can increase, and confusion and misunderstanding can decrease. These techniques can be taught and practiced in simulation drills or workshops, and include:

SBAR

This is the acronym for situation, background, assessment, and recommendation (or request) which helps facilitate fast, precise, and accurate communication with one sentence per item, for example,

Closed-loop communication

This consists of a precise conversation between a sender and receiver, whereby the sender gives clear and direct verbal information to the receiver (commonly an action request), the receiver verbally acknowledges the understanding of the information, enacts the request, and verbally confirms to the sender when the action has been completed (or explains to the sender if, and why, it has not been completed) which closes the loop.[5]

Recap

A recap is a short summary of an ongoing clinical situation and ensures that all team members understand what is happening. It can be initiated by anyone; however, it should ideally be led by a person with high situational awareness, often the team leader. The team leader briefly asks *everyone* in the room to be silent and then explains the presumed diagnosis, what has been done so far, what the current treatment plan is, and what the plan is if the current treatment plan does not work. This is followed by questions from any team member to clarify or pertinent information from any team member to add that may change the plan. Recaps should not be performed when a critical task is being accomplished, for example, when the anesthesiologist is intubating a patient or when the obstetrician is trying to surgically control a hemorrhage. A recap can be initiated more than once for the same patient; however, there is a balance between performing them too frequently (and disrupting workflow) and too infrequently (leading to lack of team situational awareness).

Team Huddles

A team huddle is a short briefing that occurs with team members before the start of a surgical case or procedure, the purpose of which is to share case-related information for coordinated care, and discuss any potential safety issues.[6] The main benefits of a team huddle include improved patient and staff safety, improved efficiency, enhanced communication, and better teamwork.[6]

Direct patient care in an emergency takes precedence, so in most emergencies, there may not be enough time to discuss detailed treatment plans beforehand. An abbreviated huddle may be used in emergency situations, summarizing salient points in less than 1 minute. When there is time, especially before a high-risk case, it is prudent for the multidisciplinary team to huddle to anticipate and plan for any critical events that may occur if the patient decompensates, or if the surgery has the potential to be complicated, especially when other teams may be on stand-by (eg, the gynecology-oncology team). Some institutions perform team huddles for high-risk patients only, but ideally, team huddles should be performed before all cases and procedures, scheduled, and unscheduled, so that it becomes common practice.

Team Debriefs

Following an acute event, it is good practice for the *whole team* to debrief to discuss what unfolded, ideally immediately after the event whereas people's memories are clear. Examples include: planned procedures when the outcome was not as expected; patient or staff harm (or near-miss); events when the outcome was as expected but involved some associated circumstance for which team members would benefit from receiving more information, and/or clarification why action A or action B was performed; sentinel, rare, or unusual events; significant system issues, including barriers to job performance and communication breakdowns. Often during an acute event, there is not enough time to adequately explain to a team member why action A or action B needs to be accomplished. Taking the time to debrief after patient care is complete can be a very worthwhile exercise to increase knowledge and understanding if the same or similar event occurs again, and it can improve team cohesiveness by making team members feel included and valued. Ideally, a team debrief should be actioned after every procedure/event, but in reality, this is not always feasible due to time constraints or other clinical responsibilities.

Debriefs, led by the team leader or trained facilitator, should include all team members and be conducted in an area that is private and quiet to allow open discussion. Adverse events can have a catastrophic impact on health care provider's well-being and debriefing is an opportunity to try and alleviate this. It is prudent to have paper copies of a debriefing tool available in a standardized location on L&D so that the location of the debrief is not restricted to a location with computer access. An effective team debrief involves covering various aspects of care using a standardized and structured approach so that all the important elements are addressed. Examples of debriefing tools include, the "Promoting Excellence And Reflective Learning in Simulation (PEARLS)" health care debriefing tool, and the "Debriefing In Situ Conversation after Emergent Resuscitation Now (DISCERN)" tool.[7–9]

WRITTEN/ELECTRONIC CARE TOOLS

Care tools encompass a broad range of resources that provide clinically relevant information that can assist in patient care and may be available in paper or electronic format. Electronic tools should have paper copies available in L&D for use during a power or Internet outage or other types of disasters that could involve the evacuation of the facility. Electronic tools can be integrated into electronic medical programs and electronic medical records (EMRs) to enhance usability and compliance by health care providers.

Cognitive Aids

Cognitive aid is a generic term that encompasses various types of resources that can be used in emergent or routine situations, and include checklists, handbooks, emergency manuals, reference cards, and pocket cards. Cognitive aids provide a structured and standardized response to accomplish appropriate tasks and optimize communication, and they can be used during an emergency, or retrospectively to check that all necessary steps/tasks have been accomplished.[10] Cognitive aids should be used during down-time for teaching purposes, and during simulations to enhance user-familiarity. A good example is the postpartum hemorrhage checklist that was developed at Stanford University School of Medicine (**Fig. 1**).

Although some types of anesthesia-related emergencies are common to an adult patient irrespective of pregnancy status, there are some emergencies specific to pregnancy or require nuances and adaptions for a pregnant patient. An example of an obstetrical-specific emergency manual is the Obstetric Anesthesia Emergency Manual, and an example of a resource aimed for a generic adult patient with adaptations for pregnancy is material for Advanced Cardiac Life Support (ACLS) training.[11,12]

Algorithms, Flowsheets/Charts, Guidelines, and Protocols

Various organizations have published algorithms, flowsheets/charts, guidelines, and protocols to assist with the delivery of safe health care during emergencies.

PPH Checklist

Recognize ⟩ Call for Help ⟩ Treat ⟩ Transfuse early

STEP 1: CALL FOR HELP!

☐ OB Rapid Response   ☐ Primary OB   ☐ OB Hospitalist   ☐ Anesthesiologist

☐ Assign nursing roles

STEP 2: IDENTIFY & TREAT CAUSE ~ Atony, Laceration, Retained Placenta, Coagulopathy

☐ Vitals q1-2 min   ☐ PPH kit + PPH cart

☐ 100% oxygen   ☐ Fundal massage

☐ IV fluids - high rate   ☐ Urinary catheter

☐ 2 wide-bore IVs   ☐ Uterotonics ⟹

		Time given:
Oxytocin	· <u>Bolus</u>: 1-2 u IV bolus, up to max 5 u IV (anesthesiologists only)	
	· <u>Infusion</u>: 30 u/500 mL normal saline @ 125 mL/h (7.5 u/h) (max rate 500 mL/h (30 u/h))	
Methylergonovine	0.2 mg IM q2-4 h	_____
Carboprost	0.25 mg IM q15 min	_____
	Repeat dose @	_____
Misoprostol	600-800 mcg SL	_____

STEP 3: ASSESS MAGNITUDE
Phase 1 (first 5 – 10 min)

☐ **Consider doing a RECAP now**

☐ Send STAT labs (ABG, CBC, PT/PTT, INR, Fibrinogen, iCa, TEG)

☐ Activate MTP   ☐ Resuscitate using rapid infuser device

☐ Assess QBL   ☐ Consider uterine balloon tamponade device

Phase 2 (10 – 15 min)

☐ Early transfer to OR (if bleeding is ongoing) or IR (if bleeding ongoing + stable)

☐ Consider fibrinogen concentrate or cryoprecipitate

☐ Consider tranexamic acid 1 g IV

☐ Treat hypocalcemia   ☐ Maintain normothermia

Fig. 1. Postpartum hemorrhage checklist. ABG, arterial blood gas; CBC, complete blood count; iCa, ionized calcium; INR, international normalized ratio; IR, interventional radiology; IV, intravenous; MTP, massive transfusion protocol; OB, obstetric; OR, operating room; PPH, postpartum hemorrhage; PT, prothrombin time; PTT, partial thromboplastin time; q, quaque (every); QBL, quantitative blood loss; STAT, statum (immediately); TEG, thromboelastography. (Figure published under Creative Commons License: Attribution-NonCommercial-NoDerivs 3.0 Unported (CCBY-NC-ND 3.0).)

Algorithms and flowsheets are a subset of cognitive aids and are intended to be simplistic diagrams, straightforward to follow and use, and are usually limited to a single problem. A good example is the Maternal Sepsis Evaluation Flow Chart published by the California Maternal Quality Care Collaborative (CMQCC) (**Fig. 2**). Guidelines and protocols are usually written text with integrated tables, algorithms, and/or flowsheets.

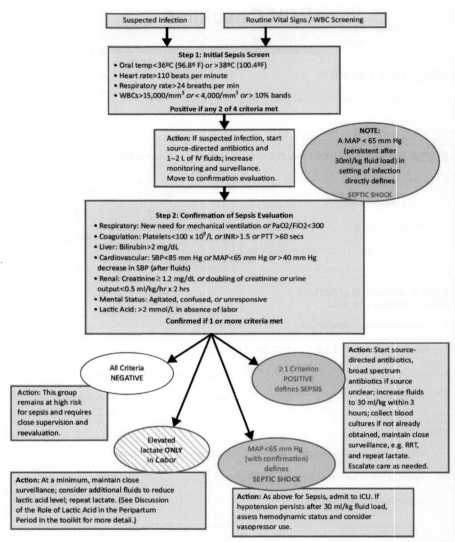

Fig. 2. California Maternal Quality Care Collaborative Maternal Sepsis Evaluation Flow Chart. ICU, intensive care unit; INR, international normalized ratio; MAP, mean arterial pressure; PTT, partial thromboplastin time; RRT, rapid response team; SBP, systolic blood pressure; WBC, white blood cell. (©2019 California Maternal Quality Care Collaborative: The material in this toolkit may be freely reproduced and disseminated for informational, educational and non-commercial purposes only. Gibbs R, Bauer M, Olvera L, Sakowski C, Cape V, Main E. Improving Diagnosis and Treatment of Maternal Sepsis: A Quality Improvement Toolkit. Stanford, CA: California Maternal Quality Care Collaborative.)

Although these are commonly evidence-based, guidelines allow for deviation by the health care provider using clinical judgment if the situation deems it necessary, whereas adherence to protocols is more stringent with deviation only acceptable in extenuating circumstances.

Consensus Statements and Practice Advisories

Consensus statements and practice advisories are evidence-based documents written by a designated group of experts to clarify the understanding of a specific topic. The purpose of these statements is to disseminate knowledge and increase awareness and understanding, not as resources for use during an emergency. The educational content in consensus statements and practice advisories can enhance the health care provider's expertise to deliver optimal care during an emergency. Examples of a consensus statement and practice advisory published by the Society of Obstetric Anesthesia and Perinatology, include "Neuraxial procedures in obstetric patients with thrombocytopenia" and "Sugammadex during pregnancy and lactation," both of which are informative for an anesthesiologist dealing with an emergency cesarean delivery (CD), for example,[13,14]

Care Bundles/Toolkits

The Alliance for Innovation on Maternal Health (AIM), which is a national quality improvement working group within the Council on Patient Safety in Women's Health Care, describe a patient safety bundle as *"a set of evidence-based guidelines, to be adapted for local circumstances, to optimally manage a medical condition and thus improve patient outcomes."*[15] The Council currently has 10 obstetric patient safety bundles (4 primary and 6 supporting) which include obstetric hemorrhage, severe hypertension in pregnancy, maternal venous thromboembolism, and 2 nonobstetrical (ie, gynecologic) patient safety bundles available for free download.[16] The bundles are divided into sections: readiness, recognition and prevention, response, and reporting/systems learning.

Toolkits are similar to care bundles and include cognitive aids for specific clinical tasks relevant to the clinic subject. For example, the CMQCC describes toolkits as *"a compendium of best practice tools and articles, care guidelines in multiple formats, hospital-level implementation guide, and professional education slide set."*[17] The CMQCC currently has 8 toolkits available for free download, which include cardiovascular disease in pregnancy and postpartum, and maternal sepsis.[17]

Surveillance Tools

Generic adult surveillance tools are suboptimal for obstetric patients (pregnant and postpartum patients) as they do not consider physiologic changes in pregnancy.[18] Obstetrical-specific surveillance tools such as a maternal early warning system (MEWS) are recommended to enhance the bedside evaluation of the obstetric patient and allow timely diagnosis and early resuscitation/treatment strategies, and ultimately reduce maternal morbidity and mortality.[18] A standardized process to alert the health care provider when a patient meets surveillance criteria is required, otherwise the tool does not achieve its purpose and is redundant. It is possible to associate MEWS criteria with an alert notification platform in the EMR, which is being advocated for by experts and national bodies (and has been undertaken at one of the authors' institutions (GA)).[19–21]

Simulation Training and Emergency Drills

Multidisciplinary (or single discipline) simulation is an excellent modality to test emergency preparedness including team responsiveness, systems issues, and to practice using the tools described in this article. Debriefing, as discussed earlier, is a process that takes extensive faculty development and practice to successfully accomplish and therefore introducing it into simulation training can make it easier to translate into clinical care.

Rapid Response and Obstetric Code Teams

When an emergency occurs, it is vital to have a rapid and coordinated response for the patient's (or staff, or visitor's) needs. This not only involves an appropriate number of responders, but necessitates responders arriving with appropriate knowledge and skills to institute correct actions/treatment. For example, appropriate team members of an "Obstetric (OB) Rapid Response Team" may include obstetricians, obstetric anesthesiologists, L&D nursing, plus a notification to a pharmacist. At one of the author's institutions (GA), the designated OB Rapid Response Team differs from an OB Code Blue Team, which includes neonatologists and neonatology nurses if delivery is anticipated during a maternal cardiac arrest or other serious events. An "OB Rapid Response" is activated for a maternal nondeliverable indication; however, if the situation unfolds to involve delivery, the neonatology team can be alerted on an ad hoc basis, which avoids alert fatigue if the neonatology team is called for every event unnecessarily. It is important to designate which members of each discipline will respond to an OB Rapid Response, especially when these may occur in locations outside of L&D. For example, there needs to be designated adequate backup coverage on L&D for ongoing patient care if the covering anesthesiologist responds to an OB Rapid Response call. This will vary for each institution depending on the layout of the hospital and proximity of other patient care areas to L&D, and with the number of anesthesiologists. One option is for a nonanesthesiologist member (eg, anesthesiology resident or fellow, certified registered nurse anesthetist, or anesthesia assistant) to respond and call for backup, if necessary. The team members need to be aware of their roles in the team, their responsibilities; the expected response time and an expectation to delegate the duty to another health care provider if responding to the alert would be detrimental to a patient already under their care.

Emergency Supplies

Preparation for emergency management includes gathering and packaging necessary supplies in easily accessible locations, and for health care providers to be aware and familiar with these specific locations. Emergency supplies may take the form of a mobile rolling cart, portable drug box, or portable kit for specific medical conditions (eg, hemorrhage cart, malignant hyperthermia (MH) box, difficult airway box, etc.). Development of resources needs to be in conjunction with physicians, nursing, and pharmacy so that appropriate storage, stocking, and drug regulations are followed. This section will cover creating emergency carts containing supplies that may be used for obstetric hemorrhage, MH, severe hypertension/eclampsia, difficult airway, local anesthetic systemic toxicity (LAST), difficult intravenous (IV) access, and perimortem cesarean delivery (PMCD). There may be additional equipment that can be bundled together for various health care settings depending on the patient population and incidence of certain emergencies.

Emergency Carts and Drug Kits

Emergency carts are portable collections of equipment, algorithm cards, and drug kits that can be deployed in preparation or response to clinical situations. They should be securely closed with a tamper-proof easily removable plastic tag to ensure they remain fully stocked in between use. One of the most recognizable equipment carts is the "crash cart" (or "code cart") that should be available in L&D units.

Hemorrhage Cart & Postpartum Hemorrhage Drug Kit

Hemorrhage occurs in 3% to 5% of obstetric patients and accounts for approximately 11% of maternal deaths in the US and 27% of maternal deaths worldwide.[1,22,23] Effective July 2020, after the review of The Joint Commission's (TJC's) Sentinel Event Database indicated maternal hemorrhage was a causal factor in 51% of maternal death or severe maternal morbidity cases, TJC mandated Joint Commission-accredited hospitals to implement specific evidence-based practices for maternal hemorrhage, and severe hypertension/preeclampsia with the aim to reduce maternal morbidity and mortality.[24]

Within AIM's obstetric hemorrhage toolkit is a recommendation to prepare an easily accessible and mobile hemorrhage cart with easy access to uterotonic drugs (eg, postpartum hemorrhage drug kit).[25] Drugs need to be housed in separate locations due to refrigeration requirements for certain second-line uterotonic drugs such as ergonovine and carboprost.

Hemorrhage carts house equipment and instruments for the management of peripartum hemorrhage due to etiologies such as uterine atony and perineal lacerations. Supplies include IV access and fluid, blood draw equipment and laboratory tubes, invasive lines such as arterial and central venous catheters, surgical instruments and sponges, retractors, Foley catheters, uterine balloon tamponade devices, B-Lynch sutures, and vaginal packing. The AIM obstetric hemorrhage bundle contains a list of recommended supplies that can be tailored to a specific institution (eg, hospital or birthing location).[25] Contents should be clearly labeled, checked daily, and replenished after every use. This cart can be moved to the bedside or operating room (OR) at certain trigger points: available for patients at high risk for hemorrhage due to comorbidities, or in response to ongoing blood loss estimated to be greater than 1000 mL, for example, It is important for health care providers and technicians to become familiar with the cart's contents and location so that it can easily be retrieved and used. Depending on institutional pharmacy regulations, tranexamic acid, shelf-stable uterotonic drugs, and vasopressors may be added to a hemorrhage cart. Research from Johns Hopkins University, MD, showed the introduction of a hemorrhage cart and drug kit significantly reduced the mean response time to hemorrhage by 77%: 11 minutes preintroduction, and 2 minutes 14 seconds postintroduction of the cart and kit.[26]

A postpartum hemorrhage drug kit (**Table 2**) can be a physical box with uterotonic drugs and an antifibrinolytic drug (optional, due to high-risk drug status), or a bundled list that automatically dispenses these drugs (eg, oxytocin, methylergonovine, carboprost, misoprostol, and tranexamic acid) from an automated drug dispensing machine. Frequently, a kit may be put together by a hospital pharmacy and stored in a refrigerator on L&D, in the main OR suite and in the Emergency Department (ED), so

Table 2
Sample postpartum hemorrhage drug kit

Drug	Dose and Quantity
Oxytocin	4 × 10 unit vial
Ergonovine	1 × 0.2 mg ampule
Carboprost	1 × 0.25 mg ampule
Misoprostol	5 × 200 mcg tablet
Tranexamic acid (optional, due to high-risk drug status)	1 × 1 g vial

that it is immediately available during hemorrhage situations. Local guidelines must be followed regarding drug labeling, storage, and refrigeration. Minimizing the number of "clicks," a health care provider has to perform to retrieve drugs is paramount for emergency accessibility. Commonly, hemorrhage drug kits are certified as "drug override" so they can be removed from a drug storage system without approval from the pharmacy for emergency use, and EMR admission order sets can include standing orders for uterotonic drugs.

Malignant Hyperthermia Cart

MH is a rare, autosomal dominant disorder that presents as a hypermetabolic response to volatile anesthetic and depolarizing neuromuscular blocking drugs. The incidence of MH in an obstetric patient undergoing CD is approximately 1:125,000,[27] and this life-threatening anesthetic-induced emergency requires immediate treatment to decrease significant morbidity and mortality associated with it. The Malignant Hyperthermia Association of the United States (MHAUS) recommends dantrolene (the drug used to treat MH) be available for administration within 10 minutes of the decision to treat[28] and MHAUS has developed a list of equipment and drugs to be stored in an MH cart.[29]

Although it is understood that an MH cart is required in locations that use volatile anesthetics and depolarizing neuromuscular blocking drugs, there is debate regarding the cost-effectiveness of maintaining an MH cart on L&D when carts are immediately available in other areas of the hospital. An economic study looked at the cost-effectiveness of maintaining an MH cart in L&D and modeling showed that a fully stocked MH cart may only be cost-effective if the general anesthetic rate is greater than 11%,[30] otherwise it may be prudent to maintain a small supply of 250 mg dantrolene vials on L&D for administration while mobilizing the MH cart from a centralized location within the hospital.

Preparation for the care of an MH-susceptible patient on L&D includes several steps: the patient should be evaluated by a multidisciplinary team including an anesthesiologist, obstetrician, and nursing; dantrolene should be stocked, available, and in-date, and the pharmacist should be alerted; the anesthesiology team needs to be familiar with the dosing regimen; anesthetic workstations should have vaporizers removed, be flushed according to manufacturer guidelines and have charcoal filters applied.

Difficult Airway Cart

Administration of general anesthesia and airway instrumentation is usually only performed in a minority of pregnant patients, for example, those undergoing emergent CD. Other indications include patients undergoing nonobstetrical surgery during pregnancy, fetal surgery, surgery in the immediate postpartum period, or patients requiring ventilatory support due to respiratory failure or critical illness. Physiologic changes in pregnancy such as increased airway edema, cephalad displacement of the diaphragm, breast enlargement, and delayed gastric emptying can contribute to difficulty in preoxygenation, rapid desaturation, poor laryngoscopic view, and increased risk of aspiration. There is significant morbidity and mortality associated with a difficult (2.3%–3.3%) or failed (0.4%) airway in an obstetric patient so it is imperative to have immediate access to difficult airway equipment, and a difficult airway cart serves this purpose during an airway emergency.[31,32] There are several difficult airway guidelines and algorithms for nonpregnant adults, and the first national obstetrical-specific guideline was published jointly by the Obstetric Anaesthetists' Association and Difficult Airway Society in the United Kingdom.[33]

A difficult airway cart should be placed in a centralized location in the L&D OR area, so that it is immediately available for an unanticipated difficult airway and brought to the bedside in preparation when anticipating a difficult airway. A difficult airway cart's contents should be institution-specific and include various endotracheal tube sizes and laryngoscope blades, supraglottic airway devices, oral/nasal airways, and front-of-neck access kits, and commonly a fiberoptic scope and video laryngoscope are included. A review by Bjurstrom and colleagues describes contents of an airway cart with each drawer serving a specific purpose and procedure, for example, mask ventilation, intubation, supraglottic airway devices, and front-of-neck access.[34] Care should be taken not to over-stock emergency carts as it can make it difficult to retrieve items in an emergency. The cart should be checked regularly and restocked after each use. Teaching difficult airway management in an obstetric patient should include familiarization with the content of the difficult airway cart, indications for use in an emergency, and review of the difficult airway algorithm with changes pertinent to pregnancy.[33]

Severe Hypertension/Eclampsia Drug Kit

Preeclampsia complicates 2% to 8% of pregnancies globally and contributes to 16% of maternal deaths in developed countries.[35,36] Blood pressure control and prevention of seizures are paramount to avoiding severe morbidity and mortality from hypertensive disorders in pregnancy. AIM has published severe hypertension in pregnancy bundle that recommends L&D units have rapid access to drugs for severe hypertension and eclampsia, including a drug administration and dosage guide.[15] It is advisable to have severe hypertension/eclampsia drug kit readily available which contains drugs for blood pressure treatment, seizure prophylaxis, and magnesium toxicity. Drugs can be stored in a mobile box that also contains infusion supplies, fluid to flush drugs, and IV access equipment, and it is prudent to include drug administration information and a hypertension treatment checklist to enable quick administration of these drugs in an emergency (**Tables 3** and **4**). A system should be used for quality assurance to track usage and ensure drug replenishment.

Local Anesthetic Systemic Toxicity Kit

LAST is a rare and life-threatening risk of local anesthetic (LA) overdose that can complicate neuraxial or regional anesthesia, with an incidence of 1.8 to 2.6 cases per 1000 regional anesthetics.[37] Pregnant patients may be at increased risk of LAST due to epidural venous engorgement causing increased uptake of LA from the epidural space, increased risk of epidural catheter migration (eg, intravascularly),[38] and hormonal changes that increase neuronal sensitivity to LAs, thereby reducing the seizure threshold.[39] Treatment of cardiopulmonary arrest from LAST differs from standard ACLS due to LA interactions with cardiac myocytes. A basic LAST rescue kit should include a LAST checklist, 20% lipid emulsion bag/vial, large syringes (eg, 50 mL) and needles, IV infusion tubing, and be available in a centralized location in L&D.[40] Ideally, a cognitive aid on the treatment of LAST should be included within the rescue kit to guide dosing regimens of lipid emulsion therapy and remind responders of altered rescue medication doses (eg, epinephrine, vasopressin, and calcium channel blockers).

IV Access Kit

Tools for rapid IV access should be readily available in all patient care units to respond to emergencies that require immediate fluid and/or drug administration. An IV access kit should include tourniquets, skin preparation solution/wipes, IV cannulas of various

Table 3	
Acute-onset, severe hypertension, and eclampsia drug box dosing guidelines	
Magnesium 20 g/500 mL bag	*Initial (Loading Dose):* 4–6 g (100 mL–150 mL) IV over 20 min *Maintenance Dose:* 1–2 g/h (25 mL/hr–50 mL/h) continuous IV infusion
Labetalol 100 mg/20 mL vial	*Initial: Draw 4 mL from the vial* *20 mg (4 mL)* IV bolus followed by *40 mg (8 mL)* IV if not effective within 10 min; followed by *80 mg (16 mL)* IV if not effective within 10 min See acute-onset, severe hypertension algorithm for further dosing
Hydralazine 20 mg/mL vial	*Initial: Draw 0.25 mL from the vial* *5–10 mg (0.25–0.5 mL)* IV bolus followed by *10 mg (0.5 mL)* IV if not effective within 20 min See acute-onset, severe hypertension algorithm for further dosing
Nifedipine 10 mg tablets	*10 mg* PO, followed by *20 mg* PO if not effective within 20 min; followed by another *20 mg* PO if not effective within 20 min See acute-onset, severe hypertension algorithm for further dosing
Esmolol 100 mg/10 mL vial *(Anesthesiologists ONLY)*	*1–2 mg/kg (0.1–0.2 mL/kg)* IV over 1 min
Propofol 10 mg/mL, 20 mL vial *(Anesthesiologists ONLY)*	*30–40 mg (3–4 mL)* IV bolus
Calcium gluconate 1000 mg/10 mL vial	*1000 mg/10 mL* IV over 2–5 min

Abbreviations: IV, intravenous; PO, per oral.

sizes (eg, 14–18 gauge), guidewires, flush syringes, gauze, and securing devices. Ultrasound-guided IV cannulation may be required in certain situations (eg, in an obese or edematous patient, or in a patient who abuses drugs), and access to an intraosseous (IO) drill or needle should also be considered as using the IO route can be life-saving in patients with collapsed vasculature, ideally in the humerus.[41] Development of a "difficult IV start" protocol with escalation to health care providers with more experience can be helpful to minimize attempts required to secure adequate IV access.

Perimortem Cesarean Delivery Kit

In the US, cardiac arrest occurs in approximately 1:12,000 admissions for delivery.[42] A PMCD is the delivery of the fetus performed during a maternal cardiac arrest, with incision at 4 minutes and the aim to deliver the fetus within 5 minutes of the cardiac arrest, which can improve outcomes for the mother and fetus.[12,43] PMCD should be considered in a pregnant patient if the fundal height is at, or above the level of the umbilicus,[12] and the resuscitation should be performed at the location of the arrest as it is not possible to achieve effective resuscitation during transportation; the patient should not be transported to the OR until return of spontaneous circulation has been

Table 4
Acute-onset, severe hypertension, and eclampsia drug box contents

Drug Name	Stock Amount
Magnesium sulfate 20 g/500 mL bag	1
Calcium GLUCONATE 1000 mg/10 mL vial	1
Labetalol 5 mg/mL, 20 mL vial	1
Hydralazine 20 mg/mL vial	1
Nifedipine 10 mg capsule	5
Esmolol 10 mg/mL, 10 mL vial (*anesthesiologist only*)	1
Propofol 10 mg/mL, 20 mL vial (*anesthesiologist only*)	1
Sodium chloride 0.9% (NS) 10 mL vial	2

Supply Name	Stock Amount
20 mL syringe	1
10 mL syringe	2
3 mL syringe	2
18 gauge needle (pink)	5
Alaris pump tubing set	1
3-port IV extension	1

Abbreviation: IV, intravenous.
Sample from Lucile Packard Children's Hospital, Stanford. Published under Creative Commons License: Attribution-NonCommercial-NoDerivs 3.0 Unported (CCBY-NC-ND 3.0).

obtained.[44] For pregnant patients admitted to locations in the hospital outside of the obstetric unit (eg, intensive care unit or coronary care unit), a PMCD tray and neonatal resuscitation equipment should be readily available in these locations.[12] An equipment list should be developed in conjunction with obstetric colleagues, and as a minimum, a scalpel with a size 10 blade and umbilical cord clamps are all that are required to start a PMCD (**Box 1**).

EMERGENCY OBSTETRIC CARE OUTSIDE OF THE OBSTETRIC UNIT

Health care providers in the ED, critical care units, and outpatient settings (ie, any patient care area that a pregnant patient may attend) need to be aware of obstetric

---

Box 1
Perimortem cesarean delivery kit[46]

- No. 10 Scalpel
- 2 Hemostat clamps
- Needle driver
- Russian forceps
- Sutures
- Suture scissors
- Retractor
- Gauze sponges

emergencies and should perform a needs assessment to determine what supplies and resources are required to effectively care for an obstetric emergency. Frequently, these resources overlap with those that are available on L&D, such as emergency toolkits, drug kits for hemorrhage or severe hypertension/eclampsia, PMCD kits, etc.

Courses are available to prepare providers in the ED and critical care units to care for obstetric emergencies and include Advanced Life Support in Obstetrics (ALSO), Managing Medical and Obstetric Emergencies and Trauma (mMOET), and the American College of Obstetricians and Gynecologists' Emergencies in Clinical Obstetrics (ECO). Most courses combine didactic teaching with hands-on simulation training.

PATIENT EDUCATION RESOURCES

Patients that experience obstetric emergencies can have significant mental and physical sequela, and recent initiatives such as toolkits for obstetric emergencies include patient resources. AIM has developed a specific patient safety bundle titled, "*Support after a severe maternal event,*" which addresses ways to support the patient, her family members, and also staff members.[45] Following an obstetric emergency or unexpected outcome, in addition to a team debrief, a debrief should be undertaken with the patient and/or family member(s) as well as patient advocates to discuss the outcome and offer support and educational resources. Communication with the Risk Management department is also prudent. Health care providers should be educated on how to recognize signs of stress or trauma in patients and their families after severe maternal events, and early intervention and trauma support should be routinely available and offered to decrease the psychological impact of such events.

SUMMARY

This article provides some of the best emergency resources currently available to obstetric anesthesiology providers. The surfeit of resources is both a benefit and a challenge. It is vital that departments craft a consistent, tested, and verifiable emergency response plan to adequately take action during critical events. Preparation involves many forms, starting with an institutional and departmental culture of safety and emergency readiness which can be established, maintained, and mobilized using drills, simulations, debriefs, and standardized communication methods. More broadly, emergency readiness means developing the correct response teams, supplies, equipment, drugs, and management algorithms to reduce variance and risk. A commitment to continual quality improvement is critical to promote the best outcomes for maternal and fetal health.

CLINICS CARE POINTS

- Familiarization and utilization of emergency resources is recommended to enhance patient care and improve patient outcomes.
- Emergency resources such as cognitive aids can be utilized before, during, or after an event, in addition to other times for educational purposes.
- Practicing communication strategies and incorporating emergency resources through simulation may reduce maternal morbidity and mortality.

DISCLOSURE

The authors have nothing to disclose.

REFERENCES

1. Pregnancy mortality surveillance system. Availabe at: https://www.cdc.gov/reproductivehealth/maternal-mortality/pregnancy-mortality-surveillance-system.htm. Accessed May 1, 2021.

2. Binyamin Y, Weiniger CF, Heesen P, et al. Israel National Obstetric Anesthesia WhatsApp group as a communication tool, before and during the COVID-19 pandemic. Int J Obstet Anesth 2021;45:154–5.

3. Dutton RP, Lee LA, Stephens LS, et al. Massive hemorrhage: a report from the anesthesia closed claims project. Anesthesiology 2014;121(3):450–8.

4. Davies Joanna M, Posner Karen L, Lee Lorri A, et al. Liability associated with obstetric anesthesia: a closed claims analysis. Anesthesiology 2009;110(1):131–9.

5. Salas E, Klein C, King H, et al. Debriefing medical teams: 12 evidence-based best practices and tips. Jt Comm J Qual Patient Saf 2008;34(9):518–27.

6. McQuaid-Hanson E, Pian-Smith MC. Huddles and debriefings: improving communication on labor and delivery. Anesthesiol Clin 2017;35(1):59–67.

7. Bajaj K, Meguerdichian M, Thoma B, et al. The PEARLS healthcare debriefing tool. Acad Med 2018;93(2):336.

8. Debrief 2 Learn. Availabe at: https://debrief2learn.org/. Accessed May 1, 2021.

9. Mullan PC, Wuestner E, Kerr TD, et al. Implementation of an in situ qualitative debriefing tool for resuscitations. Resuscitation 2013;84(7):946–51.

10. Abir G, Austin N, Seligman KM, et al. Cognitive aids in obstetric units: design, implementation, and use. Anesth Analg 2020;130(5):1341–50.

11. Abir G, Seligman KM, Chu LF. Obstetric anesthesia emergency manual. Stanford (CA): Stanford Anesthesia Informatics and Media (AIM) Lab; 2019.

12. Jeejeebhoy FM, Zelop CM, Lipman S, et al. Cardiac arrest in pregnancy: a scientific statement from the american heart association. Circulation 2015;132(18):1747–73.

13. Bauer ME, Arendt K, Beilin Y, et al. The society for obstetric anesthesia and perinatology interdisciplinary consensus statement on neuraxial procedures in obstetric patients with thrombocytopenia. Anesth Analg. Feb 4 2021;doi:10.1213/ane.0000000000005355

14. Willett B, Togioka, Bensadigh, et al, Zakowski. Society for obstetric anesthesia and Perinatology statement on Sugammadex during pregnancy and lactation. 2019. Available at: https://www.soap.org/assets/docs/SOAP_Statement_Sugammadex_During_Pregnancy_Lactation_APPROVED.pdf. Accessed May 1, 2021.

15. Bernstein PS, Martin JN, Barton JR, et al. National partnership for maternal safety: consensus bundle on severe hypertension during pregnancy and the postpartum period. Obstet Gynecol 2017;130(2):347–57.

16. Patient safety bundles. Available at: https://safehealthcareforeverywoman.org/council/patient-safety-bundles/maternal-safety-bundles/?et_fb=1&PageSpeed=off. Accessed May 18, 2021.

17. California maternal quality care collaborative toolkits. Availabe at: https://www.cmqcc.org/resources-tool-kits/toolkits. Accessed May 1, 2021.

18. Mhyre JM, D'Oria R, Hameed AB, et al. The maternal early warning criteria: a proposal from the national partnership for maternal safety. Obstet Gynecol 2014;124(4):782–6.

19. Friedman AM, Campbell ML, Kline CR, et al. Implementing obstetric early warning systems. AJP Rep 2018;8(2):e79–84.

20. Klumpner TT, Kountanis JA, Langen ES, et al. Use of a novel electronic maternal surveillance system to generate automated alerts on the labor and delivery unit. BMC Anesthesiol 2018;18(1):78.
21. Abir G, Oakeson AM, Padilla C, et al. Implementation of an electronic alert notification platform for a maternal early warning system. Abstract No. 1009303. 53rd SOAP Annual Meeting 2021. Virtual conference. May 13-16, 2021.
22. Callaghan WM, Creanga AA, Kuklina EV. Severe maternal morbidity among delivery and postpartum hospitalizations in the United States. Obstet Gynecol 2012; 120(5):1029–36.
23. Creanga AA. Maternal mortality in the united states: a review of contemporary data and their limitations. Clin Obstet Gynecol 2018;61(2):296–306.
24. Gavigan S, Rosenberg N, Hulbert J. Proactively preventing maternal hemorrhage- related dealths. The Joint Commission blog 2019. Available at: https://www.jointcommission.org/resources/news-and-multimedia/blogs/leading-hospital-improvement/2019/11/proactively-preventing-maternal-hemorrhagerelated-deaths/. Accessed March 1, 2021.
25. Main EK, Goffman D, Scavone BM, et al. National partnership for maternal safety: consensus bundle on obstetric hemorrhage. Anesth Analg 2015;121(1):142–8.
26. Kogutt BK, Will S, Ferrell J, et al. 1180: Development of an obstetric hemorrhage response intervention: the postpartum hemorrhage cart. Am J Obstet Gynecol 2020;222(1):S725–6.
27. Guglielminotti J, Rosenberg H, Li G. Prevalence of malignant hyperthermia diagnosis in obstetric patients in the United States, 2003 to 2014. BMC Anesthesiology 2020;20(1):19.
28. The malignant hyperthermia Association of the United States. Available at: https://www.mhaus.org/faqs/category/frequently-asked-questions-about/dantrolene/. Accessed March 1, 2021.
29. What should be on an MH Cart?. Available at: https://www.mhaus.org/healthcare-professionals/be-prepared/what-should-be-on-an-mh-cart/. Accessed March 1, 2021.
30. Ho PT, Carvalho B, Sun EC, et al. Cost-benefit analysis of maintaining a fully stocked malignant hyperthermia cart versus an initial dantrolene treatment dose for maternity units. Anesthesiology 2018;129(2):249–59.
31. McDonnell NJ, Paech MJ, Clavisi OM, et al. Difficult and failed intubation in obstetric anaesthesia: an observational study of airway management and complications associated with general anaesthesia for caesarean section. Int J Obstet Anesth 2008;17(4):292–7.
32. Kinsella SM, Winton AL, Mushambi MC, et al. Failed tracheal intubation during obstetric general anaesthesia: a literature review. Int J Obstet Anesth 2015; 24(4):356–74.
33. Mushambi MC, Kinsella SM, Popat M, et al. Obstetric anaesthetists' association and difficult airway society guidelines for the management of difficult and failed tracheal intubation in obstetrics. Anaesthesia 2015;70(11):1286–306.
34. Bjurström MF, Bodelsson M, Sturesson LW. The difficult airway Trolley: a narrative review and practical guide. Anesthesiology Res Pract 2019;2019:6780254–312.
35. Gestational hypertension and preeclampsia: ACOG Practice Bulletin Summary, Number 222. Obstet Gynecol 2020;135(6):1492–5.
36. von Dadelszen P, Magee LA. Pre-eclampsia: an update. Curr Hypertens Rep 2014;16(8):454.

37. Mörwald EE, Zubizarreta N, Cozowicz C, et al. Incidence of local anesthetic systemic toxicity in orthopedic patients receiving peripheral nerve blocks. Reg Anesth Pain Med 2017;42(4):442–5.

38. Bern S, Weinberg G. Local anesthetic toxicity and lipid resuscitation in pregnancy. Curr Opin Anaesthesiol 2011;24(3):262–7, 1473-6500 (Electronic)).

39. Santos AC, DeArmas PI. Systemic toxicity of levobupivacaine, bupivacaine, and ropivacaine during continuous intravenous infusion to nonpregnant and pregnant ewes. Anesthesiology 2001;95(5):1256–64, 0003-3022 (Print)).

40. Neal JM, Neal EJ, Weinberg GL. American society of regional anesthesia and pain medicine local anesthetic systemic toxicity checklist: 2020 version. Reg Anesth Pain Med 2021;46(1):81–2.

41. de Vogel J, Heydanus R, Mulders AGM, et al. Lifesaving intraosseous access in a patient with a massive obstetric hemorrhage. AJP Rep 2011;1(2):119–22.

42. Mhyre JM, Tsen LC, Einav S, et al. Cardiac arrest during hospitalization for delivery in the United States, 1998–2011. Anesthesiology 2014;120(4):810–8.

43. Einav S, Kaufman N, Sela HY. Maternal cardiac arrest and perimortem caesarean delivery: evidence or expert-based? Resuscitation 2012;83(10):1191–200.

44. Lipman SS, Daniels KI, Carvalho B, et al. Deficits in the provision of cardiopulmonary resuscitation during simulated obstetric crises. Am J Obstet Gynecol 2010; 203(2):179-e1.

45. Support after a severe maternal event. Available at: https://safehealthcareforeverywoman.org/aim/patient-safety-bundles/support-after-a-severe-maternal-event-patient-safety-bundle-aim/. Accessed March 1, 2021.

46. Kikuchi J, Deering S. Cardiac arrest in pregnancy. Semin perinatol 2018; 42(1):33–8.

Updates on Simulation in Obstetrical Anesthesiology Through the COVID-19 Pandemic

Bryan Mahoney, MD*, Elizabeth Luebbert, DO

KEYWORDS

- Obstetrical anesthesiology • High-fidelity simulation • Multidisciplinary team training
- Partial task trainers • Quality improvement • Competency assessment

KEY POINTS

- Simulation remains essential in the training and assessment of individuals and multidisciplinary teams in obstetric anesthesiology.
- Simulation plays an increasing role in evaluation of work environments, processes, and tools for patient care.
- The challenges presented to caring for obstetric patients during the COVID-19 pandemic revealed the utility of simulation in both training and workflow development.

INTRODUCTION

Simulation has played a critical role in medicine for decades as a pedagogical or assessment tool utilized at the levels of the individual, multidisciplinary team, and institution. The labor and delivery unit provides an ideal setting for leveraging the advantages provided by simulation given the variety of technical and clinical skills required by health care providers, the collaborative nature of patient care, the potential for unanticipated patient emergencies, and the consistent emphasis on quality improvement in patient care. A useful conceptual model for a survey of simulation in the field of obstetric anesthesiology discriminates the domains of training and assessment along an expanding continuum of learner cohorts: the individual, the patient care team, and the health care organization or environment. Prior reviews of this topic consistently have utilized this approach in surveying the literature on this topic.[1–6] Given rapid advances in simulation technology and education, an update of simulation in obstetric anesthesiology is in order every few years. Simulation as a tool for training and assessment, however, has proved its utility during the COVID-19 pandemic as training programs and health care systems have been forced to navigate a radically altered learning and patient care environment requiring novel approaches to training and

Department of Anesthesiology, Perioperative and Pain Medicine, Mount Sinai Morningside and West Hospitals, 1000 10th Avenue, New York, NY 10019, USA
* Corresponding author.
E-mail address: bryan.mahoney@mountsinai.org

Anesthesiology Clin 39 (2021) 649–665
https://doi.org/10.1016/j.anclin.2021.08.001
1932-2275/21/© 2021 Elsevier Inc. All rights reserved.
anesthesiology.theclinics.com

team-based care. This review continues in the tradition of surveying the newest literature on simulation training and assessment for individuals, teams, and systems while also providing a specific overview of the role of simulation in obstetric anesthesiology in the context of the COVID-19 pandemic and the shift toward the virtual learning environment accelerated by social distancing requirements during the pandemic.

SIMULATION-BASED INDIVIDUAL TRAINING AND ASSESSMENT

The practice of obstetric anesthesiology requires the acquisition of both technical skills and complex nontechnical clinical skills that extend beyond those to which anesthesiology trainees are exposed in the general practice of anesthesiology. Simulation technology can serve as a strategy for this skill acquisition. Partial task trainers (used to address a specific psychomotor or technical skill) and high-fidelity mannequin-based or virtual reality–based simulation (used to address clinical scenarios requiring complex multidomain skill acquisition) are both well described in the obstetric anesthesia simulation literature.

A variety of partial task trainers for spinal or epidural neuraxial technique training have been described and made available to educators. These have ranged from a simulator constructed from a balloon, intubation pillow, and slice of bread,[7] to anatomically accurate manikin-based or computer-driven or haptic feedback–driven models allowing for trainee practice.[8] A 2013 review comparing 17 manikin-based simulators to 14 computer-based models by Vaughan and colleagues[8] notes that although manikin-based simulators are inexpensive, portable, and maintain a higher fidelity as a physical simulation of patient anatomy, computer-based models utilizing haptics provide real-time 3-dimensional screen-based visual feedback combined with a higher fidelity in the loss of resistance technique and better simulating tactile feel of encountering the ligaments, tissues, and bone involved in neuraxial technique. The ideal partial task trainer for neuraxial technique training would combine the physical and anatomic fidelity of manikins with the visuospatial feedback advantages and tactile fidelity found in computer-based models. More recently, haptics have been incorporated with virtual reality and gamification features[9,10] in an effort to enhance skill acquisition and trainee motivation. The use of a virtual environment now can achieve a higher degree of fidelity in recreating the clinical environment while retaining the fidelity in the tactile sensation of spinal or loss of resistance technique that haptics can provide. Gamification (scoring points and achieving increasing experience levels) increasingly is incorporated into both partial task simulation training and more complex multidomain clinical skills acquisition.[11] Capogna and colleagues[12] asked novice trainees engaged in simulated epidural technique training to wear eye-tracking glasses. Although epidural procedure duration and number of attempts decreased following a simulation-based training tutorial, they also found a positive correlation between the number of needle-insertion attempts and gaze fixation counts along with a negative correlation between epidural attempts and gaze duration.

Over the past decade, an increasing volume of research has supported the use of high-fidelity manikin-based simulation for the anesthetic management of the maternal airway and obstetric emergencies. Exposure to high-fidelity simulation in conjunction with traditional lecture-based learning has been shown to enhance trainee performance in emergency management of an obstetric emergency requiring general anesthesia to the competency normally only seen in a fully trained faculty member utilizing a previously validated scoring system with significant retention 8 months following the initial assessment.[13,14] A large volume of scenarios for anesthesia training for obstetric emergencies has been published for educators, including high spinal anesthetic level,[15] maternal cardiac arrest,[16] and a variety of other conditions.[5,17,18] Clinton and Minehart provided a roadmap in 2020 for the development of comprehensive simulation curriculum for advancing clinical skills with the inclusion of sample scenarios (**Table 1**).

Simulation-based training has continued to show effectiveness in learning and retention of skills essential for the practice of obstetric anesthesiology, such as airway management during emergent cesarean delivery,[19] recognition and management of high neuraxial blockade,[20] and management of a general anesthetic for cesarean delivery.[21] The instruction of communication skills increasingly has been addressed through the use of simulation-based training. Raemer and colleagues[22] explored the role of simulation in overcoming the traditional hierarchical mode of communication within the health care workspace. To promote the ability of residents to speak up on identification of inappropriate clinical behavior on the part of faculty obstetricians, anesthesiologists, and labor and delivery nursing staff, 2 simulated clinical scenarios were provided to allow for the practice of the advocacy-inquiry and 2-challenge inquiry techniques. They found an increase in appropriate challenging behavior from 27% to 67% following post-simulation exposure.[22] More recently, Szmulewicz and colleagues[23] utilized interdisciplinary simulation-based training for the disclosure of a medical error to patients. This work showed trainees' improvement in both verbal and nonverbal communication skills with retention up to 6 months following the intervention.[23]

Table 1
Sample obstetric anesthesia simulation scenario[5]

Characters	Narrative	Vital signs	
High spinal 1. Patient (mannequin) 2. Primary registered nurse 3. Primary physician Time, 0:00–2:00 min	32-year-old healthy G2PI at 39 wk in labor, status post recent epidural placement	Blood pressure, 110/60 Heart rate, 90 Respiratory rate, 20 Spo$_2$, 98% on room air	[ ] Engage patient. [ ] Assess for pain or discomfort.
II Above, + Anesthesia Backup obstetrician Second registered nurse Resource nurse Time, 2.00–4.00 min	Patient begins to feel anxious and is having trouble breathing	Blood pressure, 100/60; dropping to blood pressure 60s/40s over 2 min Heart rate, 110; drops to 45 over 2 min Respiratory rate rises to 30 over 2 min Spo$_2$, 98%–88% Fetal late decelerations	[ ] Patient distress [ ] Call for help/backup. [ ] Verbalize hypotension, hypoxemia. [ ] Communicate critical event. [ ] Emergency manual [ ] Examination and vital signs verbalization to group [ ] Shut off epidural pump. [ ] Initiate treatment of hypotension, hypoxemia.

(*continued on next page*)

Characters	Narrative	Vital signs	
Table 1			
(continued)			
III	Patient unresponsive,	Blood pressure, 55/30	[ ] Support
Above, +	unconscious	Heart rate 45; drops	hypotension/
Additional registered	Event pause and	to 30 if not treated	anaphylaxis kit
nurse support	discuss situation	Respiratory rate falls	[ ] Ambu bag and
Second anesthesia	(mini-debrief) to	to 0 when systolic	ventilate
Second obstetric	ensure proper	blood pressure	[ ] Ventilation support/
provider	treatment	drops	hypotension
Any available	(optional)	below 60	management with
additional help		Spo$_2$, 88%; falls	epinephrine
Time, 4:00–8:00		rapidly	infusion or other
		to 40% if not bag-	appropriate
		mask	available α-/
		ventilated and	β-agonists
		then intubated	[ ] Communicate
		Fetal heart rate,	patient is
		prolonged	unconscious (to
		deceleration	team).
			[ ] Verbalize fetal
			intolerance of
			hypotension.
			[ ] Establish event
			manager.
			[ ] Communicate
			possible causes of
			loss of
			consciousness and
			initiate plan for
			immediate care.
			[ ] Code cart,
			defibrillator
			[ ] Emergency manual
IV	Recovery with support	Blood pressure, 90/60	End scenario with
All team members		Heart rate, 70	resuscitation and
Time, 8.00–10.00		Fetal recovery with	plan for supportive/
		restitution of	intensive care while
		maternal vital signs	spinal regresses

Advances in both Web-based and communication technologies increasingly have been integrated into simulation education for trainees, removing the need for both trainee and instructor to be in the same location. Telesimulation has become a tool to provide training of technical and nontechnical skills around the world. The use of telesimulation was described by educators in Canada to teach trainees in Botswana laparoscopic surgical technique with nothing more than a simple trainer box, a Web camera, and a laptop computer.[24] A randomized trial conducted by Sorenson and colleagues[25] in 2017 compared simulation-based obstetric anesthesia training in clinical management of an emergency caesarean section and a postpartum hemorrhage (PPH) scenario with in situ simulation versus off-site simulation. They found similar individual and team outcomes in patient safety attitudes, stress, motivation, perceptions of the simulations, and team performance while those receiving in situ simulation training did find a greater degree of fidelity than those receiving remote training. Given the success found in telesimulation-based training in both technical and nontechnical clinical skills acquisition, remote teaching may be an exciting frontier for the teaching of neuraxial technique or anesthetic management of obstetric emergencies by international experts to trainees around the world. Recent work by Lim and colleagues,[26] showing that mental imagery training can be used to develop epidural anesthesia technical skills as effectively as low-fidelity haptic simulators, even may suggest that effective remote education could be provided with only a Web camera.

Simulation-based skills assessment has continued in line with advances in training. Kiwalabye and colleagues[27] assessed preparedness of anesthesia interns in managing a failed obstetric intubation following their anesthesiology rotation. They observed a pass rate of only 40% despite prior exposure to an Essential Steps in Managing Obstetric Emergencies training module, leading them to propose that this gap in skill acquisition discovered by simulated scenarios can be remedied through the use of simulation-based education during their training. An additional area in which simulation increasingly has been used in assessment lies in credentialing of those who have graduated from anesthesiology training programs. Since 2018, the American Board of Anesthesiology has included Objective Structured Clinical Examinations (OSCEs) as part of the APPLIED examination, including simulated interactions with patients. Although the technical and clinical components of obstetric anesthesia practice currently are not among the topics included in the OSCEs, communication with the parturient is addressed in modules assessing informed consent and communication of medical errors. This has led many programs to integrate OSCE training into their residency curriculum to better prepare trainees for the process of credentialing. Dabbagh and colleagues[28] found an increase in the relative annual pass rate of anesthesiology residents following the integration of a preparation program, including mock OSCEs prior to the National Board of Anesthesiology certifying examination.

SIMULATION-BASED MULTIDISCIPLINARY TEAM TRAINING AND ASSESSMENT

Multidisciplinary team training for obstetric care and crisis resource management (CRM) has been well described in the simulation literature.[29] Although confidence in this approach as a means to improve patient outcomes has been shown by stakeholders, such as insurance companies, there has long been effort to link the utilization of simulation for team training to improvements in patient outcomes.[30] A recent review of simulation team training, including human factors components, has provided some insight into this long-standing goal of those engaged in the field. Five single prospective site studies investigating multidisciplinary obstetric simulation training, including CRM and reported outcomes in high-resource and low-resource countries, were identified.[31] Two showed a 34% reduction in maternal mortality and 3 a 41% to 50% reduction in blood transfusion, whereas cluster analysis revealed a 17% reduction in PPH incidence and a 37% reduction on weighted obstetrics adverse outcomes. Furthermore, there was a 15% reduction in maternal mortality in favor of trained teams and a reduction of neonatal deaths from 24 weeks during the first 24 hours of 83% in intervention sites compared with an 18% increase in control sites. Lutgendorf and colleagues[32] conducted 16 multidisciplinary simulated scenarios, including PPH over 2 days to assess team performance and operational readiness. A comparison of PPH incidents in their institution revealed a decrease in the time to prepare blood products over the course of simulation training and a trend toward a reduction in the incidence of PPH.[32] These important results only increase the need for further work exploring the impact of simulation-based team training on obstetric patient and neonatal outcomes.

Although work continues in the field of developing simulation-based team training curricula,[33] several studies have investigated team behavior through the use of simulation. A recent prospective observational study utilized individual personality testing to find associations with overall assessments of teamwork and communication in simulated management of PPH. The investigators discovered that a high degree of neuroticism among individual team members led to increased communication in a manner that was detrimental to overall team performance whereas other personality traits yielded no associations.[34] Capogna and colleagues[35] had team leaders of a simulated PPH scenario wear eye-tracking glasses to find associations between eye-tracking metrics of 27 selected areas of interest and team performance evaluated by a PPH checklist. Their group found that high-performance leader groups were associated with a greater duration of visual fixations as well as a more uniform distribution of gaze on team members compared with the low-performance leader groups. Methods of evaluating teams during obstetric emergencies, such as PPH, continue to evolve as more evidence is brought to bear on the importance of nontechnical skills, such as cognitive and social factors. Toward this end, Cheloufi and colleagues[36] employed a multidisciplinary Delphi method consisting of 4 cycles with 16 experts, including obstetricians, midwives, and anesthesiologists to create the Obstetric Team Performance Assessment Scale to be utilized during assessment of team performance during high-fidelity simulation exercises. This scale, based on expert consensus, emphasized the value of nontechnical skills, such as situational awareness and requesting help from the anesthesia team, in addition to traditionally identified checklist items, such as intravenous access and prompt activation of transfusion protocols. This work reflects the increased emphasis on the psychometric and social factors in the role of team performance being better understood through simulation.

SIMULATION-BASED ASSESSMENT OF THE WORK ENVIRONMENT AND PRACTICE METHODS

Hemorrhage remains a leading cause of death in parturients and an area of interest in developing protocols for quantification and management of blood loss. Simulation has been used effectively to assess the accuracy of different methods of blood loss quantification. The use of a pictorial guide as a means to assess blood loss during a simulated cesarean delivery was evaluated by Homcha and colleagues[37] comparing assessments of blood loss prior to and after use of the guide. Prior to use of the pictorial guide, they observed a more than 25% overestimation of blood loss, whereas use of the guide revealed an increase from 7% to 24% of accurate estimation defined as an estimate within 5% of the actual volume lost. Piekarski and colleagues[38] sought to compare a mobile colorimetric application for blood loss estimation with visual and gravimetric methods utilized by 53 anesthesiologists exposed to a simulated PPH scenario. They found the least deviation in estimates from the actual volume of blood loss among the colorimetric estimation followed by gravimetric and visual methods, whereas overestimation of blood loss occurred most in the visual estimation followed by the gravimetric and colorimetric methods.

The risk of chlorhexidine contamination of materials introduced to the neuraxial space motivated Taylor and colleagues[39] to conduct a simulated study to identify the incidence of transfer of chlorhexidine from the lumbar region to standard surgical gloves in a study simulating standard lumbar region antiseptic preparation. Their findings revealed an incidence of primary transfer above 99% up to 10 minutes following chlorhexidine application to the lumbar region of volunteers, with a 68.9% incidence of secondary transfer from gloves to another surface. To evaluate the effectiveness of current Society for Obstetric Anesthesia and Perinatology (SOAP) Patient Safety Committee proposals to utilize a cap and run approach (capping epidural and intravenous lines to prevent tangling prior to transfer) to facilitate transport of patients from the labor room to operating theater during emergency cesarean deliveries. Mhyre and colleagues[40] utilized a prospective randomized in situ simulation study. They found no statistically significant difference in the time from decision to proceed with cesarean delivery to readiness for general anesthesia between groups, although qualitative analysis during debriefing did reveal some perceived advantages, such as bed maneuverability and a decrease in tangled lines.

Efforts in low-income and middle-income nations to decrease maternal mortality hold great promise, given the ongoing discrepancy with rates observed in high-income nations. Simulation continues to play a large role in both education and developing or assessing initiatives aimed at improving maternal care. Alexander and colleagues[41] used the simulated setting to pilot test a context-relevant safe anesthesia checklist for cesarean delivery in East Africa. By comparing anesthesiologists providing care for a variety of conditions in the simulated environment with and without a checklist developed in conjunction with East African health care professionals, they found a significant increase in the completion of critical actions in the setting of preeclampsia and PPH. Gallardo and colleagues[42] utilized the simulated environment and a randomized crossover design, including 10 trainees, to compare the performance of trainees in simulated high-resource and low-resource environments managing PPH from uterine atony. They found a significant decrease in performance by those exposed to the simulated low-resource environment, including both technical and nontechnical skills, including leadership, resource utilization, and communication.

SIMULATION IN OBSTETRIC ANESTHESIOLOGY DURING THE COVID-19 PANDEMIC

The COVID-19 pandemic has radically altered the landscape for clinicians and educators across the world, and the invaluable role of simulation came to the fore in the field of obstetric anesthesiology. With direct patient contact and in-person teaching limited by social distancing requirements and infectious risk mitigation, simulation provided opportunities for medical students and anesthesiology trainees to learn both technical and nontechnical clinical skills. To accelerate education for management of critical events in the context of patients infected with COVID-19, high-fidelity simulation-based individual and team training proved invaluable. Most importantly, with the need to develop new work environments and processes, simulation technology served to test their feasibility and prepare health care systems and medical staff.

Trainees found their ability to attain obstetric anesthesiology skills and knowledge limited by the fact that patient care brought a level infectious risk not previously common to the labor and delivery unit. In-person teaching also was impacted by requirements for social distancing imposed on training programs. Although the surgical volume elsewhere in hospitals decreased profoundly by the cancellation or delay of all but the most urgent surgical procedures, such measures could not be taken in labor and delivery units, and the need for clinical care remained relatively unaffected. Training programs leveraged simulation technology, such as partial task trainers, to provide exposure to neuraxial technique given the need for personal protective equipment (PPE) during patient interactions and limited exposure to parturients with known or suspected COVID-19.[43] Simulation also was described as a mechanism for training difficult airway management, PPE protocols, aseptic technique, and airway management. Virtual reality with gamification features also was described as a tool for approaching the maternal airway.

Previously routine interactions with patients changed dramatically during the pandemic, necessitating rapid training of health care providers to mitigate the risk of infection to providers and patients. Professional societies turned to in situ multidisciplinary simulation as a resource for physicians and other health care professionals early in the pandemic. The American College of Obstetricians and Gynecologists Simulations Working Group created 4 standardized scenarios for use to guide multidisciplinary teams in patient interactions during the pandemic: (1) an obstetric patient with suspected COVID-19 presenting in labor; (2) an obstetric patient with suspected COVID-19 progressing in labor to spontaneous vaginal delivery, (3) an

COVID19 LABOR TO CESAREAN DELIVERY: CASE FLOW AND FACILITATOR'S GUIDE
Author: Rebecca D. Minehart, MD, MSHPEd
Contributors: Gill Abir, MD; Katie Arendt, MD; Erik Clinton, MD; Roxane Gardner, MD, MSHPEd, DSc; Daniel Katz, MD; Allison Lee, MD; Vanessa Torbenson, MD

Notes to facilitators:
- *Please feel free to drill any relevant part(s) of this and omit those parts that are not relevant.*
- *Please modify anything that does not align with your institutional guidelines.*
- *Consider holding small sessions (≤6 people) and/or hosting virtual sessions using filmed footage to talk through considerations with a larger team*
- *Consider prioritizing PPE when holding drills for the first time, and adding in additional components later (such as the support person, etc.)*
- *Please note that the focus of this packet of drills is not to be physiologically representative of any particular clinical situation; rather, it is meant as a platform to practice teamwork and organizational skills*

SCENARIO Synopsis to orient participants:
- Cori Vidman is a 30 yo G2P1 female at 37w2d who presents to triage in active labor after ROM.
- Her PMH includes asthma, h/o rapid first labor, and recent onset of cold-like symptoms. No known COVID19 exposures.
- She is requesting labor analgesia but has not been seen by an obstetrics/midwife provider yet (if starting in triage).
- She needs evaluation, assessment, and treatment.

Equipment needed:
- Mannequin or standardized patient/actor (for mother); (optional: standardized patient/actor for support person for Part 4)
- Neonatal mannequin/trainer (if doing neonatal scenario)
- Space for using as triage bed, labor room, OR as needed
- Plan for PPE—consider using props (e.g., handkerchiefs or facial tissues/Kleenex taped to ears for masks, patient robes worn backwards for gowns, likely can use gloves as these are not generally on shortage—otherwise, consider miming all donning/doffing or using lanyards to denote PPE items)
- Appropriate monitors for settings, appropriate equipment for OR (can mime for surgical equipment, but will likely need anesthetic equipment if possible, and airway equipment if performing intubation/extubation)

OVERALL FLOW

Time		Key Scenario Points	Ideal Actions
Pre-drill	Orient Participants to patient in triage area	• Patient is in triage bed (mannequin vs standardized patient/actor)	• Orient team members to drill environment • Discuss use of props/miming to conserve PPE and other equipment
Part 1: Triage eval	**Patient in active labor** Participants involved (as per institution): OB/CNM, RN, anesthesia provider to assess respiratory status	• Patient coughing, in active labor • (Patient may have mask on if available through regular entry points) Maternal baseline vitals: BP: 120/50 HR: 112 O2 Sat: 92% on RA (goes to 95% on any O2) RR: 21 Temp: 99.9F; FHR: Category I tracing • Relevant history: symptoms started a week ago; her toddler had a playdate around that time and maybe the other	Clinical: 1. Correct donning of PPE outside of triage room according to institutional guidelines (**consider practicing with props or having people mime steps rather than using actual PPE**) 2. (Correct contactless passing of mask to patient if she has no mask on; again, consider practicing with props or miming) 3. Confirm patient identity and perform focused history and physical exam (may discuss airway exam depending

Fig. 1. Covid 19 labor to cesarean delivery: case flow and facilitator's guide. BP: blood pressure, BPH: Beats per minute, CNM: Certified Nurse Midwives, C/D: cesarean delivery, Cm: centimeters, ETT: Endotracheal tube, EtCO2: End tidal carbon dioxide, EBL: Estimated blood loss, F: Fahrenheit, FHR: Fetal Heart Rate, GA: General Anesthesia, HR: Heart rate, NICU: Neonatal intensive care unit, NMB: Neuromuscular blocking agents, OB: obstetrician, O2 sat: Oxygen saturation, OR: operating room, O2: oxygen, PAPR: Powered Air Purifying Respirators, PPE, personal protective equipment; MP: Mallampati, RN: registered nurse, RR: Respiratory Rate, RSV: Respiratory syncytial virus, RA: Room air, TOF: Train of four.

		family has some people with colds. Otherwise, she feels her asthma is exacerbated recently, and thinks it may be due to allergies. • Relevant physical exam: cervical exam is 6cm/90%/-1 station (hand paper with written exam to OB/CNM). Airway exam (if done—this may be a point of discussion) shows MP 3, otherwise favorable airway features. Lung exam demonstrates diminished sounds at right base. Other findings normal. • During contractions, once surgical or oxygen mask is placed, patient may occasionally remove surgical/oxygen mask but will respond to replace mask if asked by staff PAUSE AND DISCUSS AT ANY POINT DURING CASE TO HIGHLIGHT GOOD BEHAVIORS OR HAVE PARTICIPANTS REDO	on institutional guidelines) 4. Apply oxygen to patient 5. Obtain influenza, RSV, coronavirus swabs Behavioral: 1. Clear communication between staff members to coordinate entry into triage room 2. Clear role delineation and plan to move patient to labor room 3. Updates to labor room to coordinate receiving patient 4. Encourage patient to keep mask on (perhaps even designate someone to watch this to limit spread) 5. Clear communication to others at an institutional level that a patient with possible COVID19 is present (per institutional policies) 6. (Optional: Team can Name/Claim/Aim to orient participants to situation and organize their team's activities)
Part 2: **Triage to** **labor room**	**Patient** **needing** **transport** Participants (as per institution): [insert appropriate participants]	• Patient being transported to labor room, needs to be counseled to keep mask on (surgical or oxygen mask, depending on what has been placed—can be discussed that oxygen mask may not protect others) • (Optional: Patient's support person arrives on labor floor, is a close contact of patient) Maternal vitals in labor room: BP: 131/72 HR: 125 O2 Sat: 92% on RA (goes to 95% on any O2) RR: 21 Temp: 99.9F; FHR: Category 2 tracing • Patient still contracting, will remove mask if not counseled • Patient arrives in labor room, requests anesthesia provider for neuraxial placement • Cervical exam on entry to room is 7cm/100%/0 station PAUSE AND DISCUSS AT ANY POINT DURING CASE TO HIGHLIGHT GOOD BEHAVIORS OR HAVE PARTICIPANTS REDO	Clinical: 1. Correct transport with minimal patient/personnel exposure in clinical environment 2. Correct donning of PPE outside of labor room with providers either awaiting placement inside room or outside room (according to institutional guidelines) 3. (Optional: Correctly giving support person a surgical mask) 4. (Abbreviated anesthesia consent is appropriate here for sake of time with the drill) Behavioral: 1. Clearly defining limited staff on entry to room 2. Encouraging patient to continue to keep mask on 3. (Optional: Team can Name/Claim/Aim to orient participants to situation and organize their team's activities)
Part 3: Fetal **brady,** **transfer to** **OR**	**Patient with** **recent** **neuraxial** **analgesia,** **getting** **comfortable,** **with** **nonreassuring** **fetal status**	• Patient now getting comfortable after neuraxial placement, still with some discomfort (low suprapubic) 5 minutes after anesthetic initiation • FHR then drops to 80 BPM with recurrent late decelerations (Category 3 tracing) without uterine hyperstimulation	Clinical: 1. Early dosing of neuraxial for C/D to avoid need for intubation 2. Correct donning of PPE for all providers necessary for care 3. Correct transport and personnel involved in moving patient into the OR while minimizing exposure of others

Fig. 1. (*continued*).

	Participants (as per institution): [insert appropriate participants]	Maternal vitals at this time: BP: 108/50 HR: 126 O2 Sat: 92% on RA (goes to 95% on any O2) RR: 21 Temp: 99.9F; FHR Category 2→3 • Cervical exam is 8cm/100%/0 station PAUSE AND DISCUSS AT ANY POINT DURING CASE TO HIGHLIGHT GOOD BEHAVIORS OR HAVE PARTICIPANTS REDO	4. Consider the role of preparing to use N95/PAPR for the entire team in case of general anesthesia/intubation Behavioral: 1. Clear communication to teams to ready equipment in the OR 2. Clear role delineation when organize to move patient 3. (Optional: Team can Name/Claim/Aim to orient participants to situation and organize their team's activities)
Part 4: STAT C/D and conversion to GA with intubation	**Patient with inadequate level of anesthesia, needing to convert to GA with intubation** Participants (as per institution): [insert appropriate participants]	• Patient in OR, fails level (level at T10 bilaterally) *or* patient with adequate level but complains of pain with incision Maternal vitals at this time: BP: 108/50 HR: 126 (goes to 100 with any phenylephrine) O2 Sat: 92% on RA (goes to 95% on any O2→can go to 99% on 100% O2 with preoxygenation, over 8 breaths) RR: 21 Temp: 99.9F; FHR Category 3 (still 80 BPM if checked) • Cervical exam is 8cm/100%/+1 station • (Optional, depending on institutional policies): Patient's support person needs a plan—whether this person is already in the OR by now, or whether this person needs to be updated is up to the facilitators PAUSE AND DISCUSS AT ANY POINT DURING CASE TO HIGHLIGHT GOOD BEHAVIORS OR HAVE PARTICIPANTS REDO	Clinical: 1. Correct PPE of ALL TEAM MEMBERS prior to preoxygenation (according to institutional guidelines) 2. Correct equipment ready to prepare for any difficulty in intubation (e.g., videolaryngoscopy) 3. Preoxygenation with lowest O2 flows possible, and with HEPA filter 4. ETT cuff inflated prior to positive pressure ventilation Behavioral: 1. Clear communication around the time of intubation to coordinate help and steps 2. Clear role delineation when initiating general anesthesia 3. Clear communication of now-contaminated areas, with steps to minimize further contamination of personnel 4. (Optional: Description of conversation with support person, and clear communication to support person in labor room, or removal of support person from OR) 5. (Optional: Clear communication with support person of isolation protocols for neonate, per institutional guidelines) 6. (Optional: Team can Name/Claim/Aim to orient participants to situation and organize their team's activities)
Part 5: Neonatal resuscitation and transport	**Patient under general anesthesia, neonate requiring resuscitation and transport to NICU/isolation (per institution)** Participants (as	• Patient stable during delivery, under general anesthesia Maternal vitals at this time: BP: 108/50 HR: 107 (goes to 100 with any phenylephrine) O2 Sat: 97% on 100% O2→ 94% if nitrous oxide used RR: (set by ventilator)—can be 15, EtCO2 is 28 Temp: 99.9F EBL: 800mL, good uterine tone	Clinical: 1. Correct PPE of all team members in OR and caring for neonate 2. Correct neonatal resuscitation personnel available in OR 3. Correct equipment and isolation procedures demonstrated while preparing to transport neonate (per institutional guidelines) 4. Correct transport out of OR while minimizing contact with neonate (per institutional guidelines)

Fig. 1. (*continued*).

	per institution): [insert appropriate participants]	Neonate at delivery: Color: Blue/dusky color Heart rate: 80 Reflex irritability: No response Muscle tone: Limp Respiration: Absent APGARs at 1 & 5 minutes (with any resuscitation): Color: Acrocyanotic Heart rate: 130 Reflex irritability: Grimace Muscle tone: Some flexion Respiration: Weak Cry/Hypoventilation • Neonate needs transportation/isolation (per institutional guidelines) PAUSE AND DISCUSS AT ANY POINT DURING CASE TO HIGHLIGHT GOOD BEHAVIORS OR HAVE PARTICIPANTS REDO	Behavioral: 1. Clear communication within neonatal team regarding care of neonate 2. Clear role delineation when caring for neonate 3. (Optional: Team can Name/Claim/Aim to orient participants to situation and organize their team's activities)
Part 6: Extubation, recovery, and disposition of patient	**Procedure complete, patient stable** Participants (as per institution): [insert appropriate participants]	• Cesarean delivery completed <u>Maternal vitals at this time:</u> BP: 128/70 HR: 125 O2 Sat: 97% on 100% O2 RR: (breathing spontaneously)—can be 21, EtCO2 is 28 Temp: 99.9F TOF: 0.9 (if additional nondepolarizing NMBs used) • At start of Part 6, all anesthetic agents are turned off, patient is making some movements indicative of emergence (but not following commands yet) • Patient then emerges normally, needs extubation (vitals do not change dramatically after extubation—SpO2 can drop to 95% on 100% O2 by oxygen mask) PAUSE AND DISCUSS AT ANY POINT DURING CASE TO HIGHLIGHT GOOD BEHAVIORS OR HAVE PARTICIPANTS REDO	Clinical: 1. Minimize personnel who are unnecessary during extubation 2. Correct PPE use (with N95/PAPR) 3. Consider decreasing oxygen flows during extubation or placing anesthesia machine on standby (per institutional guidelines) 4. Correct limiting of spreading contamination on surfaces related to anesthesia workstation 5. Correct moving of patient to appropriate recovery area (per institutional guidelines) Behavioral: 1. Clear communication and organization of team during extubation with warning others to stay back in case of patient coughing 2. Anticipating and planning for gathering all equipment needed for extubation and sequestering it prior to extubation 3. Clear communication of plan in case of airway obstruction 4. Clear communication of recovery and disposition plan with team (per institutional guidelines) 5. (Optional: Team can Name/Claim/Aim to orient participants to situation and organize their team's activities)
Post-drill	End Case	Clearly state, "Thank you so much—we are concluding this drill and will now focus on our debrief of the whole session."
<u>**COVID19 Debriefing (suggested structure)**</u>		
Location: can be *in situ* or	**DEBRIEF Case:** • Reactions Phase	

Fig. 1. (*continued*).

in a separate location	o "one word" to describe elicited emotion • Move to "Plus/Delta" debrief o Two columns to discuss: Under "Plus" column are things that the team feel they did well, and under "Delta" column are things that the team could change or improve o Facilitators should find a few things that the teams did well to highlight to them, as participants are usually hard on themselves (and under a great deal of stress right now) o Facilitators can also make a column of "unanswered/new questions" that need to be addressed at an institutional level, with a promise to circle back with participants • Move to "Take-aways" phase o Ask participants what they are taking away from the session today (this will serve as useful feedback for facilitators, and identify anything about the session that should be changed for the future) o **Thank participants for joining** • Finally, pass out evaluations and collect them once everyone fills them out
End debrief	**Thank them for participating!**

References:
• Podovei M, Bernstein K, George R, Habib A, Kacmar R, Bateman B, Landau R. Interim Considerations for Obstetric Anesthesia Care related to COVID19. Accessed 3/17/20 at: https://soap.org/wp-content/uploads/2020/03/SOAP_COVID-19_Obstetric_Anesthesia_Care_031620-2.pdf.
• Clinton E. COVID-19 simulation script. Department of Obstetrics & Gynecology, Massachusetts General Hospital, Boston, MA, USA.
• Torbenson V. OB Simulation Emergency Drill 2020. Department of Obstetrics & Gynecology, Mayo Clinic, Rochester, MN, USA
• Chan A, Lau V, Wong H. Covid-19 Sample Scenario Script for Airway Management in OT. Department of Anaesthesia and Intensive Care, Prince of Wales Hospital, Hong Kong.
• ACOG Committee Opinion 644. The Apgar Score. Accessed 3/17/20 at: https://www.acog.org/Clinical-Guidance-and-Publications/Committee-Opinions/Committee-on-Obstetric-Practice/The-Apgar-Score?IsMobileSet=false.
• World Health Organization. Infection prevention and control during health care when novel coronavirus (nCoV) infection is suspected. Accessed 3/17/20 at: https://www.who.int/publications-detail/infection-prevention-and-control-during-health-care-when-novel-coronavirus-(ncov)-infection-is-suspected-20200125.
• Zhou F, Yu T, Du R, Fan G, Liu Y, Liu Z, et al. Clinical course and risk factors for mortality of adult inpatients with COVID-19 in Wuhan, China: a retrospective cohort study. The Lancet. 3/15/20 at: https://www.thelancet.com/journals/lancet/article/PIIS0140-6736(20)30566-3/fulltext.
• Fauci AS, Lane C, Redfield RR. Covid-19—Navigating the Uncharted. NEJM. Accessed 3/15/20 at: https://www.nejm.org/doi/full/10.1056/NEJMe2002387

Fig. 1. (*continued*).

obstetric patient with suspected COVID-19 in labor requiring cesarean delivery; and (4) an obstetric patient with suspected COVID-19 requiring intensive care unit transfer due to worsening respiratory symptoms.[44] SOAP provided a scripted simulation scenario designed to guide teams through meeting a parturient with suspected COVID-19 team in triage, transport to a labor room and placement of a labor epidural, emergency cesarean delivery, induction, and recovery from a general anesthetic (**Fig. 1**).[18] Simulation has been proposed as a mechanism for addressing novel scenarios brought about the pandemic, such as donning and doffing of PPE, transport of infected obstetric patients, management of a second obstetric emergency when the team currently is caring for an obstetric patient, approaches to the delay of an emergency cesarean delivery due to infection prevention and control measures, and communication with patients or families about visitation policies impacted by infection prevention and control measures.[45] Simulation scenarios also have been described to include not only multidisciplinary care of the obstetric patient but also neonatal care based on variable maternal COVID-19 status and symptomatology and gestational age at the time of delivery.[46,47]

The COVID-19 pandemic required major changes to not only workflow but also patient care areas in efforts to maximize infection prevention and control while providing patient care. Simulation served as the means for testing and revising these changes in real time throughout the world. Lie and colleagues[48] reported the use of plan-do-study-act cycles incorporating simulation to identify process threats, infection control threats, and equipment or PPE issues and then modified their COVID-19 patient care workflow based on their findings. Wong and colleagues[49] utilized simulated drills to test the feasibility of changes to their operating room setup and workflow. Findings based on these drills led to the designation of an operating room coordinator to ensure adherence to the protocol they had developed. Muhsen and colleagues[50] describe major changes made to their maternity ward floor plan, introduction of radio communications, and increases in staffing following simulation training sessions in preparation for care of COVID-19 infected obstetric patients. Other groups describe the use of simulation as part of the development of anesthetic care–specific checklists and protocols, including labor analgesia, neuraxial anesthesia for cesarean delivery, conversion of a labor epidural to cesarean delivery, and general anesthesia for the obstetric patient.[51] One group incorporated actual obstetric patients into live simulation drills by providing their care as if they were patients infected with COVID-19, to test preliminary protocols designed for care of obstetric patients infected with COVID-19, and cited positive reactions from the patients involved.[52]

THE FUTURE OF SIMULATION IN OBSTETRIC ANESTHESIOLOGY

Although the COVID-19 pandemic served as a crisis that showcased the value simulation brings to education, training, and preparedness in the field of obstetric anesthesiology, the limits placed on human interaction due to social distancing requirements accelerated the shift in learning and communicating to the virtual environment. The seeds of this evolution in the world of simulation existed prior to the pandemic, and recent literature provides a rough sketch of the world of simulation that may come into existence in the future. A recent review of alternatives to high-fidelity simulation by Delisle and colleagues[53] describes many of the modalities that do not require in-person training with partial task trainers or high-fidelity manikin-based simulation. Telesimulation allows for remote observation of a simulation scenario with live remote debriefing extending the geographic reach of a single simulation session for learners separated by vast distances. Screen-based simulation removes the need for a live instructor through the use automated facilitation and feedback mechanisms. Game-based simulation, much like screen-based simulation, removes the requirement of a live instructor but also incorporates motivational aspects that exist in popular single-player or multiplayer videogames and can incorporate both technical and nontechnical skills. Improvements in virtual reality technology will allow game-based simulation increasingly to approach or surpass the fidelity of existing manikin-based simulation technology. Benda and colleagues[54] utilized an obstetric scenario to compare the educational effectiveness of serious game training to high-fidelity manikin-based training. Groups randomized to manikin-based or serious game-based training prior to an assessment of performance in a high-fidelity manikin-based simulation scenario showed no difference in overall performance.

SUMMARY

Although the role of simulation in training and assessment of individuals, multidisciplinary teams, and the work environment in obstetric anesthesiology continued at the end of the second decade of the twenty-first century, the COVID-19 pandemic provided the ideal circumstances to reveal the unparalleled value simulation brings to training and preparation for emergencies, both locally and globally. Ironically, this turbulent period of pandemic health care, in which high-fidelity, team-based simulation has shone so brightly, likely will accelerate the transition toward alternative modes of simulation-based training and assessment through the increased use and capability of virtual platforms and screen-based learning environments.

CLINICS CARE POINTS

- Simulation in obstetrical anesthesia should continue to be utilized to teach and to assess the competencies of the individual, the group and the institution at large.
- The COVID-19 pandemic showcased the ability of simulation in obstetrical anesthesiology to evolve and to address new and unprecedented emergencies within the obstetric unit.
- Simulation in obstetrical anesthesia will continue to evolve as technology advances and as the world encounters new medical challenges.

DISCLOSURE

The authors have nothing to disclose.

REFERENCES

1. Pratt SD. Simulation in obstetric anesthesia. Anesth Analg 2012;114(1):186–90.
2. Pratt SD. Recent trends in simulation for obstetric anesthesia. Curr Opin Anaesthesiol 2012;25(3):271–6.
3. Wenk M, Pöpping DM. Simulation for anesthesia in obstetrics. Best Pract Res Clin Anaesthesiol 2015;29(1):81–6.
4. Schornack LA, Baysinger CL, Pian-Smith MCM. Recent advances of simulation in obstetric anesthesia. Curr Opin Anaesthesiol 2017;30(6):723–9.
5. Clinton E, Minehart RD. Simulation in obstetrics. In: Mahoney B, Minehart RD, Pian-Smith MCM, editors. Comprehensive healthcare simulation: anesthesiology. Switzerland: Springer International Publishing; 2020. p. 221–9.
6. Marynen F, Van Gerven E, Van de Velde M. Simulation in obstetric anesthesia: an update. Curr Opin Anaesthesiol 2020;33(3):272–6.
7. Leighton BL. A greengrocer's model of the epidural space. Anesthesiology 1989. https://doi.org/10.1097/00000542-198902000-00038.
8. Vaughan N, Dubey VN, Wee MYK, et al. A review of epidural simulators: where are we today? Med Eng Phys 2013;35(9):1235–50.
9. Brazil AL, Conci A, Clua E, et al. Haptic forces and gamification on epidural anesthesia skill gain. Entertain Comput 2018;25:1–13.
10. Moo-Young J, Weber TM, Kapralos B, et al. Development of unity simulator for epidural insertion training for replacing current lumbar puncture simulators. Cureus 2021;13(2):e13409.
11. A. L. Brazil, A. Conci, E. Clua, et al. "Force modeling and gamification for Epidural Anesthesia training." In: IEEE international Conference on serious games and applications for health (SeGAH). IEEE; 2016. p. 1–8.
12. Capogna E, Salvi F, Vecchio A Del, et al. Changes in gaze behavior during the learning of the epidural technique with a simulator in anesthesia novices. Open J Anesthesiol 2020;10(11):361–70.
13. Ortner CM, Richebé P, Bollag LA, et al. Repeated simulation-based training for performing general anesthesia for emergency cesarean delivery: long-term retention and recurring mistakes. Int J Obstet Anesth 2014;23(4):341–7.
14. Scavone BM, Sproviero MT, McCarthy RJ, et al. Development of an objective scoring system for measurement of resident performance on the human patient simulator. Anesthesiology 2006. https://doi.org/10.1097/00000542-200608000-00008.

15. Eason M, Olsen ME. High spinal in an obstetric patient: a simulated emergency. Simul Healthc 2009;4(3):179–83.
16. Lee A, Sheen JJ, Richards S. Intrapartum maternal cardiac arrest: a simulation case for multidisciplinary providers. Mededportal J Teach Learn Resour 2018; 14:10768.
17. Obr C, Mueller A. Diabetic ketoacidosis in the obstetric population: a simulation scenario for anesthesia providers. MedEdPORTAL 2016;12(1):1–5.
18. Minehart R, Abir G, Arendt K, et al. COVID19 labor to Cesarean delivery: case flow and facilitator ' s guide. Available at: https://soap.memberclicks.net/covid-19-toolkit. Accessed May 24, 2021.
19. Sree Kumar EJ, Purva M, Chander MS, et al. Impact of repeated simulation on learning curve characteristics of residents exposed to rare life threatening situations. BMJ Simul Technol Enhanc Learn 2020;6(6):351–5.
20. Kariya N, Kawasaki Y, Okutani H, et al. Effects of simulation study of high neuraxial block during epidural analgesia for labor pain on pre/posttest evaluation in junior clinical trainees. Anesthesiol Pain Med 2020;10(1):3–7.
21. Teixeira JARM, Alves C, Martins C, et al. General anesthesia for emergency cesarean delivery: simulation-based evaluation of residents. Braz J Anesthesiol 2021. https://doi.org/10.1016/j.bjane.2021.02.059.
22. Raemer DB, Kolbe M, Minehart RD, et al. Improving anesthesiologists' ability to speak up in the operating room: a randomized controlled experiment of a simulation-based intervention and a qualitative analysis of hurdles and enablers. Acad Med 2016;91(4):530–9.
23. Szmulewicz C, Rouby P, Boyer C, et al. Communication of bad news in relation with surgery or anesthesia: an interdisciplinary simulation training program. J Gynecol Obstet Hum Reprod 2021;50(7):102062.
24. Okrainec A, Henao O, Azzie G. Telesimulation: an effective method for teaching the fundamentals of laparoscopic surgery in resource-restricted countries. Surg Endosc 2010;24(2):417–22.
25. Sorensen JL, Van der Vleuten C, Rosthoj S, et al. Simulation-based multiprofessional obstetric anesthesia training conducted in situ versus off-site leads to similar individual and team outcomes: a randomized educational trial. BMJ Open 2015;5(10):e008344-e008344.
26. Lim G, Krohner RG, Metro DG, et al. Low-fidelity haptic simulation versus mental imagery training for epidural anesthesia technical achievement in novice anesthesiology residents: a randomized comparative study. Anesth Analg 2016; 122(5):1516–23.
27. Kiwalabye I, Cronjé L, Schoeman S, et al. A simulation-based study evaluating the preparedness of interns' post-anaesthesia rotation in managing a failed obstetric intubation scenario: Is our training good enough? South Afr Med J 2021; 111(3):265–70.
28. Dabbagh A, Elyassi H, Sabouri AS, et al. The role of integrative educational intervention package (Monthly ITE, mentoring, mocked OSCE) in improving successfulness for anesthesiology residents in the national board exam. Anesthesiol Pain Med 2020;10(2):e98566.
29. Calvert KL, McGurgan PM, Debenham EM, et al. Emergency obstetric simulation training: how do we know where we are going, if we don't know where we have been? Aust N Z J Obstet Gynaecol 2013;53(6):509–16.
30. Arriaga AF, Gawande AA, Raemer DB, et al. Pilot testing of a model for insurer-driven, large-scale multicenter simulation training for operating room teams. Ann Surg 2014;259(3):403–10.

31. Bogne kamdem valery, Daelemans C, Englert Y, Morin F, et al. Using simulation team training with human's factors components in obstetrics to improve patient outcome: a review of the literature. Eur J Obstet Gynecol Reprod Biol 2021; 260:159–65.

32. Lutgendorf MA, Spalding C, Drake E, et al. Multidisciplinary in situ simulation-based training as a postpartum hemorrhage quality improvement project. Mil Med 2017;182(3):e1762–6.

33. Austin N, Goldhaber-Fiebert S, Daniels K, et al. Building comprehensive strategies for obstetric safety: simulation drills and communication. Anesth Analg 2016;123(5):1181–90.

34. Dillon SJ, Kleinmann W, Seasely A, et al. How personality affects teamwork: a study in multidisciplinary obstetrical simulation. Am J Obstet Gynecol 2021; 3(2):100303.

35. Capogna E, Capogna G, Raccis D, et al. Eye tracking metrics and leader's behavioral performance during a post-partum hemorrhage high-fidelity simulated scenario. Adv Simul 2021;6(1):1–12.

36. Cheloufi M, Picard J, Hoffmann P, et al. How to agree on what is fundamental to optimal teamwork performance in a situation of postpartum hemorrhage? A multidisciplinary Delphi French study to develop the Obstetric Team Performance Assessment Scale (OTPA Scale). Eur J Obstet Gynecol Reprod Biol 2021; 256:6–16.

37. Homcha BE, Mets EJ, Goldenberg MDF, et al. Development and assessment of pictorial guide for improved accuracy of visual blood loss estimation in cesarean delivery. Simul Healthc 2017;12(5):314–8.

38. Piekarski F, Gerdessen L, Schmitt E, et al. Quantification of intraoperative blood loss in a simulated scenario using a novel device. Shock 2020;55(6): 759–65.

39. Taylor J, Chau A, Gunka V, et al. The incidence of dry chlorhexidine gluconate transfer from skin to surgical gloves: a simulation and in vitro study. Int J Obstet Anesth 2021;45:111–4.

40. Mhyre J, Ward N, Whited TM, et al. Randomized controlled simulation trial to compare transfer procedures for emergency cesarean. J Obstet Gynecol Neonatal Nurs 2020;49(3):272–82.

41. Alexander LA, Newton MW, McEvoy KG, et al. Development and pilot testing of a context-relevant safe anesthesia checklist for cesarean delivery in East Africa. Anesth Analg 2019;128(5):993–8.

42. Gallardo AR, Meneghetti G, Franc JM, et al. Comparing resource management skills in a high- versus low-resource simulation scenario: a pilot study. Prehosp Disaster Med 2020;35(1):83–7.

43. Lee JSE, Chan JJI, Ithnin F, et al. Resilience of the restructured obstetric anaesthesia training programme during the COVID-19 outbreak in Singapore. Int J Obstet Anesth 2020;43:89–90.

44. Eubanks A, Thomson B, Marko E, et al. Obstetric simulation for a pandemic. Semin Perinatol 2020;44(6):151294.

45. Kiely DJ, Posner GD, Sansregret A. Health Care team training and simulation-based education in obstetrics during the COVID-19 pandemic. J Obstet Gynaecol Can 2020;42(8):1017–20.

46. Rastogi S. Simulations of deliveries of SARS-CoV-2 positive pregnant women and their newborn babies: plan to implement a complex and ever-changing protocol. Am J Perinatol 2020;37(10):1061–5.

47. Benlolo S, Nensi A, Campbell DM, et al. The use of in situ simulation to enhance COVID-19 pandemic preparedness in obstetrics. Cureus 2021;13(1):1–6.
48. Lie SA, Wong LT, Chee M, et al. Process-oriented in situ simulation is a valuable tool to rapidly ensure operating room preparedness for COVID-19 outbreak. Simul Healthc 2020;15(4):225–33.
49. Wong J, Goh QY, Tan Z, et al. Preparing for a COVID-19 pandemic: a review of operating room outbreak response measures in a large tertiary hospital in Singapore. Can J Anesth 2020;67(6):732–45.
50. Muhsen WS, Marshall-Roberts R. Simulation-guided preparations for the management of suspected or confirmed COVID-19 cases in the obstetric emergency theater. J Matern Neonatal Med 2020;0(0):1–4.
51. Li Y, Ciampa EJ, Zucco L, et al. Adaptation of an obstetric anesthesia service for the severe acute respiratory syndrome coronavirus-2 pandemic: description of checklists, workflows, and development tools. Anesth Analg 2021; 132(1):31–7.
52. Cegielski D, Darling C, Noor C, et al. Patients as partners in readiness for COVID-19: using 'live simulation' to implement infection prevention and control procedures in the maternity operating theatre. Anaesth Rep 2020;8(2):191–5.
53. Delisle M, Hannenberg AA. Alternatives to high-fidelity simulation. Anesthesiol Clin 2020;38(4):761–73.
54. Benda NC, Kellogg KM, Hoffman DJ, et al. Lessons learned from an evaluation of serious gaming as an alternative to mannequin-based simulation technology: Randomized controlled trial. JMIR Serious Games 2020;8(3):1–12.

Escalating Care on Labor and Delivery

Elisa C. Walsh, MD, Emily E. Naoum, MD*

KEYWORDS

- Maternal mortality • Severe maternal morbidity • Maternal health
- Levels of maternal care • Escalation of care / Escalating care • Critical care
- Intensive care

KEY POINTS

- Maternal morbidity and mortality remain a significant global issue.
- For patients with known high-risk pregnancies, it is essential for them to be triaged to an appropriate level of care facility to optimize outcomes.
- A significant number of maternal adverse events are potentially preventable with improved recognition of illness and protocolized pathways.
- Obstetrical-specific risk assessments have been developed to escalate care early and predict morbidity and mortality while accounting for the normal physiologic changes in pregnancy.
- For patients requiring intensive care, telemedicine may represent a unique opportunity to provide appropriate care for critical illness while remaining on a labor and delivery floor.

CASE

A 33-year-old G1P0 at 35-weeks gestation is admitted for the induction of labor in the setting of elevated blood pressures and a persistent headache due to concern for pre-eclampsia. She has a history of chronic kidney disease with a baseline creatinine of 1.2 mg/dL. She has been admitted for cervical ripening and has had a prolonged induction of labor with artificial rupture of membranes more than 24 hours ago. The team is alerted by her bedside nurse that the patient has a fever of 40.1°C. She has an epidural in place for labor analgesia that is working well; however, she seems diaphoretic and states that she feels exhausted. Her vital signs are significant for a respiratory rate of 32 bpm, a heart rate of 120 bpm, BP 105/45 mm Hg, and oxygen saturation of 96% on room air. Additionally, she has had minimal urine output for the last 3 hours after Foley catheter placement. Her laboratories are significant for a white blood cell count of 19,000 cells/μL, hemoglobin of 8.6 g/dL, platelet count of 73,000/μL, creatinine of 1.9 mg/dL, and a lactate of 5.3 mmol/L. Blood cultures are

Department of Anesthesia, Critical Care and Pain Medicine, Massachusetts General Hospital, 55 Fruit Street, GRB 444, Boston, MA 02114, USA
* Corresponding author.
E-mail address: Enaoum@mgh.harvard.edu

Anesthesiology Clin 39 (2021) 667–685
https://doi.org/10.1016/j.anclin.2021.08.002   anesthesiology.theclinics.com

drawn and sent, and she is started on ampicillin and gentamicin for presumed chorioamnionitis. She is given a 2 L of fluid bolus with lactated ringers; however, her mean arterial pressure (MAP) remains 58 to 60 mm Hg for the next hour and she is persistently tachycardic (heart rate 110s) and tachypneic to the high 20s. Her cervical examination continues to be unchanged on the last examination at 8 cm dilated, 100% effaced, and −1 station. The fetal heart tracing is significant for fetal tachycardia with an average rate of 180 bpm and lack of variability.

INTRODUCTION

Despite advances in medical care over the past century, maternal morbidity and mortality remain a significant global issue. The United States (US) is the only developed nation whereby maternal mortality has increased since 1990, from 7.2 per 100,000 live births in 1986 to 17.3 per 100,000 live births in 2017.[1,2] Although this can be partially attributed to improved identification and data collection, numerous studies have corroborated that the maternal mortality rate is rising.[3] Pregnancy-related mortality increases with maternal age; other predominant causes that have been identified include cardiovascular disease (26.5%), preexisting illnesses (14.5%), sepsis (12.7%), and hemorrhage (11.4%).[1] Overall, mortality due to hemorrhage, hypertensive disorders of pregnancy, and anesthetic complications has declined in the United States, whereas mortality due to cardiovascular and chronic illness has increased.[1,4] The latter category includes conditions such as chronic hypertension, underlying maternal obesity, pregestational diabetes, human immunodeficiency virus (HIV), and pulmonary hypertension.[5]

The Centers for Disease Control and Prevention (CDC) has established a list of severe maternal morbidity (SMM) diagnostic indicators associated with unanticipated outcomes of labor and delivery that result in significant short- or long-term health consequences.[6] SMM in the US has more than doubled from 49.5 per 10,000 deliveries in 1993 to 144 in 2014, predominantly driven by women requiring a blood transfusion and less often by hysterectomy and ventilation or temporary tracheostomy.[7] In one state-level study, the incidence of SMM ranged from 0.05% to 1.13%.[8] Similar to maternal mortality, this surge is also likely driven by increasing maternal age and chronic medical conditions.

Significant racial and ethnic disparities in maternal mortality and SMM are also present. This gap exists in every racial and ethnic minority category compared with deliveries among non–Hispanic white women.[9–11] Non–Hispanic black women are particularly affected, with SMM occurring in 231.1 per 10,000 delivery hospitalizations compared to only 139.2 in non–Hispanic white women.[11] If racial and ethnic minority women experienced SMM at the same rate as non–Hispanic white women, it is estimated that this would result in a 28% reduction in cases of SMM among racial and ethnic minority women and a 15% overall reduction in SMM.[11] In addition to racial and ethnic minority status, public or absent health insurance as well as lower education levels have also been associated with an increased incidence of maternal mortality and morbidity.[12]

The rising incidence and complexity in maternal illness demand that providers have familiarity with potential complications as well as protocols in place to prevent, identify, and properly manage those complications. Although the implementation of care bundles has already shown a tremendous benefit in improving maternal outcomes, triage to facilities with appropriate capabilities, prompt intensive care consultation, obstetrical-specific risk assessment tools, and provider awareness are also necessary to recognize early signs of decompensation and allow rapid escalation of care.

LEVELS OF MATERNAL CARE

Perinatal regionalization is an approach that classifies institutions by capabilities and personnel to ensure women and infants receive care at a facility that aligns with their risk. The Society for Maternal-Fetal Medicine and the American College of Obstetricians and Gynecologists (ACOG) define 4 levels of maternal care based on available clinicians and resources as basic care (Level I), specialty care (Level II), subspecialty care (Level III), and regional perinatal health centers (Level IV) **(Table 1)**.[13] Accredited birth centers, freestanding facilities that are not hospitals, represent an important resource for patients with low-risk pregnancies as well as those in rural and underserved communities but are separately governed. All levels of care should be capable of initial stabilization and develop collaborative relationships with higher acuity centers to facilitate maternal transport when appropriate.[13] The CDC created a web-based voluntary Levels of Care Assessment Tool (CDC LOCATe), which produces a standardized tool for participating hospitals to assess their capabilities and personnel to identify any gaps and areas for improvement.[14]

Although guidelines regarding levels of maternal care have been in place since 2015, there has been variable adoption of its principles and there remains a significant gap between idea and implementation. In a cross-sectional study of 7 states, only a small fraction (2.4%) of high-risk patients warranted delivery in a level III or IV hospital and the majority (97.6%) of all patients delivered at a hospital with an appropriate level of maternal care. However, 43.4% of the high-risk patients (n = 19,988) were delivered at a level I or II hospital. Rates of delivery at inappropriate centers were highest for women with a placenta previa and prior uterine surgery (37.7%) and those with chronic medical conditions such as maternal cardiac disease (68.2%).[15] In a national retrospective study, the adjusted risk ratio for SMM in a high-risk population was 9.55 in low-acuity hospitals compared with 6.50 in high-acuity hospitals.[16]

If transfer to a higher-level facility is indicated, ACOG and the American Academy of Pediatrics have defined standard guidelines for perinatal transfer for the escalation of care.[17,18] Minimum monitoring standards include continuous pulse oximetry, electrocardiography, and regular assessment of vital signs. Additionally, venous access must be established and secured. Patients with preexisting arterial or central venous catheters must continue invasive hemodynamic monitoring during transport. Patients requiring mechanical ventilation must have the position of the endotracheal tube confirmed and secured before transport and must be monitored for adequate oxygenation and ventilation. There are no standards on fetal monitoring during transport, but routine left uterine displacement and supplemental oxygen are often provided.

EPIDEMIOLOGY OF MATERNAL INTENSIVE CARE UNIT ADMISSION

Overall estimates suggest that 1% to 3% of pregnant women require intensive care unit (ICU) admission or critical care services (corresponding to a Level IV facility) in the US each year.[19] This is comparable to rates in other developed nations.[20,21] The exact epidemiology of maternal critical care is complicated due to the lack of consistency in definition and is likely underestimated due to confounders such as the exclusion of women over 6 weeks postpartum, exclusion of women who were critically ill but were not ultimately admitted to an ICU, or exclusion of women who did not suffer organ failure (eg, massive hemorrhage with appropriate resuscitation and no subsequent organ failure).

Causes of maternal ICU admission may be classified as obstetric (eg, hemorrhage, hypertensive disorders of pregnancy, puerperal sepsis, thromboembolic disease) and nonobstetrical (eg, preexisting medical conditions, nonpuerperal sepsis). The most

Table 1
Levels of maternal care and relevant capabilities

	Definition	Capabilities	Health Care Providers
Accredited Birth Center	Care for low-risk women with uncomplicated singleton vertex pregnancies who are expected to have an uncomplicated birth	Basics	
Level I (Basic Care)	Care for low- to moderate-risk pregnancies with the ability to detect, stabilize, and initiate management for unanticipated antepartum, intrapartum, or postpartum issues until transport to facility with specialty maternal care is available	Basics	Qualified birthing professional (midwife, family physician, or OB) present at birth, readily available physician with the ability to perform cesarean delivery, appropriately trained and qualified RN
Level II (Specialty Care)	Level I *plus* care of appropriate moderate- to high-risk antepartum, intrapartum, or postpartum conditions	**Level I** + additional imaging available	**Level I** + OB readily available, OB leadership qualifications, MFM, anesthesiologist MD available, internal medicine and general surgical specialists available
Level III (Subspecialty Care)	Level II *plus* care of more complex maternal medical conditions, obstetric complications, and fetal conditions	**Level II** + blood availability, imaging available at all times, fetal imaging availability, IR available at all times, ICU transfer capability	**Level II** + ICU provider availability, MFM ICU consultant, nursing leadership expertise, board-certified OB present + OB leadership qualifications, OB anesthesia expertise, full specialist availability
Level IV (Regional Perinatal Health Care Centers)	Level III *plus* on-site medical and surgical care for highest complexity maternal conditions and critically ill parturients/fetuses throughout antepartum, intrapartum, and postpartum care	**Level III** + ICU capability	**Level III** + co-management of MFM and ICU teams, perinatal system leadership, MFM readily available always, nursing leadership, RN experience, OB anesthesia expertise always present, subspecialty consult availability

common causes for ICU admission in the US are hypertensive disorders of pregnancy and hemorrhage, followed by sepsis, cardiovascular conditions, and embolic phenomenon. **Fig. 1** summarizes the described literature regarding the rates of maternal ICU admission and the most common diagnoses for maternal ICU admission in developed countries.[21–28] Hemorrhage and hypertensive disorders of pregnancy continue to account for most maternal ICU admissions in developed countries, although the exact case mix differs widely in each country and even within different regions of certain countries. This is likely multifactorial and related to differences in preconception counseling and prenatal care, socioeconomic factors, environmental factors, surgical practices, and regional ICU admission guidelines. The causes of ICU admission do not differ significantly in developing versus developed countries, although there is a significantly higher maternal mortality rate in developing countries (3.3% vs 14.0%).[29]

CARE OF THE CRITICALLY ILL PARTURIENT

Regardless of the cause of maternal critical illness, it is important to differentiate between obstetric and nonobstetrical disease, identify and treat organ dysfunction, and determine maternal and fetal risk from continuing pregnancy, proceeding to delivery if necessary.[30] A thorough discussion of maternal and neonatal intensive care and outcomes is beyond the scope of this article.

Multidisciplinary teams of obstetricians, neonatologists, anesthesiologists, and intensivists are essential in the care of critically ill obstetric patients. In the antepartum patient, opportunities for obstetric input include maternal side effects of common obstetric medications (eg, cardiac and respiratory depression from magnesium for preeclampsia), potential teratogenicity and placental transfer of medications, antenatal steroids for fetal lung development, fetal surveillance, and careful choice of imaging modalities limiting fetal radiation if possible. Additionally, obstetric input is essential to assess the anticipated course of disease as well as the plan for delivery if necessary, including location, mode (vaginal, vaginal assisted, or cesarean delivery), analgesic and anesthetic management, and neonatal considerations. Postpartum, obstetric input is essential in the evaluation of vaginal or intraabdominal bleeding, potential obstetric sources of infection, duration of specific therapies such as magnesium for eclampsia, need for surgical intervention, and feasibility of breastfeeding and bonding time with the mother and her newborn.

One important consideration for critically ill obstetric patients with imminent delivery is the physical location of their care. The advantages of delivering on the labor floor are increased physical space, team familiarity with obstetric interventions, and reduced

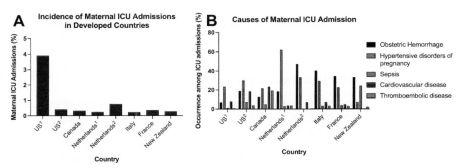

Fig. 1. Aggregate data of (*A*) maternal ICU admission rates and (*B*) cause of maternal ICU admission in developed nations.

risk of nosocomial infections.[31] The Association of Women's Health, Obstetric, and Neonatal Nurses (AWHONN) guidelines recommend 1:1 specialized perinatal nurse to patient staffing during labor and childbirth.[31] Conversely, the advantages of delivering in the ICU are immediate availability of ICU providers, advanced monitoring, and higher-level interventions. The choice depends on the degree of patient instability and interventions required, with emphasis on maternal wellbeing as the primary goal. The COSMIC paradigm is a 4-step system of early multidisciplinary consultation, automated surveillance, monitoring, and intensive care that seeks to identify high-risk and clinically deteriorating parturients and triage them to the appropriate care setting. In this paradigm, deteriorating patients are best managed on the labor and delivery floor with a remote ICU telemedicine service except in extraordinary cases.[32] Of note, there are innovative units that specialize in critically ill obstetric patients, such as the Pavilion for Women at Texas Children's Hospital and the Magee-Women's Hospital ICU at the University of Pittsburgh, but these are rare.[33,34]

Patients requiring the following interventions likely merit admission to a physical ICU instead of relying on ICU telemedicine[19]:

1. respiratory support, including endotracheal intubation, need for mechanical ventilation, and treatment of pneumothorax;
2. aggressive hemodynamic support, including vasopressors, or continuous vasodilators;
3. requirement for invasive monitoring, including arterial, central venous, and/or pulmonary artery catheter placement, maintenance, and interpretation;
4. electrical instability requiring continuous interpretation and/or intervention with cardioversion or defibrillation;
5. ongoing severe hemorrhage and coagulopathy requiring a rapid infusion of appropriate products and interpretation of laboratory results;
6. requirement for extracorporeal membrane oxygenation (ECMO);
7. acute liver failure requiring intervention including assessment for transplant eligibility; and
8. cerebrovascular disease requiring frequent neurologic assessments

In the event of cardiopulmonary arrest during management, teams should follow typical BLS/ACLS protocol with the following modifications:

1. continuous manual left uterine displacement;
2. if relevant, discontinuation of intravenous magnesium and empiric administration of calcium chloride or gluconate;
3. use of most experienced provider for airway management due to 8-fold risk of the difficult airway; and
4. perimortem cesarean delivery should be considered for maternal and fetal benefit with the goal to deliver approximately 4 minutes after cardiopulmonary arrest in the third trimester.[35]

RISK ASSESSMENTS FOR MATERNAL CRITICAL ILLNESS

One of the key principles in preventing severe morbidity and mortality in all critical illnesses is the early recognition and rapid escalation of care. In one study of 401 nonpregnant general ward patients requiring ICU admission, each hour of delay in admission was associated with a 1.5% increase in the risk of ICU death and a 1% increase in-hospital mortality.[36] However, this must be balanced with the high cost and time burden associated with inappropriate escalation of care. Most of the obstetric patients admitted to an ICU ultimately do not require high-level intervention.[19]

There are several existing scoring systems to identify patients at the risk of mortality and ICU admission in the general population. These tools aid providers in identifying signs of decompensation and avoiding delays in the assessment and implementation of appropriate interventions. However, the application of general scoring systems is often challenging in the peripartum population due to the normal physiologic changes in pregnancy and their overlap with systemic inflammatory response syndrome (SIRS). Several maternal early warning systems and risk assessment tools have emerged to address this problem. **Table 2** reviews the purpose and definition of several of these predictive tools, including those developed specifically for use in the peripartum population.

General Assessments

Scoring systems used to predict ICU mortality in the general population have had variable prognostic value in peripartum patients based on the etiology for ICU admission. The total sequential organ failure assessment (SOFA) score predicts ICU mortality based on several laboratory results and patient signs.[37] Initial scores of 11 or mean scores of greater than 5 correspond to a mortality rate greater than 80% in patients admitted to the ICU. Regardless of the initial score, an unchanged or increasing score is associated with an increased mortality rate.[38] A recent retrospective cohort study found that the SOFA score had a good overall performance for predicting SMM from hypertensive disease for obstetric patients admitted to the ICU (AUC 0.86) but was inferior to the APACHE-II score for predicting SMM from hemorrhage (AUC 0.75).[39]

The acute physiologic assessment and chronic health evaluation (APACHE) score is calculated based on several physiologic measurements, age, and prior health conditions and was developed to estimate ICU mortality for general patients. An APACHE-II score of greater than 34 is associated with 85% nonoperative and 88% postoperative in-hospital mortality.[40] Pregnant and obstetric patients were not specifically identified in this study but were likely included. In one literature review, the median APACHE-II score for obstetric patients admitted to the ICU was found to be 10.9 corresponding to a median predicted mortality of 16.6%. Actual mortality was found to be 4.6%, suggesting that the APACHE-II score overestimated mortality risk for obstetric patients in the ICU.[41] Conversely, a retrospective single-center analysis of obstetric patients requiring critical care found a mean APACHE-II score of 9.8 ± 5.6 and suggested that the APACHE-II scores were artificially low for predicting SMM due to the lack of inclusion of liver enzymes and platelet count in the APACHE-II score.[42]

The SIRS and "quick" sequential organ failure assessment (qSOFA) criteria were developed to predict in-hospital mortality but are frequently used as screening tools to identify patients with potential sepsis outside of the ICU.[43] Unfortunately, neither performs well in an obstetric population. One meta-analysis of healthy pregnant women demonstrated that, with the exception of temperature, SIRS criteria fell within the normal range of physiologic changes in pregnancy.[44] Similarly, qSOFA demonstrated low sensitivity (~50%) in obstetric patients with maternal sepsis due to low incidence of mental status changes.[45]

Obstetrical-Specific Assessments

The use of maternal early warning systems has promise in reducing preventable mortality and morbidity in the pregnant population.[22,26,46] A perfect set of abnormal vitals and laboratory findings in the obstetric population has yet to be defined; however, obstetric early warning systems are highly sensitive and reasonably specific in predicting maternal morbidity and the need for ICU care and serve as valuable screening tools.[47]

Table 2
Comparison of risk assessment tools for inpatient mortality and/or morbidity developed for the general and obstetric populations

Tool	Application	Included Variables	Comments
SOFA[43,45]	Scoring tool (24 points) to identify patients with suspected infection who are at risk of sepsis and in-hospital mortality	Physiologic data from 6 different organ systems within the first 24 h of admission	Better predictive value for patients admitted to the ICU for in-hospital mortality than SIRS or qSOFA. Poor specificity for maternal sepsis due to physiologic changes in pregnancy
APACHE-II-IV[40,42,67,68]	Scoring system using physiologic variables, age, and chronic health conditions to predict ICU mortality	12 physiologic variables within the first 24 h of ICU admission as well as age, chronic health conditions, admission information, admission diagnosis, and need for thrombolysis	May overestimate mortality for peripartum ICU admission
SIRS[43]	Physiologic criteria used to identify patients with suspected infection who are at risk of sepsis and in-hospital mortality	Two or more of temperature >38 or <36° Celsius, respiratory rate >20 breaths per minute or $Paco_2$ < 32 mm Hg, pulse >90 beats per minute, and white blood cell (WBC) count >12,000 cells/mm3 or <4000 cells/mm3, or bands >10%	Previously used as the criteria in the Sepsis 1 to define sepsis. Poor specificity for maternal sepsis due to physiologic changes in pregnancy
qSOFA[43,45]	Simple scoring tool (3 points) to identify patients with suspected infection who are at risk of sepsis and in-hospital mortality	Hypotension (SBP<100 mm Hg), high respiratory rate (>22 breaths per minute), and altered mental status (GCS<14)	Better predictive validity in patients outside of the ICU for in-hospital mortality than SOFA. Low sensitivity (~50%) in obstetric patients with maternal sepsis due to low incidence of mental status changes and unreliable reporting in the respiratory rate
OB-CMI[15]	Scoring tool to quantify maternal comorbidities and predict SMM	Weighted presence of 20 maternal comorbidities associated with SMM as defined by the CDC and maternal age	Excellent prediction of SMM

MEWC[45,49,50]	Scoring tool of abnormal physiologic parameters that indicate urgent clinical evaluation for diagnosis, intervention, and potential escalation of care in obstetric and nonobstetrical complications	One "red" trigger: Systolic BP <90 or >160 Diastolic BP >100 Heart rate <50 or >120 Respiratory rate <10 or >30 Oxygen saturation <95% on room air Oliguria <35/mL/h for > 2 h Neurologic: Maternal agitation, confusion, or unresponsiveness; Patient with preeclampsia reporting a nonremitting headache or shortness of breath	Recurrent abnormal criteria in a patient with normal baseline values or an accumulation of more than one criterion should prompt increases in the frequency and intensity of monitoring. Reported sensitivity 89% and specificity 79% with incidence of 13% SMM PPV 39%, NPV 98%
MEOWS[51-53]	" "	One "red" trigger or 2 "yellow" triggers for provider evaluation: "Yellow" Systolic BP 90–100 or 150–160 Diastolic BP 90–100 Heart rate 40–50 or 100–120 Respiratory rate 21–30 Temperature 35–36 Responds to voice Pain score 2–3 "Red" Systolic BP <90 or >160 Diastolic BP >100 Heart rate <40 or >120 Respiratory rate <10 or >30 Oxygen saturation <95% on room air Temperature <35 or >38 Unresponsive or severe pain	The original MEOWS criteria were highly sensitive for the prediction of ICU admission (89%) but had low specificity. There were no universally defined entry criteria for ICU admission; however, all cases experienced either organ failure or shock that precipitated ICU admission In 676 admissions on labor and delivery, 200 women triggered MEOWS and 86 women fit the criteria for morbidity (defined in the paper, not CDC defined). The women who triggered MEOWS were more likely to have or develop morbidity (sensitivity 89%, specificity 79%) and have a longer median length of stay

(continued on next page)

Table 2
(continued)

Tool	Application	Included Variables	Comments
MEWT[48]	" "	One "red" "trigger or 2 "yellow" triggers for provider evaluation: "Yellow" Systolic BP <80 or 156–160 Diastolic BP <45 or 106–110 Heart rate <50 or 111–130 Respiratory rate <12 or 25–30 Temperature <36 Oxygen saturation 90%–93% on room air Altered mental status "Red" Nursing discomfort Systolic BP >160 Diastolic BP >110 Heart rate >130 Respiratory rate >30 Temperature >38 Oxygen saturation <90% on room air MAP <55	Compared with MEWC/MEOWS, MEWT further defines decision support and clinical guidance based on the most common obstetric and nonobstetrical complications
SOS[56,57]	Scoring tool to identify pregnant and postpartum patients with sepsis at risk for ICU admission	8 physiologic variables (temperature, blood pressure, heart rate, respiratory rate, oxygen saturation, white blood cell count, % immature neutrophils, and lactic acid) rated on a scale of abnormally low to abnormally high	Modified scoring based on the physiologic changes in pregnancy. Better positive and negative predictive value of maternal sepsis than qSOFA or MEWS

Abbreviations: SMM, severe maternal morbidity; qSOFA, quick sequential organ failure assessment; ICU, intensive care unit; MAP, mean arterial pressure; CDC, Centers for Disease Control and Prevention; MEOWS, modified early warning score.

It is likely that this benefit is derived from more reliable routine vital sign measurement, reduced time from the recognition of abnormal vital signs to physician bedside assessment, and more rapid corrective action. Coupling screening tools with pathway-specific recommendations for the assessment and management for the most common maternal indications for ICU admission have been shown to reduce maternal morbidity.[48]

Comprehensive early warning systems developed specifically for obstetric patients include the maternal early warning criteria (MEWC), maternal early warning trigger (MEWT), and modified early warning score (MEOWS), which have been studied and implemented across the world.[48–50] The MEWC require one or more of several physiologic alterations to trigger the evaluation and possible escalation of care. It has demonstrated a sensitivity of 82% and a specificity of 87% for maternal sepsis.[45] The MEWT and MEOWS are similar but account for tiered critical ("red") and subcritical ("yellow") variables in the assessment.[48,51,52] A case-control validation study of a modified MEOWS revealed a high sensitivity (96%) but low specificity (54%) for maternal ICU admissions using greater than 1 "red" trigger or greater than 2 "amber" triggers, although using greater than 1 "red" trigger alone improved specificity to 73% while maintaining sensitivity (96%).[53]

The obstetric comorbidity index (CMI) includes 20 maternal conditions and maternal age based on an analysis of 854,823 pregnancies maternal end-organ injury or death through 30-days postpartum from 2000 to 2007 to quantify maternal risk and predict SMM.[54] A single-center retrospective study found that the CMI ranged from 0 to 15, with a median CMI of 1 for all women and a median CMI of 5 for women who experienced SMM. The frequency of SMM increased from 0.41% for those with a score of 0% to 18.75% for those with a score of $\geq$9. For every 1-point increase in the score, patients experienced a 1.55 increase in odds of SMM.[15] There remains significant unpredictability even with this assessment, however. Although women with an CMI score of 0 had the lowest rate of SMM (22.8/10,000 deliveries), a third of all women with SMM had an CMI of 0.[55]

Finally, the Sepsis in Obstetrics Score (SOS) was developed as a modified version of the SIRS criteria to account for the physiologic changes in pregnancy and serves as a scoring tool to predict women at risk for ICU admission from sepsis. It has an AUC of 0.85 for predicting ICU admission for sepsis, superior to that of qSOFA or MEWS in maternal patients. A score of 6 or greater had a sensitivity of 64%, specificity of 88%, positive predictive value of 15%, and negative predictive value of 98.6% for ICU admission for maternal sepsis.[56,57]

Automatic Electronic Surveillance Systems

As the tools for predicting maternal morbidity and SMM continue to be perfected, there is increasing interest in applying these tools as automated electronic surveillance systems in the obstetric population. The University of Michigan published findings of a novel maternal surveillance system using a combination of selected MEWC that demonstrated value in identifying patients at risk for postpartum hemorrhage and enhanced the communication of abnormal vital signs and clinical parameters to the care team.[58,59]

PREVENTABILITY OF MATERNAL CRITICAL ILLNESS AND COGNITIVE BIASES

Despite advances in care, it is likely that a significant number of maternal adverse outcomes are preventable. ICU admissions were deemed potentially avoidable in a significant number of cases (48%) by a multidisciplinary review team in a recent cohort.[26] A statewide review of maternal mortality found that 40% of cases were deemed potentially preventable with improved medical care, particularly in hemorrhage (93%), chronic preexisting medical conditions (89%), hypertensive disorders of pregnancy (60%), and infection (43%).[60] A recent UK review of maternal mortality and morbidity identified opportunities to improve the care that may have changed the outcome in the majority (68%) of cases of maternal sepsis.[61] A validation study of the SOS found poor adherence (<10%) with the best practices recommendation of antibiotics within 1 hour of sepsis diagnosis.[56] This is consistent with another statewide study that determined delays in antibiotic therapy and escalation of care affected 73% and 53% of patients with maternal sepsis, respectively.[62] Furthermore, mortality was doubled for obstetric patients who received antibiotics after greater than 1 hour of sepsis diagnosis compared with those who received antibiotics within 1 hour (8.3 vs 20%).[45]

As we continue to hone tools to prospectively identify maternal patients at risk for critical illness, it is equally important to address the human and systems factors that often contribute to preventable maternal adverse outcomes. In a UK review, at least one reviewer felt that "failure to escalate" occurred in 36% of cases due to the lack of awareness of deterioration or need to escalate, or communication breakdown in the process of attempted escalation. Providers often rely on heuristics and prior experience to rapidly assess and manage multiple patients, which can place them at significant risk for cognitive biases that can interrupt appropriate escalation of care. Common cognitive biases affecting maternal care include fixation bias (narrowed focus on a single aspect of case to the exclusion of the entire clinical picture), diagnostic momentum (acceptance of a prior diagnosis without sufficient skepticism), and confirmation bias (selective acceptance of evidence conforming to one's prior beliefs or diagnosis). Loss of situational awareness is often also present in urgent or emergent situations—particularly the passage of time—leading to the loss or delay of escalation. These individual problems are further exacerbated by workplace factors such as time limitations, fatigue, burnout, lack of physical space, perceived lack of psychological safety, frequent handovers, and understaffing.[63]

Safety huddles, embedded checklists, formal introductions of all team members, dedicated hand-off periods without interruption, and clear emergency protocols all aim to address these factors and improve the quality of care. Clinical care pathways and bundles provide a cognitive framework to facilitate more timely diagnosis, aid with management, enhance team coordination of care, and align expectations across providers.

SPECIFIC BUNDLES FOR MATERNAL CRITICAL ILLNESS

To combat preventable causes of maternal mortality and morbidity, coalitions such as the California Maternal Quality Care Collaborative (CMQCC),[64] the Safe Motherhood Initiative (SMI),[65] and the National Partnership for Maternal Safety (NPMS)[66] have identified the most common causes of adverse maternal outcomes and created several toolkits or "bundles" to help standardize an approach to care. Bundles provide evidence-based recommendations in a concise, organized format that allows each center to tailor the bundle to their individual needs. Common to all the bundles is screening and preparedness, early recognition of decompensation, rapid escalation with evidence-based interventions, and formal systems for QI assessment at the site. Implementation of a comprehensive protocol for the management of maternal hemorrhage has been shown to reduce SMM.[8,48]

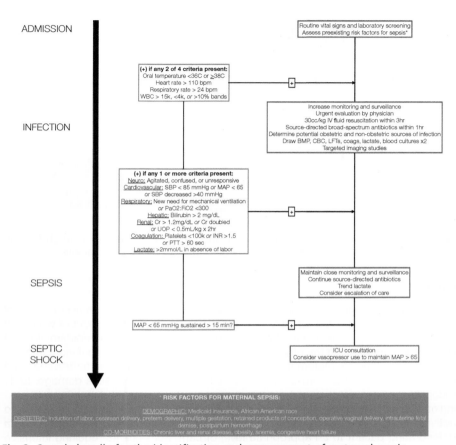

Fig. 2. Sample bundle for the identification and management of maternal sepsis.

Bundles are currently available for the diagnosis and management of the most common causes for maternal decompensation: hemorrhage, sepsis, venous thromboembolism, hypertensive disorders of pregnancy, and cardiovascular conditions. **Fig. 2** demonstrates a sample bundle for maternal sepsis, a common and preventable cause of critical illness. This bundle takes advantage of an initial screening assessment that is highly sensitive and triggers an urgent evaluation and initiation of goal-directed therapeutics with early antibiotics and fluid resuscitation, followed by a second assessment that is more specific for evidence of end-organ damage across several organ systems and triggers further escalation of care including potential ICU admission. A simplified flowchart of maternal evaluation and escalation of care for the most common causes of maternal decompensation based on obstetrical-specific risk assessments is demonstrated in **Fig. 3**. Once maternal critical illness has been identified, the team is expected to identify the most likely etiology of maternal decompensation and pursue the bundle associated with that diagnosis to expedite additional evaluation and therapies. Notably, it is beneficial to identify potential at-risk patients during preconception counseling or in the antepartum period such that the patient is admitted to a facility that can support an appropriate level of maternal care.

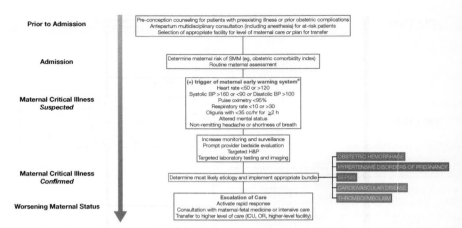

Fig. 3. Simplified flowchart of maternal evaluation and escalation of care with obstetrical-specific risk assessment tools. [a]MEWC criteria used as a representative example.

SUMMARY

Women of child-bearing age have increasing medical complexity with rising maternal comorbidities and associated morbidity and mortality. The management of women in the peripartum period is nuanced and requires a familiarity with the epidemiology of illness and alterations in the physiology and management of this population. In order to optimize outcomes, maternal critical illness must be identified and addressed at an early stage, before it becomes life-threatening or causes irreversible damage. Early recognition of deterioration, aided by improved monitoring and staff training addressing human factors as well as medical knowledge and procedural familiarity, systems to activate help, and effective escalation responses are essential to promptly triage a deteriorating patient to an appropriate level of care. For patients requiring intensive care, telemedicine may represent a unique opportunity to provide appropriate care for critical illness while remaining on a labor and delivery floor.

CASE CONTINUED

The patient is taken to the operating room for a primary cesarean delivery under epidural anesthesia given the nonreassuring fetal heart tracing and failure to progress. A male neonate is delivered with Apgar scores of 3 and 8. The patient remains febrile throughout the case and the procedure is complicated by a postpartum hemorrhage due to atony with an estimated blood loss of 2 L requiring 15-methyl-PGF2α, tranexamic acid, and transfusion of 4 units of pRBCs. At the end of the procedure, she remains on high dose phenylephrine at 100 mcg/min, develops worsening somnolence, and an oxygen requirement of 4 L via nasal cannula to maintain oxygen saturation greater than 92%. The decision is made to transfer her to the ICU for ongoing hemodynamic support and monitoring. In the ICU, a radial arterial line is placed for continuous blood pressure monitoring and central venous access is obtained via the right internal jugular vein. A norepinephrine infusion is started to maintain a MAP greater than 65 mm Hg. Antibiotic coverage is expanded to vancomycin and piperacillin–tazobactam, and further fluid resuscitation is given based on trending central venous pressure and using noninvasive arterial waveform analysis to estimate cardiac output and stroke volume variation. Over the next 12 hours, the patient's condition improves with decreased somnolence, decreased white blood cell count to 13,000/µL, decreased lactate to 1.9 mmol/L, decreased creatinine to 1.3 mg/dL, and increased urine output to 1.2 mL/kg/h. Her vital signs are now significant for a respiratory rate of 18 bpm, a heart rate of 85 bpm, BP 118/61 mm Hg off vasopressor support, and oxygen saturation of 98% on room air. Her antibiotics are deescalated to ampicillin, gentamicin, and clindamycin for 48 hours following her last fever. She remains monitored for 36 hours postpartum in the ICU before being transferred back to the postpartum floor and is discharged on postpartum day 6.

CLINICS CARE POINTS

- High-risk obstetrical patients are more likely to deliver at a center with an inappropriately low level of maternal care and have a higher rate of severe maternal morbidity (SMM) in lower-acuity hospitals.
- The obstetric comorbidity index (OB-CMI) predicts SMM and helps providers to identify at-risk patients.
- Maternal early warning systems including the maternal early warning criteria (MEWC), maternal early warning trigger (MEWT), and modified early obstetric warning system (MEOWS) may improve early recognition of maternal critical illness and prevent SMM.
- A significant number of maternal adverse outcomes have been deemed preventable in retrospective studies, including delay in antibiotics for maternal sepsis (78-90%), ICU admissions (48%), and mortality (48%).

DISCLOSURE

The authors have nothing to disclose.

REFERENCES

1. Creanga AA, Syverson C, Seed K, et al. Pregnancy-related mortality in the United States, 2011-2013. Obstet Gynecol 2017;130(2):366–73.
2. Kassebaum NJ, Bertozzi-Villa A, Coggeshall MS, et al. Global, regional, and national levels and causes of maternal mortality during 1990–2013: a systematic analysis for the Global Burden of Disease Study 2013. Lancet 2014;384(9947): 980–1004.
3. MacDorman MF, Declercq E, Thoma ME. Trends in maternal mortality by sociodemographic characteristics and cause of death in 27 States and the District of Columbia. Obstet Gynecol 2017;129(5):811–8.
4. Berg CJ, Callaghan WM, Syverson C, et al. Pregnancy-related mortality in the United States, 1998 to 2005. Obstet Gynecol 2010;116(6):1302–9.
5. Campbell KH, Savitz D, Werner EF, et al. Maternal morbidity and risk of death at delivery hospitalization. Obstet Gynecol 2013;122(3):627–33.
6. Centers for Disease Control and Prevention. Severe Maternal Morbidity in the United States. Available at: https://www.cdc.gov/reproductivehealth/maternalinfanthealth/severematernalmorbidity.html. Accessed May 21, 2021.
7. Callaghan WM, Creanga AA, Kuklina EV. Severe maternal morbidity among delivery and postpartum hospitalizations in the United States. Obstet Gynecol 2012; 120(5):1029–36.
8. Main EK, Abreo A, McNulty J, et al. Measuring severe maternal morbidity: validation of potential measures. Am J Obstet Gynecol 2016;214(5):643.e1–10.

9. Howland RE, Angley M, Won SH, et al. Determinants of severe maternal morbidity and its racial/ethnic disparities in New York City, 2008–2012. Matern Child Health J 2019;23(3):346–55.

10. Leonard SA, Main EK, Scott KA, et al. Racial and ethnic disparities in severe maternal morbidity prevalence and trends. Ann Epidemiol 2019;33:30–6.

11. Admon LK, Winkelman TNA, Zivin K, et al. Racial and ethnic disparities in the incidence of severe maternal morbidity in the United States, 2012-2015. Obstet Gynecol 2018;132(5):1158–66.

12. Wang E, Glazer KB, Sofaer S, et al. Racial and ethnic disparities in severe maternal morbidity: a qualitative study of women's experiences of peripartum care. Womens Health Issues 2021;31(1):75–81.

13. Kilpatrick SJ, Menard MK, Zahn CM, et al. Obstetric care consensus #9: levels of maternal care. Am J Obstet Gynecol 2019;221(6):B19–30.

14. Catalano A, Bennett A, Busacker A, et al. Implementing CDC's level of care assessment tool (LOCATe): a national collaboration to improve maternal and child health. J Womens Health 2017;26(12):1265–9.

15. Easter SR, Bateman BT, Sweeney VH, et al. A comorbidity-based screening tool to predict severe maternal morbidity at the time of delivery. Am J Obstet Gynecol 2019;221(3):271.e1–10.

16. Clapp MA, James KE, Kaimal AJ. The effect of hospital acuity on severe maternal morbidity in high-risk patients. Am J Obstet Gynecol 2018;219(1):111.e1–7.

17. Warren J, Fromm RE, Orr RA, et al. American College of Critical Care Medicine. Guidelines for the inter- and intrahospital transport of critically ill patients. Crit Care Med 2004;32(1):256–62.

18. Kilpatrick SJ, Papile, LA, Macones, GA. eds. Guidelines for perinatal care. 8th edition. Elk Grove Village (IL): American Academy of Pediatrics; 2017. p. 113–30.

19. ACOG Practice Bulletin No. 211 summary: critical care in pregnancy. Obstet Gynecol 2019;133(5):1063–6.

20. Senanayake H, Dias T, Jayawardena A. Maternal mortality and morbidity: epidemiology of intensive care admissions in pregnancy. Best Pract Res Clin Obstet Gynaecol 2013;27(6):811–20.

21. Aoyama K, Park AL, Davidson AJF, et al. Severe maternal morbidity and infant mortality in Canada. Pediatrics 2020;146(3):e20193870.

22. Zwart JJ, Richters JM, Ory F, et al. Severe maternal morbidity during pregnancy, delivery and puerperium in The Netherlands: a nationwide population-based study of 371,000 pregnancies. BJOG Int J Obstet Gynaecol 2008;115(7):842–50.

23. Keizer JL, Zwart JJ, Meerman RH, et al. Obstetric intensive care admissions: a 12-year review in a tertiary care centre. Eur J Obstet Gynecol Reprod Biol 2006;128(1–2):152–6.

24. Chantry AA, Deneux-Tharaux C, Bonnet M-P, et al. Pregnancy-related ICU admissions in France: trends in rate and severity, 2006-2009. Crit Care Med 2015;43(1):78–86.

25. Donati S, Maraschini A, Lega I, et al. Maternal mortality in Italy: Results and perspectives of record-linkage analysis. Acta Obstet Gynecol Scand 2018;97(11):1317–24.

26. Sadler LC, Austin DM, Masson VL, et al. Review of contributory factors in maternity admissions to intensive care at a New Zealand tertiary hospital. Am J Obstet Gynecol 2013;209(6):549.e1–7.

27. Oud L. Epidemiology of pregnancy-associated ICU utilization in Texas: 2001 - 2010. J Clin Med Res 2017;9(2):143–53.

28. Wanderer JP, Leffert LR, Mhyre JM, et al. Epidemiology of obstetric-related ICU admissions in Maryland: 1999-2008*. Crit Care Med 2013;41(8):1844–52.

29. Pollock W, Rose L, Dennis C-L. Pregnant and postpartum admissions to the intensive care unit: a systematic review. Intensive Care Med 2010;36(9):1465–74.

30. Guntupalli KK, Hall N, Karnad DR, et al. Critical illness in pregnancy: part I: an approach to a pregnant patient in the ICU and common obstetric disorders. Chest 2015;148(4):1093–104.

31. Simpson KR, Lyndon A, Spetz J, et al. Adherence to the AWHONN staffing guidelines as perceived by labor nurses. Nurs Womens Health 2019;23(3):217–23.

32. Lockhart EM, Hincker A, Klumpner TT, et al. Consultation, surveillance, monitoring, and intensive care (COSMIC): a novel 4-tier program to identify and monitor high-risk obstetric patients from the clinic to critical care. Anesth Analg 2019;128(6):1354–60.

33. Texas children's hospital pavilion for women: intensive care unit. 2021. Available at: https://women.texaschildrens.org/program/labor-and-delivery/intensive-care-unit. Accessed May 21, 2021.

34. University of Pittsburgh Magee-womens hospital intensive care unit. 2021. Available at: https://ccm.pitt.edu/content/upmc-magee-womens-hospital-icu. Accessed May 21, 2021.

35. American Heart Association. Cardiac arrest in pregnancy in-hospital ACLS algorithm 2020. Available at: https://cpr.heart.org/-/media/cpr-files/cpr-guidelines-files/algorithms/algorithmacls_ca_in_pregnancy_inhospital_200612.pdf?la=en. Accessed May 21, 2021.

36. Vincent J-L. The continuum of critical care. Crit Care 2019;23(S1):122.

37. Vincent J-L, Moreno R, Takala J, et al. The SOFA (Sepsis-related Organ Failure Assessment) score to describe organ dysfunction/failure: On behalf of the Working Group on Sepsis-Related Problems of the European Society of Intensive Care Medicine (see contributors to the project in the appendix). Intensive Care Med 1996;22(7):707–10.

38. Ferreira FL, Bota DP, Bross A, et al. Serial evaluation of the SOFA score to predict outcome in critically ill patients. JAMA 2001;286(14):1754–8.

39. Oliveira-Neto AF, Parpinelli MA, Costa ML, et al. Prediction of severe maternal outcome among pregnant and puerperal women in obstetric ICU. Crit Care Med 2019;47(2):e136–43.

40. Knaus WA, Draper EA, Wagner DP, et al. APACHE II: a severity of disease classification system. Crit Care Med 1985;13(10):818–29.

41. Ryan HM, Sharma S, Magee LA, et al. The usefulness of the APACHE II score in obstetric critical care: a structured review. J Obstet Gynaecol Can 2016;38(10):909–18.

42. Yuqi L, Tan G, Chengming S, et al. The ICU Is becoming a main battlefield for severe maternal rescue in China: an 8-year single-center clinical experience. Crit Care Med 2017;45(11):e1106–10.

43. Seymour CW, Liu VX, Iwashyna TJ, et al. Assessment of clinical criteria for sepsis: for the third international consensus definitions for sepsis and septic shock (Sepsis-3). JAMA 2016;315(8):762.

44. Bauer ME, Bauer ST, Rajala B, et al. Maternal physiologic parameters in relationship to systemic inflammatory response syndrome criteria: a systematic review and meta-analysis. Obstet Gynecol 2014;124(3):535–41.

45. Bauer ME, Housey M, Bauer ST, et al. Risk factors, etiologies, and screening tools for sepsis in pregnant women: a multicenter case-control study. Anesth Analg 2019;129(6):1613–20.

46. Austin DM, Sadler L, McLintock C, et al. Early detection of severe maternal morbidity: a retrospective assessment of the role of an Early Warning Score System. Aust N Z J Obstet Gynaecol 2014;54(2):152–5.
47. Umar A, Ameh CA, Muriithi F, et al. Early warning systems in obstetrics: a systematic literature review. PLoS One 2019;14(5):e0217864.
48. Shields LE, Wiesner S, Klein C, et al. Use of maternal early warning trigger tool reduces maternal morbidity. Am J Obstet Gynecol 2016;214(4):527.e1–6.
49. Mhyre JM, D'Oria R, Hameed AB, et al. The maternal early warning criteria: a proposal from the national partnership for maternal safety. Obstet Gynecol 2014; 124(4):782–6.
50. Lewis G. Confidential enquiries into maternal deaths in the United Kingdom, confidential enquiry into maternal and child health. Saving mothers' lives: reviewing maternal deaths to make motherhood safer - 2003-2005: the seventh report of the confidential enquiries into maternal deaths in the United Kingdom. London: CEMACH; 2007.
51. Singh A, Guleria K, Vaid NB, et al. Evaluation of maternal early obstetric warning system (MEOWS chart) as a predictor of obstetric morbidity: a prospective observational study. Eur J Obstet Gynecol Reprod Biol 2016;207:11–7.
52. Singh S, McGlennan A, England A, et al. A validation study of the CEMACH recommended modified early obstetric warning system (MEOWS)*: A validation study of MEOWS. Anaesthesia 2012;67(1):12–8.
53. Ryan HM, Jones MA, Payne BA, et al. Validating the performance of the modified early obstetric warning system multivariable model to predict maternal intensive care unit admission. J Obstet Gynaecol Can 2017;39(9):728–33.e3.
54. Bateman BT, Mhyre JM, Hernandez-Diaz S, et al. Development of a comorbidity index for use in obstetric patients. Obstet Gynecol 2013;122(5):957–65.
55. Somerville NJ, Nielsen TC, Harvey E, et al. Obstetric comorbidity and severe maternal morbidity among Massachusetts Delivery Hospitalizations, 1998-2013. Matern Child Health J 2019;23(9):1152–8.
56. Albright CM, Has P, Rouse DJ, et al. Internal validation of the sepsis in obstetrics score to identify risk of morbidity from sepsis in pregnancy. Obstet Gynecol 2017; 130(4):747–55.
57. Albright CM, Ali TN, Lopes V, et al. The Sepsis in Obstetrics Score: a model to identify risk of morbidity from sepsis in pregnancy. Am J Obstet Gynecol 2014; 211(1):39.e1–8.
58. Klumpner TT, Kountanis JA, Langen ES, et al. Use of a novel electronic maternal surveillance system to generate automated alerts on the labor and delivery unit. BMC Anesthesiol 2018;18(1):78.
59. Klumpner TT, Kountanis JA, Meyer SR, et al. Use of a novel electronic maternal surveillance system and the maternal early warning criteria to detect severe postpartum hemorrhage. Anesth Analg 2020;131(3):857–65.
60. Berg CJ, Harper MA, Atkinson SM, et al. Preventability of pregnancy-related deaths: results of a state-wide review. Obstet Gynecol 2005;106(6):1228–34.
61. Knight M, Bunch K, Tuffnell D, et al, editors. Saving lives, improving mothers' care - lessons learned to inform maternity care from the UK and Ireland confidential enquiries into maternal deaths and morbidity 2016-18. Oxford: National Perinatal Epidemiology Unit, University of Oxford; 2020.
62. Bauer ME, Lorenz RP, Bauer ST, et al. Maternal deaths due to sepsis in the State of Michigan, 1999-2006. Obstet Gynecol 2015;126(4):747–52.
63. Royal College of Obstetricians and Gynaecologists. Each baby counts: 2019 progress report. London: RCOG; 2020.

64. CMQCC. California Maternal Quality Care Collaborative (CMQCC) toolkits. 2021. Available at: https://www.cmqcc.org/resources-tool-kits/toolkits. Accessed May 21, 2021.
65. American College of Obstetricians and Gynecologists. Safe motherhood initiative 2021. Available at: https://www.acog.org/community/districts-and-sections/district-ii/programs-and-resources/safe-motherhood-initiative. Accessed May 21, 2021.
66. Banayan JM, Scavone BM. National partnership for maternal safety: maternal safety bundles. Curr Anesthesiol Rep 2017;7(1):67–75.
67. Zimmerman JE, Kramer AA, McNair DS, et al. Acute Physiology and Chronic Health Evaluation (APACHE) IV: hospital mortality assessment for today's critically ill patients. Crit Care Med 2006;34(5):1297–310.
68. Knaus WA, Wagner DP, Draper EA, et al. The APACHE III prognostic system. Risk prediction of hospital mortality for critically ill hospitalized adults. Chest 1991; 100(6):1619–36.

Postpartum Respiratory Depression

Rebecca S. Himmelwright, MD, Jennifer E. Dominguez, MD, MHS*

KEYWORDS

- Pregnancy • Postpartum • Respiratory depression • Respiratory failure • Obesity
- Opioid-induced respiratory depression (OIRD)
- Acute respiratory distress syndrome (ARDS)

KEY POINTS

- Modern, ultra-low, and low-doses of neuraxial morphine for postcesarean delivery analgesia are safe and effective, and carry a low risk of respiratory depression for the most obstetric patients.
- For selected comorbidities and conditions acquired in pregnancy, careful consideration of the patient's unique risks and benefits should be undertaken when using neuraxial morphine for postcesarean analgesia, particularly in combination with other drugs that depress respiration.
- The etiologies of postpartum respiratory depression/failure are numerous. Preexisting diseases such as obstructive sleep apnea (OSA), obesity hypoventilation syndrome (OHS), and cardiopulmonary diseases may interact with conditions acquired during pregnancy or peripartum, as well as drugs administered peripartum, to compound the risk of respiratory compromise in vulnerable patients.
- The detection of respiratory compromise in obstetric patients is complicated by the significant overlap between or confounding by normal maternal physiologic changes. It is important to modify or develop specific alert criteria and algorithms for this population.
- The incidence of severe pulmonary complications such as acute respiratory distress syndrome (ARDS) is on the rise. Novel respiratory viral infections pose a unique risk to pregnant and postpartum patients. The recent H1N1 and COVID-19 pandemics have helped demonstrate the value and safety of mechanical ventilatory support, including ECMO, in this population.

INTRODUCTION

No accepted definition of respiratory depression in studies of obstetric patients exists. Studies have variously defined thresholds for clinically significant respiratory depression including the following: need for airway intervention; hypoxia (SpO2 <90%) or bradypnea (respiratory rate (RR) <8 breaths/min) that requires supplemental oxygen; excessive sedation that requires more than verbal stimulation to maintain adequate

Duke University Medical Center, DUMC 3094, MS#9, 2301 Erwin Road, Durham, NC 27710, USA
* Corresponding author.
E-mail address: jennifer.dominguez@duke.edu

Anesthesiology Clin 39 (2021) 687–709
https://doi.org/10.1016/j.anclin.2021.08.003   anesthesiology.theclinics.com
1932-2275/21/© 2021 Elsevier Inc. All rights reserved.

respiration; or the use of pharmacologic therapy to reverse opioid or benzodiazepine narcosis.[1–3] When available, some studies have also included measures of hypercapnia or low tidal volumes.[4,5]

In the obstetric population, the incidence of respiratory depression has been best studied following the administration of neuraxial morphine, but has varied due to differences in study designs, definitions of respiratory depression, and neuraxial morphine doses. A recent systematic review of published reports of clinically significant respiratory depression in women that received neuraxial morphine or diamorphine for postcesarean delivery analgesia reviewed more than 18,000 cases and found a low prevalence of respiratory depression in this population (5.96–8.67 per 10,000).[1] Furthermore, at contemporary, low-doses of neuraxial morphine or diamorphine, clinically significant respiratory depression was even more rare (1.08–1.63 per 10,000).[1] They reported no permanent harm or death in this population, even after studying closed claims data.[6] Although reassuring for healthy obstetric patients, the recent consensus statement endorsed by the Society for Obstetric Anesthesia and Perinatology recommends increased monitoring following neuraxial morphine administration for certain patients at higher risk of respiratory depression, but studies elucidating these risk factors in obstetric patients have been scant, and clinical standards have been largely extrapolated from the general surgical population.[7]

Certainly, neuraxial morphine administration is not the only potential cause of postpartum respiratory depression or failure. Clinicians should be familiar with the differential diagnosis of respiratory depression/failure in the obstetric population to guide management and to prevent adverse outcomes in vulnerable patients. Although rare, the morbidity associated with postpartum respiratory depression can be significant. From prolonged hospital stays to the need for extracorporeal membrane oxygenation (ECMO) to death, the cost/harm/risk to affected individuals and institutions can be devastating. A retrospective database study by Callaghan *and colleagues* in 2012 studied severe maternal morbidity during delivery and postpartum hospitalizations between 1998 and 2009 in the United States and the study showed that the rate of adult respiratory distress syndrome (ARDS) in pregnant and recently postpartum women markedly increased during this 12-year period.[8]

RISK FACTORS FOR POSTPARTUM RESPIRATORY DEPRESSION

There are numerous etiologies of postpartum respiratory depression/failure that result in clinically significant outcomes. Preexisting diseases such as obstructive sleep apnea (OSA), obesity hypoventilation syndrome (OHS), and cardiopulmonary diseases may interact with conditions acquired during pregnancy or peripartum, or drugs administered peripartum, to compound the risk of respiratory compromise in vulnerable patients (**Fig. 1**).[9]

The normal physiologic changes in the respiratory system during pregnancy can complicate characterizing and detecting respiratory depression (**Table 1**).[10] Confounding variables can interact to mask certain key diagnostic parameters. For example, pregnant women experience a normal increase in RR that is mediated by relatively higher progesterone levels; a pregnant patient may seem to have a "normal" RR (for a nonpregnant woman) while actually having depressed respirations (for a pregnant woman). Similarly, when the hypercarbia expected with respiratory depression is combined with the chronic respiratory alkalosis of pregnancy, the Pco_2 laboratory value may appear "normal." Given all this, it is important for providers to be aware of pregnancy physiology and use normal vital signs and laboratory values *of pregnancy* to evaluate pregnant patients.

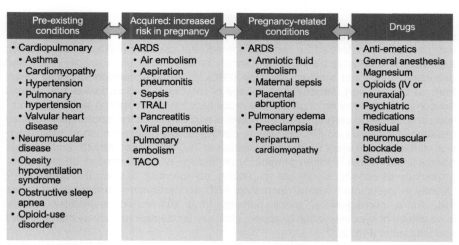

Pre-existing conditions	Acquired: increased risk in pregnancy	Pregnancy-related conditions	Drugs
• Cardiopulmonary • Asthma • Cardiomyopathy • Hypertension • Pulmonary hypertension • Valvular heart disease • Neuromuscular disease • Obesity hypoventilation syndrome • Obstructive sleep apnea • Opioid-use disorder	• ARDS • Air embolism • Aspiration pneumonitis • Sepsis • TRALI • Pancreatitis • Viral pneumonitis • Pulmonary embolism • TACO	• ARDS • Amniotic fluid embolism • Maternal sepsis • Placental abruption • Pulmonary edema • Preeclampsia • Peripartum cardiomyopathy	• Anti-emetics • General anesthesia • Magnesium • Opioids (IV or neuraxial) • Psychiatric medications • Residual neuromuscular blockade • Sedatives

Fig. 1. Risk factors and causes of postpartum respiratory depression/failure. ARDS (acute respiratory distress syndrome); TRALI (Transfusion-related acute lung injury); TACO (Transfusion-associated circulatory overload). (*Adapted from* Lapinsky, S.E., Management of Acute Respiratory Failure in Pregnancy. Semin Respir Crit Care Med. 2017 Apr;38(2):201-207.)

Each pregnant patient is unique and the risk of respiratory depression in an individual postpartum woman will vary with their specific risk factors. As in the general population, obstetric patients with underlying cardiovascular, neurologic, renal, and pulmonary comorbidities are more likely to suffer opioid-induced respiratory depression (OIRD) and respiratory compromise from other etiologies.[2,7] Next, we will review some common preexisting as well as pregnancy-related conditions to consider when evaluating a pregnant patient's risk for respiratory depression.

Preexisting conditions

Obesity
Obesity has been cited as a common risk factor for all-cause maternal morbidity and mortality,[11] as well as anesthesia-related maternal mortality.[12,13] When compared with

Table 1 Physiologic changes in pregnancy	
Upper Airway	
Edema	Tissues friable/epistaxis
Thoracic Cage: "Barrel Chest"	
Ligaments of the rib cage relax→ Increased diameter (about 5 cm) ↑40% in tidal volume	Diaphragm is displaced cephalad Decreased vertical dimension (about 4 cm) ↓25% in end residual volume ↓15% in residual volume ↓20% in functional residual capacity
Respiratory Drive and Chronic Hyperventilation	
Progesterone → ↑tidal Volumes + ↑respiratory Rate ↑20%–40% minute Ventilation (term)	Respiratory alkalosis ↑pH 7.44 ↓$Paco_2$ 28–32 mm Hg ↓HCO3 20 mmol/L ↑Pao_2 104–108 mm Hg

Data from Hines RL, Marschall KE. Stoelting's anesthesia and co-existing disease. In: Seventh edition. ed. Philadelphia, PA: Elsevier; 2018: Chapter 31.

individuals with normal body mass, obese patients present with a restrictive respiratory pattern characterized by reduced forced vital capacity (FVC), reduced forced expiratory volume after 1 s (FEV_1), potentially reduced total lung capacity (TLC), and decreased functional residual capacity (FRC).[14] These spirometry changes result from, at least in part, structural alterations of the thorax and abdomen that reduce the compliance of the rib cage and the mobility of the diaphragm. A similar phenomenon is observed in pregnancy as the gravid uterus displaces the diaphragm cephalad resulting in a decreased FRC. However, compensatory changes such as the expansion of the ribcage allow for the preservation of TLC and spirometry to remain within normal limits overall.[15] When pregnancy physiology is superimposed on the pathophysiology of obesity, significant respiratory compromise can result (**Table 2**).[14,15] Obesity is associated with a decreased FRC and pregnancy further exacerbates this. As a consequence, these patients have diminished respiratory reserve in situations of hypoventilation or apnea, and this can complicate airway management and intubation (**Fig. 2**).[16]

This interaction has become increasingly relevant in the care of obstetric patients as obesity rates have increased in many countries. The Centers for Disease Control and Prevention (CDC) reports that, of the women who gave birth in the United States in 2014, more than 50% were categorically overweight (body mass index (BMI): 25.0–29.9 kg/m^2) or obese (BMI: >29.9 kg/m^2) before pregnancy.[17] The prevalence of super obesity (defined as BMI >50 kg/m^2) is increasing at a faster rate than other classes of obesity in the US population.[18] Women with obesity, especially super obesity, have a higher rate of peripartum complications and postpartum intensive care unit (ICU) admissions than nonobese women.[19–21] In one recent study, the most common indication for postpartum ICU admission among obese women was cardiopulmonary complications.[20]

The recent consensus statement endorsed by the Society for Obstetric Anesthesia and Perinatology recommends increased monitoring following neuraxial morphine administration for patients with BMI $\geq$40 kg/m^2, but studies to guide monitoring strategies for these higher risk patients have been scant.[7] Single-center retrospective studies that have examined the incidence of respiratory depression events in postpartum women that have received low-dose neuraxial morphine have demonstrated a very low prevalence of adverse events even among obese postpartum women.[22,23] Neuraxial morphine is an effective form of postcesarean delivery analgesia and should not be withheld from obese women out of concern for

Table 2		
Lung volumes and spirometry		
	Pregnancy	**Obesity**
FEV_1	↔	↓
FVC	↔	↓
FEV_1/FVC	↔	↔
TLC	↔	↔/↓[a]
FRC	↓	↓

Abbreviations: FVC, forced vital capacity; FEV_1, forced expiratory volume after 1 s; TLC, total lung capacity; FRC, functional residual capacity.
[a] Decreased with morbid obesity BMI greater than 40 kg/m^2.
Adapted from: Melo LC, Silva MA, Calles AC. Obesity and lung function: a systematic review. Einstein (Sao Paulo). 2014;12(1):120-125.; LoMauro A, Aliverti A. Respiratory physiology of pregnancy: Physiology masterclass. Breathe (Sheff). 2015;11(4):297-301.

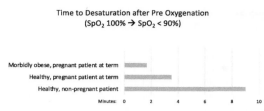

Fig. 2. Differences in time to desaturation after preoxygenation reflect the compound effect of pregnancy and obesity on functional residual capacity. A healthy, nonpregnant patient can tolerate approximately 9 minutes of apnea before desaturation. That time is reduced by 60% in a healthy, pregnant patient at term (3–4 minutes), and 80% in a morbidly obese, pregnant patient at term (98 seconds). (*Data from* Baraka AS, Hanna MT, Jabbour SI, et al. Preoxygenation of pregnant and nonpregnant women in the head-up versus supine position. Anesth Analg. 1992;75(5):757-759; Hines RL, Marschall KE. Stoelting's anesthesia and co-existing disease. In: Seventh edition. ed. Philadelphia, PA: Elsevier; 2018: Chapter 31.)

respiratory depression if ultra-low (ie, < 0.05 mg intrathecal or ≤1 mg epidural morphine) or low (ie, > 0.05 and ≤0.15 mg intrathecal, or >1 and ≤3 mg epidural morphine) doses are used with multi-modal analgesia, along with appropriate monitoring strategies (**Fig. 3**), and the avoidance of multiple sedating medications.[7]

Sleep-disordered breathing

A strong association exists between obesity and sleep-disordered breathing conditions such as snoring, OSA, and OHS. The prevalence of OSA among obese pregnant persons has been reported as 12% to 28% in various small prospective studies.[24–27] Maternal OSA has been linked to increased peripartum morbidity and mortality[28–30] and adverse fetal outcomes.[31,32] When compared with those without OSA, pregnant persons with OSA have a significantly higher risk of hypertensive disorders of pregnancy, gestational diabetes, cardiomyopathy, congestive heart failure, pulmonary edema, hysterectomy, prolonged hospital stays, and admissions to the ICU.[28,30,33]

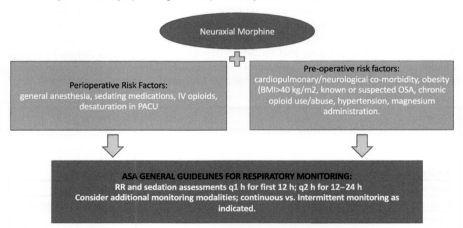

Fig. 3. Recommended respiratory monitoring algorithm for high-risk patients following neuraxial morphine administration. RR, respiratory rate. (*Adapted from* Bauchat, J.R., et al., Society for Obstetric Anesthesia and Perinatology Consensus Statement: Monitoring Recommendations for Prevention and Detection of Respiratory Depression Associated With Administration of Neuraxial Morphine for Cesarean Delivery Analgesia. Anesth Analg, 2019. 129(2): p. 458-474.)

In nonobstetrical postsurgical patients, OSA is associated with an increased risk of postoperative respiratory failure.[34] Longitudinal studies on OSA during pregnancy suggest that airway obstruction worsens as pregnancy progresses, particularly if patients develop preeclampsia.[35–37]

The Society for Obstetric Anesthesia and Perinatology guidelines recommend increased monitoring following neuraxial morphine administration for high-risk patients such as those with OSA, but no studies have been conducted in this population to guide postoperative monitoring strategies and guidance is extrapolated from the nonobstetrical literature.[7] However, obstetric patients with OSA should be carefully monitored, and noninvasive ventilation should be continued in the hospital and adjusted as needed; sedating medications should be avoided when possible and used judiciously with appropriate monitoring when unavoidable as in the case of magnesium (**Table 3**).

Restrictive and obstructive lung diseases

Obstetric patients with underlying lung disease are at increased risk for pulmonary complications and respiratory depression in the postpartum period. Restrictive lung disease is a risk factor for hypoxic or hypercapnic respiratory failure in pregnancy and the postpartum period and may manifest varied pathologic conditions during the peripartum period. A retrospective case series of 15 pregnancies in 12 women with significant interstitial lung disease or chest wall abnormalities found that patients with restrictive lung disease had high rates of premature delivery (60%) and of cesarean delivery (67%).[38] Many required supplemental oxygen or ventilatory support during labor or postpartum (40%).[38] Although pregnancy may be well tolerated by these patients, increased metabolic demands and work of breathing during labor and delivery may lead to acute decompensation and so appropriate resources should be readily available. Adequate labor analgesia is important to help control pain and work of breathing.

Patients with obstructive lung disease may also experience worsening chronic pulmonary dysfunction during pregnancy with an increased risk of postpartum respiratory depression. Asthma is common among pregnant women and its rates are increasing; approximately 1 in 10 pregnant women has asthma.[39–41] An association exists between asthma and obstetric complications such as preeclampsia, placental abruption, placenta previa, hemorrhage, and cesarean delivery.[39,40,42] Asthma seems to confer additional vulnerability to respiratory viral infections as well as more serious complications from them.[39] A prospective study of 285 pregnant patients found that 71% of

Table 3			
Common medications associated with sedation and respiratory depression			
Anesthetics & Analgesics	**Anxiolytics & Hypnotics**	**Antiemetics & Antihistamines**	**Antihypertensives & Anticonvulsants**
Opioids	Benzodiazepines (midazolam)	Promethazine	Magnesium sulfate
Propofol	Sleep-aids (zolpidem)	Diphenhydramine	Barbiturates (phenobarbital)
Clonidine	Antipsychotics (olanzapine)		

Data from Toledano RD, Kodali BS, Camann WR. Anesthesia drugs in the obstetric and gynecologic practice. Rev Obstet Gynecol. Spring 2009;2(2):93-100.; Bauchat JR, Weiniger CF, Sultan P, et al. Society for Obstetric Anesthesia and Perinatology Consensus Statement: Monitoring Recommendations for Prevention and Detection of Respiratory Depression Associated With Administration of Neuraxial Morphine for Cesarean Delivery Analgesia. Anesth Analg. Aug 2019;129(2):458-474. https://doi.org/10.1213/ANE.0000000000004195

women with asthma reported at least one "common cold" during pregnancy versus 46% of women without asthma.[43] Apart from the risk of respiratory compromise from an asthma exacerbation or status asthmaticus, the comorbidities associated with asthma may increase a patient's overall risk of postpartum respiratory complications.

Careful consideration of the risks and benefits of uterotonics for managing postpartum hemorrhage (PPH) is crucial for all patients, but especially those with asthma. Carboprost is a synthetic analog of prostaglandin F2-alpha commonly used to induce abortion or treat PPH secondary to uterine atony. The medication has several common side effects including nausea, vomiting, diarrhea, fever, and bronchoconstriction. Although all patients are at risk for bronchospasm with the administration of carboprost, patients with a history of asthma are more likely to suffer severe or life-threatening reactions.[44,45] For this reason, the carboprost material safety data sheet caution against its use in patients with a history of reactive airway disease.

Neuromuscular disorders

Pregnant patients with neuromuscular disorders are also at increased risk for respiratory compromise.[46–48] Although the physiologic changes to respiratory mechanics in pregnancy may offset some of the pulmonary compromise seen in these patients at baseline, the compensation is often overwhelmed and may manifest as worsening, chronically poor pulmonary function. With some conditions such as spinal muscular atrophy (SMA), pulmonary function will improve shortly after delivery,[49,50] whereas with other conditions, such as myasthenia gravis (MG), the presentation may be more variable.[46–48]

SMA is an autosomal recessive disease caused by the degeneration of the anterior horn cells in the spinal cord and brain stem that results in generalized muscle weakness and atrophy including the thoracoabdominal wall which leads to severe restrictive lung disease and reduced lung volumes.[46–49] SMA presents at birth, during childhood, or young adulthood. Pregnancy in patients with SMA can cause chronic alveolar hypoventilation to further deteriorate and result in acute-on-chronic respiratory failure.[49,50] This tends to improve after delivery, but these patients are best managed with close specialist monitoring throughout pregnancy.

Patients with MG experience skeletal muscle weakness and easy fatigability due to the autoimmune attack of neuromuscular junction acetylcholine receptors.[46–48] MG can first present in pregnancy or the postpartum period and is diagnosed in an estimated 1 in 20,000 pregnancies.[51] For those patients diagnosed with MG before conception, their pregnancy course can vary and some may even note improved MG symptoms.[52] When postpartum MG exacerbations do occur they are often sudden and associated with respiratory failure.[47] MG patients are especially sensitive to certain medications. Some medications, such as nondepolarizing neuromuscular blocking drugs, can be used with caution[52]; others, such as magnesium sulfate, should be avoided.[53] Magnesium sulfate is commonly administered in pregnancy for preterm fetal neuroprotection[54] and seizure prophylaxis in mothers with pre-eclampsia.[53,55] Unfortunately, studies have shown that therapeutic magnesium administration can trigger a myasthenic crisis so it has been historically contraindicated for eclampsia prophylaxis in MG patients.[56,57] In a case report, by Ozcan and colleagues, the authors describe a patient diagnosed with both MG and term pre-eclampsia who was safely managed and delivered without magnesium through the cooperation of obstetric, neurology, and anesthesiology teams.[53]

Acute inflammatory demyelinating polyradiculoneuropathy (AIDP), or Guillain–Barre syndrome, is a rare, acute neuropathy characterized by progressive, ascending weakness that can result in respiratory compromise.[46,48] Although studies have shown no difference in risk of developing AIDP during pregnancy than the general population, postpartum risk is increased. Within the first month postpartum, the risk of AIDP is tripled over the general population.[58]

Opioid use and misuse

Opioid use during pregnancy has increased over the last 2 decades, mirroring the opioid epidemic in the general population.[59,60] In a 2010 national survey of reproductive age women, 4.4% pregnant women and 11% nonpregnant women reported illicit drug use or opioid misuse in the last month.[59] This spans all racial/ethnic, socioeconomic, and geographic populations.[59–61] The American College of Obstetricians and Gynecologists (ACOG) advocates for substance use screening as a part of standard, comprehensive obstetric care for all patients.[60] Screening tools should differentiate between medical therapy, opioid misuse, and opioid use disorder to direct appropriate treatment. Treatment is essential as substance use during pregnancy is a major risk factor for pregnancy-associated deaths.[60,61] Importantly, the postpartum period is a vulnerable time for relapse and continuity of care should be maintained so patients are supported during their times of transition.[60]

Broadly, opioid use is associated with dose-dependent respiratory depression.[2,6,7,62,63] Patients who chronically use or abuse opioids are at risk for opioid tolerance and may require higher doses of opioids—increasing their risk of respiratory depression—to achieve the same degree of analgesia.[2,63] Multi-modal analgesia with nonsedating medications is essential for safe and effective analgesia in this population. As discussed in several sections of this article, appropriate monitoring is a key to minimize the risk of OIRD in the postpartum patient (see **Fig. 3**).[7]

Pregnancy-related conditions

In a 2017 retrospective analysis of obstetric patients admitted to the ICU requiring intubation and mechanical ventilation, Hung and colleagues found that PPH (28%, n = 20/71) and severe preeclampsia (18%, n = 13/71) were leading causes of respiratory failure.[64] ICU admission is a rare but significant peripartum complication (0.7–8.8 per 1000 deliveries[64,65]) that warrants reviewing the most common causes of maternal respiratory failure: preeclampsia, peripartum cardiomyopathy (PPCM), hemorrhage, amniotic fluid embolism (AFE), and infection.[8,9,64–66]

Preeclampsia

Preeclampsia is a hypertensive disorder of pregnancy characterized by elevated blood pressure and end-organ damage and/or dysfunction (eg, renal, hepatic, pulmonary, central nervous system; **Table 4**).[9,67,68] Preeclampsia is associated with abnormal placental vascular development which contributes to generalized endothelial dysfunction and a systemic proinflammatory state.[67,68] A patient with preeclampsia is at an increased risk of respiratory failure secondary associated with pulmonary edema, altered mental status, and therapeutic side effects.[67] Pulmonary edema interferes with gas exchange and can cause a range of symptoms from mild dyspnea to severe hypoxia and cardiopulmonary collapse. Seizures associated with eclampsia can compromise the upper airway with loss of protective reflexes, obstruction, and aspiration all contributing to potential respiratory insufficiency.[69] Postictal states can also cause respiratory depression through central apnea and decreased arousability.[69]

Definitive treatment for preeclampsia is delivery due to placental pathologic condition, but preeclampsia can also present in the postpartum period. Although no curative medical therapy exists, antihypertensives and magnesium sulfate are key for

Table 4
Diagnostic criteria for preeclampsia

In Patients After 20-Wk Gestation:

Elevated Blood Pressure

Systolic blood pressure >160 mm Hg or diastolic blood pressure >110 mm Hg and at least one of the following:

Proteinuria (>300 mg per 24 hr urine collection)	*Thrombocytopenia* (platelet count <100,000/μL)	*Liver dysfunction* (AST/ALT twice normal concentration)
Renal Insufficiency (elevated serum creatinine >1.1 mg/dL or doubling of baseline)	*Pulmonary edema*	*Cerebral or visual disturbances* (new onset)

Per the 2013 ACOG Task Force: Hypertension in pregnancy. Report of the American College of Obstetricians and Gynecologists' Task Force on Hypertension in Pregnancy. Obstet Gynecol. Nov 2013;122(5):1122-1131. https://doi.org/10.1097/01.AOG.0000437382.03963.88

managing pathophysiologic perturbations associated with preeclampsia.[67,68] Magnesium sulfate is currently the most effective antiepileptic drug in patients with preeclampsia with severe features, reducing the rate of seizures from 3.4% to 0.3%.[67,70,71] Accumulation of excess magnesium at neuromuscular junctions competes with calcium at acetylcholine binding sites, and thus inhibits presynaptic acetylcholine release and postsynaptic membrane excitability.[53,72] Magnesium therapy may also cause sedation, neuromuscular weakness, hypotension, uterine atony, postpartum hemorrhage, pulmonary edema, and respiratory depression.[53,67] Magnesium has been designated as a high-alert medication due to potential toxicity and has been implicated in cases of iatrogenic harm to mothers.[73] Patients on magnesium therapy should be assigned appropriate nursing ratios to ensure close, regular monitoring with vital signs, deep tendon reflexes, levels of sedation, and urine output; magnesium levels should be checked for patients with impaired renal function or concern for magnesium toxicity based on clinical signs. Calcium gluconate or carbonate should be readily available to treat patients with magnesium toxicity.[73,74]

Peripartum cardiomyopathy

PPCM is a rare (1 in 2000 US births[75]) complication that presents in late pregnancy through the early postpartum period.[76,77] PPCM is characterized by left ventricular systolic dysfunction (left ventricular ejection fraction (LVEF) <45%) that develops in patients without preexisting cause for heart failure. In 2010 the European Society of Cardiology (ESC) revised the prior diagnostic timeline set out in the 1990s by the US National Heart, Lung, and Blood Institute—heart failure that develops in the last month of pregnancy or up to 5-months postpartum—to be less restrictive and to include patients who would otherwise meet diagnostic criteria for PPCM.[76,78,79] The cause of PPCM is not entirely understood; however, research suggests a multifactorial etiology that includes genetics, hormone-mediated vascular dysfunction, or the intersection of the two.[80,81] Risk factors for PPCM include Black ancestry, advanced maternal age, preeclampsia, and multiple gestation pregnancy.[76] With pharmacologic treatment, more than half of women suffering from PPCM will recover to a normal systolic function within the first 6 months to a year; those who are left with chronic cardiomyopathy may require mechanical support or heart transplantation.[76,81–83]

Patients with PPCM present with classic heart failure symptomatology: dyspnea on exertion, paroxysmal nocturnal dyspnea, orthopnea, chest pain, lower extremity edema, and fatigue.[76,80,81] These symptoms commonly overlap with those of normal pregnancy and this may delay diagnosis.[76] For some patients, the diagnosis of PPCM will follow a catastrophic presentation of acute, severe respiratory distress, and cardiogenic shock.[76,80] Regardless of presentation, postpartum patients with new respiratory distress should be evaluated for PPCM.[84] BNP levels have been shown to be reliable and predictive of short- and long-term outcomes in pregnant women with PPCM.[85,86]

Postpartum hemorrhage

PPH is a leading cause of maternal mortality worldwide and occurs in about 6% of all childbirths.[87,88] Approximately 3% of all postpartum patients require a blood product transfusion, whereas greater than 50% of patients with PPH require a transfusion—often massive transfusions (ie, >10 units in 24 hours).[87–90] Transfusion-related acute lung injury (TRALI) and transfusion-associated cardiac overload (TACO) are significant complications associated with blood product transfusion and resuscitation.[91–94]

TRALI is a specific manifestation of acute respiratory distress syndrome (ARDS). The incidence of TRALI, while decreasing since 2006, is approximately 1 per 5000 units of transfused blood product.[91,95–97] TRALI is the most common lethal posttransfusion complication at 30% to 40% with a mortality rate of 5% to 10%.[91–94,98,99] TRALI presents with rapidly deteriorating hypoxemia, bilateral pulmonary edema, and hemodynamic instability within 6 hours of transfusion in patients without a history of pulmonary trauma or alternative etiology for acute lung injury.[91,100,101] TRALI is a diagnosis of exclusion and the differential should include alternative causes of ARDS, TACO, cardiogenic shock, venous thromboembolism, and AFE.[91,92] If a postpartum patient presents with acute, rapid respiratory decompensation after receiving a blood transfusion TRALI must be considered, and appropriate supportive therapies initiated to minimize morbidity.

Amniotic fluid embolism

AFE is a rare (2–8 cases per 100,000 deliveries)[102] but serious obstetric complication that can present with an abrupt cardiopulmonary collapse, although AFE presentation can vary considerably and no diagnostic criteria have been developed to date.[103,104] The syndrome can occur during labor, delivery, or early postpartum (up to 48 hrs) and is characterized by symptoms including hypoxia, hypotension, generalized seizures, and disseminated intravascular coagulopathy (DIC).[102,104–106] The etiology remains largely unknown. AFE is thought to be caused by the introduction of amniotic components (amniotic fluid, fetal cells, hair, or other debris) into the maternal circulation triggering an abnormal immunologic response sometimes called the "anaphylactoid syndrome of pregnancy."[105–107] Although a rare cause of postpartum respiratory depression, maintaining high clinical suspicion for AFE can increase the likelihood of early detection and effective treatment; see **Table 5** for cardiopulmonary symptoms associated with AFE.[102,105–108]

Sepsis and acute respiratory distress syndrome

Sepsis is a life-threatening medical condition defined by acute organ dysfunction that is the result of abnormal host response to infection.[109] Sepsis and septic shock are major, preventable causes of maternal morbidity and mortality.[110–112] Historically, in the preantibiotic era, nearly half of maternal deaths were due to infection; now, an estimated 4 to 10 in 10,000 live births are complicated by sepsis.[112] Early recognition and treatment are essential to improve maternal outcomes.

The Sequential Organ Failure Assessment (SOFA) score[113] is used to help identify patients at risk for sepsis/septic shock. Varied parameters assessing respiratory,

Table 5
Amniotic fluid embolism: cardiopulmonary manifestations

Cardiovascular	Pulmonary
Hypotension	Acute tachypnea and dyspnea
Tachycardia	Cough
Arrhythmia	Hypoxemia
Right heart failure	Pulmonary edema/ARDS
Left heart failure	Acute pulmonary hypertension
Cardiogenic shock	V:Q mismatch
→ *Cardiac arrest*	→ *Respiratory arrest*

Abbreviation: ARDS, acute respiratory distress syndrome.
Data from Fong A, Chau CT, Pan D, Ogunyemi DA. Amniotic fluid embolism: antepartum, intrapartum and demographic factors. J Matern Fetal Neonatal Med. May 2015;28(7):793-8. doi:10.3109/14767058.2014.932766; Kaur K, Bhardwaj M, Kumar P, Singhal S, Singh T, Hooda S. Amniotic fluid embolism. J Anaesthesiol Clin Pharmacol. Apr-Jun 2016;32(2):153-9. doi:10.4103/0970-9185.173356; Clark SL, Hankins GD, Dudley DA, Dildy GA, Porter TF. Amniotic fluid embolism: analysis of the national registry. Am J Obstet Gynecol. Apr 1995;172(4 Pt 1):1158-67; discussion 1167-9. https://doi.org/10.1016/0002-9378(9591474-9)

coagulation, hepatic, cardiovascular, central nervous, and renal system dysfunction are scored.[113] The quick SOFA (qSOFA) is a set of 3 clinical criteria that can be used for bedside assessments with 2 or more positive criteria that suggest an increased risk of adverse sepsis-related outcomes.[112] A significant overlap exists between these sepsis criteria cutoffs and normal maternal physiologic parameters, as such the Society of Obstetric Medicine Australia and New Zealand (SOMANZ) introduced modified guidelines and SOFA parameters for the obstetric population in 2017 (**Table 6**).[112,114]

As suggested by its inclusion in the SOFA and qSOFA scoring systems, respiratory compromise is an important but variable manifestation of sepsis. Studies of the recent respiratory virus pandemics (2009 H1N1 and 2019 SARS-CoV-2) provide a unique insight into sepsis, ARDS, and respiratory failure in the obstetric population.[115–118]

In a prospective cohort study of 675 women that presented for delivery in 3 New York City hospitals, Prabhu *and colleagues* reported that women with COVID-19 were more likely to deliver via a cesarean section and have an increased risk of postpartum complications. One in 10 women admitted tested positive for SARS-CoV-2 (10.4%; 78.6% were asymptomatic.) The rate of cesarean delivery in women with symptomatic COVID-19 (46.7%) was significantly higher than those without COVID-

Table 6
Quick Sequential organ failure assessment (qSOFA) score

	General Population	Obstetric Population
Systolic blood pressure	<100 mm Hg	<90 mm Hg
Respiratory rate	>22 breaths per minute	>25 breaths per minute
Altered Mental Status	Present	Present

Adapted from Society for Maternal-Fetal Medicine. Electronic address pso, Plante LA, Pacheco LD, Louis JM. SMFM Consult Series #47: Sepsis during pregnancy and the puerperium. Am J Obstet Gynecol. 2019;220(4):B2-B10. Bowyer L, Robinson HL, Barrett H, et al. SOMANZ guidelines for the investigation and management sepsis in pregnancy. Aust N Z J Obstet Gynaecol. Oct 2017;57(5):540-551. https://doi.org/10.1111/ajo.12646

19 (30.9%)[118] and historical national averages (31.7%, 2019).[119] Although the rate of postpartum complications, defined as fever, hypoxia, and readmission, was 3 times higher in the COVID-19 cohort (12.9% vs 4.5%) none of the women in the study required mechanical ventilation.[118] Similar findings have been reported by others.[117]

In the event of more serious infections and severe ARDS, women may require mechanical ventilatory support or ECMO.[8,66,115] In a systematic review of case reports, Ong *and colleagues* found approximately 40% of ECMO deployments in the peripartum or postpartum patient are for respiratory failure; more than 90% of these cases are due to ARDS.[66] The remaining 60% of ECMO cases are for cardiovascular indications of which 23.7% were cases of pulmonary embolism and 16.9% were due to PPCM.[66] A retrospective observational study by Nair *and colleagues* looked at the use of ECMO support in twelve critically ill pregnant and postpartum patients with ARDS in Australia and New Zealand during the 2009 H1N1 pandemic.[115] In their review, they found that most patients required veno-venous (VV) ECMO.[115] Bleeding was the most common complication and the use of ECMO for severe ARDS in this population was associated with a 66% survival rate (comparable to 63%–75% survival rate for ECMO patients overall).[115] Similarly, in their case series published in 2021, Barrantes *and colleagues* report on the 9 pregnant and peripartum patients with severe COVID-19 ARDS who required ECMO support.[116] In this patient subset, the survival rate was 100% and these patients also suffered minor bleeding but did not otherwise suffer any significant ECMO complications.[116] Moore *and colleagues* reviewed all cases of ECMO use during pregnancy between 1991 and 2007 (n = 45) and found an overall maternal survival rate of 78%.[120] The review by Ong *and colleagues* included the use of ECMO in both pregnant and postpartum patients between 1972 and 2017 (n = 97) with an increase in the maternal survival rate to 91%.[66]

Even with these reassuring reports on the effectiveness of ECMO as a rescue treatment for obstetric patients with severe ARDS, the treatment modality remains a limited resource that is not available or feasible for all patients. This is especially concerning given the findings of the retrospective study by Callaghan *and colleagues* that used ICD-9CM diagnosis codes and data from the National Inpatient Sample to study trends in maternal morbidity and mortality between 1998 and 2009.[8]

The study[8] made several sobering observations over the 10-year span:

- The rate of ARDS increased 75% during delivery hospitalizations and 181% during postpartum hospitalizations.
- 8 in 100,000 women died during their delivery hospitalization (0.008%, n = 4012/48,346,974).
  - Of these deaths:
    - 60.6% required mechanical ventilation (n = 2430/4012) and
    - 33.2% were diagnosed with ARDS (n = 1332/4012)
- 2 in 1000 women died during their postpartum hospitalization (0.2%, n = 1592/738,124).
  - Of these deaths:
    - 76.5% required mechanical ventilation (n = 1218/1592) and
    - 53.3% were diagnosed with ARDS (n = 848/1592).

Peripartum medications

Neuraxial opioids
Neuraxial opioid analgesia is the bedrock of obstetric anesthesia due to its effectiveness for postoperative analgesia and favorable risk-benefit profile for pregnant and lactating women. Most parturients receive epidural or intrathecal opioids via single injection, continuous or intermittent infusions and, of those who do not, many will receive systemic

opioids. As such the exposure to opioids, and the associated risk of opioid-induced respiratory depression as described above, is present for many postpartum patients.

Respiratory drive originates in the brainstem and is a culmination of inputs from central and peripheral chemoreceptors and the cerebral cortex.[121,122] Opioid receptors are present throughout the respiratory control centers. Respiratory rhythm generation in the brainstem (medulla and pons) is the most sensitive to the effects of opioids with changes in the respiratory pattern seen at lower doses than those required to manifest changes in tidal volume.[122,123] With higher opioid doses, the reduction in tidal volume is thought to be caused by a decrease in tonic inputs from opioid-sensitive chemoreceptors—both centrally and peripherally.[62] In conjunction, opioids can cause respiration to slow and become irregular resulting in hypercapnia and hypoxemia.

The incidence of respiratory depression following neuraxial opioid administration in the nonobstetrical population is also poorly defined. Opioid-induced respiratory depression more broadly is well summarized by Gupta *and colleagues* in their 2018 systematic review and metanalysis in which they report the incidence of ORID as 0.04% to 0.5% using naloxone administration as the clinical indication of ORID and 23%–41% using hypoxemia or bradypnea.[2] In the same review, Gupta *and colleagues* reported on the prevalence of certain underlying comorbidities in patients with OIRD:

- Cardiac disease 45%[124–126]
- Diabetes mellitus 23%[125–127]
- Respiratory disease 17%[124,126,127]
  - COPD 81%[124–127]
- OSA 18%[124–128]
- Renal disease 17%[124,126,127]

Similarly, Ramachandran *and colleagues* reported the presence of underlying cardiac or respiratory disease was independently associated with an increased risk of respiratory complications postoperatively[129] and a closed claims analysis by Lee *and colleagues* found OSA or suspected OSA in 24% of patients with postoperative OIRD.[6]

The low incidence of adverse events reported in the literature with modern, ultra-low, and low-doses of neuraxial morphine for postcesarean delivery analgesia suggest a high-degree of safety and efficacy in most obstetric patients.[1,7,22,23] For the selected comorbidities and conditions acquired in pregnancy that we have reviewed here, obstetric anesthesiologists should undertake careful consideration of the patient's unique risks and benefits. In particular, neuraxial opioid use in combination with other medications that depress respiration should be avoided to the extent possible, and careful postpartum monitoring strategies should be used. More research is needed to better understand and elucidate safe practices to optimize the postcesarean delivery analgesic options and monitoring strategies for patients at greater risk of postpartum respiratory depression and adverse events (see **Fig. 1**).

Sedatives

Many analgesic adjuncts, sedatives, anxiolytics, and antiemetics can compromise respiratory drive. These agents when used in combination with opioids can potentiate respiratory depression and should be used judiciously. Some common medications associated with respiratory depression used by obstetric patients are summarized in **Table 3**.[7,130]

Anesthetic complications

In addition to the effects of opioids, neuraxial analgesia can result in respiratory depression or failure in the event of a "high" or "total" spinal level blockade (spread of local anesthetic that affects spinal nerves above T4). A "high spinal" causes paralysis of the muscles involved in active exhalation (abdominals, intercostals) leading to reduced expiratory reserve volume, peak expiratory flow, and maximum minute ventilation. This can manifest as dyspnea in parturients with normal pulmonary function but, in patients with underlying obstructive pulmonary disease, the loss of accessory respiratory muscle function can be significant. Further, although rare, a "total spinal" to a cervical level can compromise the phrenic nerve and preganglionic sympathetic nerves resulting in diaphragm paralysis, hypotension, bradycardia, and subsequent hypoperfusion of the medullary respiratory center (central apnea). This results in profound respiratory failure that requires prompt intubation and supportive positive pressure ventilation as well as circulatory support.

Despite the aforementioned risks of respiratory depression with neuraxial analgesia, it is held to be the preferred anesthetic technique for cesarean delivery. General anesthesia is avoided when possible due to an increased risk for aspiration, bleeding, failed intubation, and intraoperative awareness.[131,132] A general anesthetic for cesarean delivery can also increase a patient's risk of postpartum respiratory depression due to depressant effects of anesthetic agents, residual neuromuscular blockade (NMB), and intravenous opioids.

NMB is a risk factor for postoperative respiratory compromise in the postpartum patient just as in the general population. In some cases, the risk may be even more significant and weight-based dosing of neuromuscular blockade agents should be carefully considered. Total body weight (TBW), lean body weight (LBW), and ideal body weight (IBW) are all mass measurements used in the dosing of anesthetics. In normal-weight persons, LBW and IBW are similar; however, in obese persons, the LBW increases with increasing TBW.[133] Commonly, an obstetric patient's TBW (and LBW) will increase throughout pregnancy and remain increased during the postpartum period while their IBW remains constant. Weight-based dosing during this dynamic time can result in inconsistent responses to medications. A small study by Gin *and colleagues*[134] examining the duration of rocuronium neuromuscular blockade in recently postpartum patients found that dosing by TBW resulted in a prolonged block when compared with control (and similar block duration when dosed by LBW.) Additionally, the use of agents known to prolong neuromuscular blockade, such as magnesium sulfate, is common in the obstetric population. Hypermagnesemia is desirable in situations of preterm delivery and in patients with preeclampsia for its neuroprotective qualities;[135] however, the subsequent administration of nondepolarizing NMB in the event of cesarean delivery under general anesthesia can result in profoundly deep and prolonged neuromuscular blockade.[136] Notably, magnesium sulfate therapy itself has been associated with respiratory depression at a rate of 0% to 8.2%.[55] There has been little research to guide the use of sugammadex for the antagonism of NMBs in obstetric and lactating patients, as such their use has been limited in this population.[137] Sugammadex seems to be safe for use in term and postpartum lactating women and its use should not be withheld when it may improve maternal safety. The Society for Obstetric Anesthesia and Perinatology issued a statement on its use in these populations in 2019.[138]

SUMMARY

The peripartum period is a vulnerable time for many patients. Several of the conditions discussed here in the context of respiratory depression can have far-reaching ramifications including disability and death. Postpartum respiratory depression is a complex, multifactorial issue that encompasses a patient's baseline preexisting conditions, certain pregnancy-specific conditions, or complications, as well as the iatrogenic effects of medications given during the peripartum period. Importantly, while the etiologies of postpartum respiratory depression/failure are numerous, certain patients are more vulnerable than others to respiratory compromise. The detection of respiratory compromise in these patients can be complicated by the significant overlap between or confounding by normal maternal physiologic changes. For this reason, it is important to modify or develop specific alert criteria and algorithms for the obstetric population.

The use of opioids, specifically neuraxial morphine, for postcesarean delivery analgesia at modern, ultra-low, and low dosages is safe and effective, and carries a low risk of respiratory depression for most obstetric patients. For those patients at higher risk for respiratory depression given select co-morbidities or conditions, careful consideration of each patient's unique risks and benefits should be undertaken before the administration of neuraxial morphine or any other drug that may depress respiration, and further research is needed to better elucidate these risk factors.

Over the last decade, there has been an increase in the incidence of severe peripartum pulmonary complications resulting in ARDS and severe respiratory failure. The recent, novel H1N1 and COVID-19 viral respiratory pandemics have taken this to an extreme and, in the process, helped to demonstrate the value and safety of mechanical ventilatory support, including ECMO, in pregnant and postpartum patients.

Ultimately, each patient and pregnancy is unique. The care of each postpartum patient should be individualized and consider their specific risk factors and their risk for postpartum respiratory depression.

CLINICS CARE POINTS

- Pre-existing diseases such as obstructive sleep apnea, obesity hypoventilation syndrome, and cardiopulmonary diseases may interact with conditions acquired during pregnancy or postpartum, or with drugs administered peripartum, to compound the risk of respiratory compromise in vulnerable patients.

- When pregnancy physiology is superimposed on the pathophysiology of obesity, significant respiratory compromise can result.

- Neuraxial morphine is an effective form of post-cesarean delivery analgesia and should not be withheld from obese women out of concern for respiratory depression if ultra-low or low doses are utilized with multi-modal analgesia, along with appropriate monitoring strategies and care plans.

- Obstetrical patients with obstructive sleep apnea should be carefully monitored, and non-invasive ventilation should be continued in hospital and adjusted as needed; sedating medications should be avoided when possible and used judiciously with appropriate monitoring when unavoidable as in the case of magnesium.

- Restrictive lung disease is a risk factor for hypoxic or hypercapnic respiratory failure in pregnancy and the postpartum period and may manifest varied pathology during the peripartum period.

- While all patients are at risk for bronchospasm with the administration of carboprost, patients with a history of asthma are more likely to suffer severe or life-threatening reactions.

- Patients who chronically use or abuse opioids are at risk for opioid tolerance and may require higher doses of opioids— increasing their risk of respiratory depression— to achieve the same degree of analgesia.

- Magnesium has been designated as a high-alert medication due to potential toxicity, and has been implicated in cases of iatrogenic harm to mothers.

- BNP levels have been shown to be reliable and predictive of short- and long-term outcomes in pregnant women with peripartum cardiomyopathy.

- If a postpartum patient presents with acute, rapid respiratory decompensation after receiving a blood transfusion TRALI must be considered, and appropriate supportive therapies initiated to minimize morbidity.

DISCLOSURE

The authors have nothing to disclose.

REFERENCE

1. Sharawi N, Carvalho B, Habib AS, et al. A systematic review evaluating neuraxial morphine and diamorphine-associated respiratory depression after cesarean delivery. Anesth Analg 2018;127(6):1385–95.
2. Gupta K, Nagappa M, Prasad A, et al. Risk factors for opioid-induced respiratory depression in surgical patients: a systematic review and meta-analyses. BMJ Open 2018;8(12):e024086.
3. Cashman JN, Dolin SJ. Respiratory and haemodynamic effects of acute postoperative pain management: evidence from published data. Br J Anaesth 2004; 93(2):212–23.
4. Dahan A, Aarts L, Smith TW. Incidence, reversal, and prevention of opioid-induced respiratory depression. Anesthesiology 2010;112(1):226–38.
5. Ko S, Goldstein DH, VanDenKerkhof EG. Definitions of "respiratory depression" with intrathecal morphine postoperative analgesia: a review of the literature. Can J Anaesth 2003;50(7):679–88.
6. Lee LA, Caplan RA, Stephens LS, et al. Postoperative opioid-induced respiratory depression: a closed claims analysis. Anesthesiology 2015;122(3):659–65.
7. Bauchat JR, Weiniger CF, Sultan P, et al. Society for obstetric anesthesia and perinatology consensus statement: monitoring recommendations for prevention and detection of respiratory depression associated with administration of neuraxial morphine for cesarean delivery analgesia. Anesth Analg 2019;129(2):458–74.
8. Callaghan WM, Creanga AA, Kuklina EV. Severe maternal morbidity among delivery and postpartum hospitalizations in the United States. Obstet Gynecol 2012;120(5):1029–36.
9. Lapinsky SE. Management of acute respiratory failure in pregnancy. Semin Respir Crit Care Med 2017;38(2):201–7.
10. Hines RL, Marschall KE. Stoelting's anesthesia and co-existing disease. 7th edition. Elsevier; 2018. p. xi, 724. Available at: https://login.proxy.lib.duke.edu/login?url=https://www.clinicalkey.com/dura/browse/bookChapter/3-s2.0-C20150003987.
11. Lisonkova S, Muraca GM, Potts J, et al. Association between prepregnancy body mass index and severe maternal morbidity. JAMA 2017;318(18):1777–86.
12. Mhyre JM, Riesner MN, Polley LS, et al. A series of anesthesia-related maternal deaths in Michigan, 1985-2003. Anesthesiology 2007;106(6):1096–104.
13. McAuliffe FM, Killeen SL, Jacob CM, et al. Management of prepregnancy, pregnancy, and postpartum obesity from the FIGO Pregnancy and Non-Communicable Diseases Committee: a FIGO (International Federation of Gynecology and Obstetrics) guideline. Int J Gynaecol Obstet 2020;151(Suppl 1):16–36.
14. Melo LC, Silva MA, Calles AC. Obesity and lung function: a systematic review. Einstein (Sao Paulo) 2014;12(1):120–5.
15. LoMauro A, Aliverti A. Respiratory physiology of pregnancy: physiology masterclass. Breathe (Sheff) 2015;11(4):297–301.

16. Baraka AS, Hanna MT, Jabbour SI, et al. Preoxygenation of pregnant and nonpregnant women in the head-up versus supine position. Anesth Analg 1992;75(5):757–9.
17. Branum AM, Kirmeyer SE, Gregory EC. Prepregnancy body mass index by maternal characteristics and state: data from the birth certificate, 2014. Natl Vital Stat Rep 2016;65(6):1–11.
18. Sturm R. Increases in clinically severe obesity in the United States, 1986-2000. Arch Intern Med 2003;163(18):2146–8.
19. Smid MC, Kearney MS, Stamilio DM. Extreme obesity and postcesarean wound complications in the maternal-fetal medicine unit cesarean registry. Am J Perinatol 2015;32(14):1336–41.
20. Smid MC, Dotters-Katz SK, Vaught AJ, et al. Maternal super obesity and risk for intensive care unit admission in the MFMU Cesarean Registry. Acta Obstet Gynecol Scand 2017;96(8):976–83.
21. Stamilio DM, Scifres CM. Extreme obesity and postcesarean maternal complications. Obstet Gynecol 2014;124(2 Pt 1):227–32.
22. Ende HB, Dwan RL, Freundlich RE, et al. Quantifying the incidence of clinically significant respiratory depression in women with and without obesity class III receiving neuraxial morphine for post-cesarean analgesia: a retrospective cohort study. Int J Obstet Anesth 2021;7:103187.
23. Crowgey TR, Dominguez JE, Peterson-Layne C, et al. A retrospective assessment of the incidence of respiratory depression after neuraxial morphine administration for postcesarean delivery analgesia. Anesth Analg 2013;117(6):1368–70.
24. Louis J, Auckley D, Miladinovic B, et al. Perinatal outcomes associated with obstructive sleep apnea in obese pregnant women. Obstet Gynecol 2012; 120(5):1085–92.
25. Dominguez JE, Grotegut CA, Cooter M, et al. Screening extremely obese pregnant women for obstructive sleep apnea. Am J Obstet Gynecol 2018;219(6):613.e1-10.
26. Facco FL, Ouyang DW, Zee PC, et al. Development of a pregnancy-specific screening tool for sleep apnea. J Clin Sleep Med 2012;8(4):389–94.
27. Lockhart EM, Ben Abdallah A, Tuuli MG, et al. Obstructive sleep apnea in pregnancy: assessment of current screening tools. Obstet Gynecol 2015;126(1):93–102.
28. Bourjeily G, Danilack VA, Bublitz MH, et al. Obstructive sleep apnea in pregnancy is associated with adverse maternal outcomes: a national cohort. Sleep Med 2017;38:50–7.
29. Li L, Zhao K, Hua J, et al. Association between sleep-disordered breathing during pregnancy and maternal and fetal outcomes: an updated systematic review and meta-analysis. Front Neurol 2018;9:91.
30. Louis JM, Mogos MF, Salemi JL, et al. Obstructive sleep apnea and severe maternal-infant morbidity/mortality in the United States, 1998-2009. Sleep 2014;37(5):843–9.
31. Bourjeily G, Danilack VA, Bublitz MH, et al. Maternal obstructive sleep apnea and neonatal birth outcomes in a population based sample. Sleep Med 2020; 66:233–40.
32. Hawkins M, Parker CB, Redline S, et al. Objectively assessed sleep-disordered breathing during pregnancy and infant birthweight. Sleep Med 2021;81:312–8.
33. Dominguez JE, Krystal AD, Habib AS. Obstructive sleep apnea in pregnant women: a review of pregnancy outcomes and an approach to management. Anesth Analg 2018;127(5):1167–77.
34. Hai F, Porhomayon J, Vermont L, et al. Postoperative complications in patients with obstructive sleep apnea: a meta-analysis. J Clin Anesth 2014;26(8):591–600.

35. Pien GW, Pack AI, Jackson N, et al. Risk factors for sleep-disordered breathing in pregnancy. Thorax 2014;69(4):371–7.
36. Facco FL, Parker CB, Reddy UM, et al. Association between sleep-disordered breathing and hypertensive disorders of pregnancy and gestational diabetes mellitus. Obstet Gynecol 2017;129(1):31–41.
37. Dominguez JE, Habib AS, Krystal AD. A review of the associations between obstructive sleep apnea and hypertensive disorders of pregnancy and possible mechanisms of disease. Sleep Med Rev 2018;42:37–46.
38. Lapinsky SE, Tram C, Mehta S, et al. Restrictive lung disease in pregnancy. Chest 2014;145(2):394–8.
39. Bonham CA, Patterson KC, Strek ME. Asthma outcomes and management during pregnancy. Chest 2018;153(2):515–27.
40. Kwon HL, Triche EW, Belanger K, et al. The epidemiology of asthma during pregnancy: prevalence, diagnosis, and symptoms. Immunol Allergy Clin North Am 2006;26(1):29–62.
41. Murphy VE, Jensen ME, Gibson PG. Asthma during pregnancy: exacerbations, management, and health outcomes for mother and infant. Semin Respir Crit Care Med 2017;38(2):160–73.
42. Mendola P, Laughon SK, Mannisto TI, et al. Obstetric complications among US women with asthma. Am J Obstet Gynecol 2013;208(2):127, e1–e8.
43. Murphy VE, Powell H, Wark PAB, et al. A prospective study of respiratory viral infection in pregnant women with and without asthma. Chest 2013;144(2):420–7.
44. Cooley DM, Glosten B, Roberts JR, et al. Bronchospasm after intramuscular 15-methyl prostaglandin F2 alpha and endotracheal intubation in a nonasthmatic patient. Anesth Analg 1991;73(1):87–9.
45. Harber CR, Levy DM, Chidambaram S, et al. Life-threatening bronchospasm after intramuscular carboprost for postpartum haemorrhage. BJOG 2007;114(3):366–8.
46. Edmundson C, Guidon AC. Neuromuscular disorders in pregnancy. Semin Neurol 2017;37(6):643–52.
47. Sax TW, Rosenbaum RB. Neuromuscular disorders in pregnancy. Muscle Nerve 2006;34(5):559–71.
48. Guidon AC, Massey EW. Neuromuscular disorders in pregnancy. Neurol Clin 2012;30(3):889–911.
49. Abati E, Corti S. Pregnancy outcomes in women with spinal muscular atrophy: a review. J Neurol Sci 2018;388:50–60.
50. Rudnik-Schoneborn S, Breuer C, Zerres K. Stable motor and lung function throughout pregnancy in a patient with infantile spinal muscular atrophy type II. Neuromuscul Disord 2002;12(2):137–40.
51. Pijnenborg JM, Hansen EC, Brolmann HA, et al. A severe case of myasthenia gravis during pregnancy. Gynecol Obstet Invest 2000;50(2):142–3.
52. Batocchi AP, Majolini L, Evoli A, et al. Course and treatment of myasthenia gravis during pregnancy. Neurology 1999;52(3):447–52.
53. Ozcan J, Balson IF, Dennis AT. New diagnosis myasthenia gravis and pre-eclampsia in late pregnancy. BMJ Case Rep 2015;26:2015.
54. Chollat C, Sentilhes L, Marret S. Fetal neuroprotection by magnesium sulfate: from translational research to clinical application. Front Neurol 2018;9:247.
55. Smith JM, Lowe RF, Fullerton J, et al. An integrative review of the side effects related to the use of magnesium sulfate for pre-eclampsia and eclampsia management. BMC Pregnancy Childbirth 2013;13:34.
56. Bashuk RG, Krendel DA. Myasthenia gravis presenting as weakness after magnesium administration. Muscle Nerve 1990;13(8):708–12.

57. Cohen BA, London RS, Goldstein PJ. Myasthenia gravis and preeclampsia. Obstet Gynecol 1976;48(1 Suppl):35S–7S.

58. Chan LY, Tsui MH, Leung TN. Guillain-Barre syndrome in pregnancy. Acta Obstet Gynecol Scand 2004;83(4):319–25.

59. Administration SAaMHS. Results from the 2010 National Survey on Drug Use and Health: Summary of National Findings. Vol. NSDUH Series H-41, HHS Publication No. (SMA) 11-4658.

60. Committee Opinion No. 711: opioid use and opioid use disorder in pregnancy. Obstet Gynecol 2017;130(2):e81–94.

61. Health VDo. Pregnancy-associated deaths from drug overdose in Virginia, 1999-2007. In: A report from the Virginia maternal mortality review team. 2015.

62. Bouillon T, Bruhn J, Roepcke H, et al. Opioid-induced respiratory depression is associated with increased tidal volume variability. Eur J Anaesthesiol 2003; 20(2):127–33.

63. Quinlan J, Cox F. Acute pain management in patients with drug dependence syndrome. Pain Rep 2017;2(4):e611.

64. Hung CY, Hu HC, Chiu LC, et al. Maternal and neonatal outcomes of respiratory failure during pregnancy. J Formos Med Assoc 2018;117(5):413–20.

65. Pollock W, Rose L, Dennis CL. Pregnant and postpartum admissions to the intensive care unit: a systematic review. Intensive Care Med 2010;36(9):1465–74.

66. Ong J, Zhang JJY, Lorusso R, et al. Extracorporeal membrane oxygenation in pregnancy and the postpartum period: a systematic review of case reports. Int J Obstet Anesth 2020;43:106–13.

67. Mahendra V, Clark SL, Suresh MS. Neuropathophysiology of preeclampsia and eclampsia: a review of cerebral hemodynamic principles in hypertensive disorders of pregnancy. Pregnancy Hypertens 2021;23:104–11.

68. Hypertension in pregnancy. Report of the American College of Obstetricians and Gynecologists' Task Force on Hypertension in Pregnancy. Obstet Gynecol 2013;122(5):1122–31.

69. Sowers LP, Massey CA, Gehlbach BK, et al. Sudden unexpected death in epilepsy: fatal post-ictal respiratory and arousal mechanisms. Respir Physiol Neurobiol 2013;189(2):315–23.

70. Belfort MA, Anthony J, Saade GR, et al. A comparison of magnesium sulfate and nimodipine for the prevention of eclampsia. N Engl J Med 2003;348(4):304–11.

71. Coetzee EJ, Dommisse J, Anthony J. A randomised controlled trial of intravenous magnesium sulphate versus placebo in the management of women with severe pre-eclampsia. Br J Obstet Gynaecol 1998;105(3):300–3.

72. Fawcett WJ, Haxby EJ, Male DA. Magnesium: physiology and pharmacology. Br J Anaesth 1999;83(2):302–20.

73. McDonnell NJ, Muchatuta NA, Paech MJ. Acute magnesium toxicity in an obstetric patient undergoing general anaesthesia for caesarean delivery. Int J Obstet Anesth 2010;19(2):226–31.

74. Safe Medication Administration: Magnesium Sulfate.

75. Mielniczuk LM, Williams K, Davis DR, et al. Frequency of peripartum cardiomyopathy. Am J Cardiol 2006;97(12):1765–8.

76. Honigberg MC, Givertz MM. Peripartum cardiomyopathy. BMJ 2019;364:k5287.

77. !!! INVALID CITATION !!! 73.

78. Sliwa K, Hilfiker-Kleiner D, Petrie MC, et al. Current state of knowledge on aetiology, diagnosis, management, and therapy of peripartum cardiomyopathy: a position statement from the Heart Failure Association of the European Society

of Cardiology Working Group on peripartum cardiomyopathy. Eur J Heart Fail 2010;12(8):767–78.

79. Pearson GD, Veille JC, Rahimtoola S, et al. Peripartum cardiomyopathy: National Heart, Lung, and Blood Institute and Office of Rare Diseases (National Institutes of Health) workshop recommendations and review. JAMA 2000;283(9):1183–8.

80. Arany Z, Elkayam U. Peripartum cardiomyopathy. Circulation 2016;133(14): 1397–409.

81. Cunningham FG, Byrne JJ, Nelson DB. Peripartum cardiomyopathy. Obstet Gynecol 2019;133(1):167–79.

82. Elkayam U. Clinical characteristics of peripartum cardiomyopathy in the United States: diagnosis, prognosis, and management. J Am Coll Cardiol 2011;58(7): 659–70.

83. McNamara DM, Elkayam U, Alharethi R, et al. Clinical outcomes for peripartum cardiomyopathy in North America: Results of the IPAC Study (Investigations of Pregnancy-Associated Cardiomyopathy). J Am Coll Cardiol 2015;66(8):905–14.

84. Hameed AB, Lawton ES, McCain CL, et al. Pregnancy-related cardiovascular deaths in California: beyond peripartum cardiomyopathy. Am J Obstet Gynecol 2015;213(3):379 e1–10.

85. Resnik JL, Hong C, Resnik R, et al. Evaluation of B-type natriuretic peptide (BNP) levels in normal and preeclamptic women. Am J Obstet Gynecol 2005; 193(2):450–4.

86. Blatt A, Svirski R, Morawsky G, et al. Short and long-term outcome of pregnant women with preexisting dilated cardiomypathy: an NTproBNP and echocardiography-guided study. Isr Med Assoc J 2010;12(10):613–6.

87. Kolin DA, Shakur-Still H, Bello A, et al. Risk factors for blood transfusion in traumatic and postpartum hemorrhage patients: analysis of the CRASH-2 and WOMAN trials. PLoS One 2020;15(6):e0233274.

88. Collaborators WT. Effect of early tranexamic acid administration on mortality, hysterectomy, and other morbidities in women with post-partum haemorrhage (WOMAN): an international, randomised, double-blind, placebo-controlled trial. Lancet 2017;389(10084):2105–16.

89. Thurn L, Wide-Swensson D, Hellgren-Wangdahl M. [Postpartum hemorrhage and need of blood transfusions]. Lakartidningen 2021;118:20147, 118Postpartumblodningar med blodtransfusioner har okat.

90. Thurn L, Wikman A, Westgren M, et al. Massive blood transfusion in relation to delivery: incidence, trends and risk factors: a population-based cohort study. BJOG 2019;126(13):1577–86.

91. Toy P, Lowell C. TRALI–definition, mechanisms, incidence and clinical relevance. Best Pract Res Clin Anaesthesiol 2007;21(2):183–93.

92. Michala L, Madhavan B, Win N, et al. Transfusion-related acute lung injury (TRALI) in an obstetric patient. Int J Obstet Anesth 2008;17(1):66–9.

93. Pietrzak B, Bobrowska K, Luterek K, et al. Transfusion-related acute lung injury in a patient diagnosed with hypofibrinogenemia after a cesarean section–case report and review of the literature. Ginekol Pol 2014;85(8):635–8.

94. Sachs UJ. Pathophysiology of TRALI: current concepts. Intensive Care Med 2007;33(Suppl 1):S3–11.

95. Meyer DE, Reynolds JW, Hobbs R, et al. The incidence of transfusion-related acute lung injury at a large, urban tertiary medical center: a decade's experience. Anesth Analg 2018;127(2):444–9.

96. Eder AF, Dy BA, Perez JM, et al. The residual risk of transfusion-related acute lung injury at the American Red Cross (2008-2011): limitations of a predominantly male-donor plasma mitigation strategy. Transfusion 2013;53(7):1442–9.

97. Eder AF, Herron RM Jr, Strupp A, et al. Effective reduction of transfusion-related acute lung injury risk with male-predominant plasma strategy in the American Red Cross (2006-2008). Transfusion 2010;50(8):1732–42.

98. Kleinman S, Caulfield T, Chan P, et al. Toward an understanding of transfusion-related acute lung injury: statement of a consensus panel. Transfusion 2004; 44(12):1774–89.

99. Stainsby D, Jones H, Asher D, et al. Serious hazards of transfusion: a decade of hemovigilance in the UK. Transfus Med Rev 2006;20(4):273–82.

100. Goldman M, Webert KE, Arnold DM, et al. Proceedings of a consensus conference: towards an understanding of TRALI. Transfus Med Rev 2005;19(1):2–31.

101. Bernard GR, Artigas A, Brigham KL, et al. Report of the American-European Consensus conference on acute respiratory distress syndrome: definitions, mechanisms, relevant outcomes, and clinical trial coordination. Consensus Committee. J Crit Care 1994;9(1):72–81.

102. Fong A, Chau CT, Pan D, et al. Amniotic fluid embolism: antepartum, intrapartum and demographic factors. J Matern Fetal Neonatal Med 2015;28(7):793–8.

103. Bonnet MP, Zlotnik D, Saucedo M, et al. Maternal death due to amniotic fluid embolism: a national study in France. Anesth Analg 2018;126(1):175–82.

104. Ponzio-Klijanienko A, Vincent-Rohfritsch A, Girault A, et al. Evaluation of the 4 diagnosis criteria proposed by the SMFM and the AFE foundation for amniotic fluid embolism in a monocentric population. J Gynecol Obstet Hum Reprod 2020;49(9):101821.

105. Kaur K, Bhardwaj M, Kumar P, et al. Amniotic fluid embolism. J Anaesthesiol Clin Pharmacol 2016;32(2):153–9.

106. Tamura N, Farhana M, Oda T, et al. Amniotic fluid embolism: pathophysiology from the perspective of pathology. J Obstet Gynaecol Res 2017;43(4):627–32.

107. Sultan P, Seligman K, Carvalho B. Amniotic fluid embolism: update and review. Curr Opin Anaesthesiol 2016;29(3):288–96.

108. Clark SL, Hankins GD, Dudley DA, et al. Amniotic fluid embolism: analysis of the national registry. Am J Obstet Gynecol 1995;172(4 Pt 1):1158–67 [discussion 1167–9].

109. Rhodes A, Evans LE, Alhazzani W, et al. Surviving sepsis campaign: international guidelines for management of sepsis and septic shock: 2016. Crit Care Med 2017;45(3):486–552.

110. Burlinson CEG, Sirounis D, Walley KR, et al. Sepsis in pregnancy and the puerperium. Int J Obstet Anesth 2018;36:96–107.

111. Galvao A, Braga AC, Goncalves DR, et al. Sepsis during pregnancy or the postpartum period. J Obstet Gynaecol 2016;36(6):735–43.

112. Society for Maternal-Fetal Medicine. Electronic address pso, Plante LA, Pacheco LD, Louis JM. SMFM Consult Series #47: Sepsis during pregnancy and the puerperium. Am J Obstet Gynecol 2019;220(4):B2–10.

113. Vincent JL, Moreno R, Takala J, et al. The SOFA (Sepsis-related Organ Failure Assessment) score to describe organ dysfunction/failure. On behalf of the Working Group on Sepsis-Related Problems of the European Society of Intensive Care Medicine. Intensive Care Med 1996;22(7):707–10.

114. Bowyer L, Robinson HL, Barrett H, et al. SOMANZ guidelines for the investigation and management sepsis in pregnancy. Aust N Z J Obstet Gynaecol 2017; 57(5):540–51.

115. Nair P, Davies AR, Beca J, et al. Extracorporeal membrane oxygenation for severe ARDS in pregnant and postpartum women during the 2009 H1N1 pandemic. Intensive Care Med 2011;37(4):648–54.

116. Barrantes JH, Ortoleva J, O'Neil ER, et al. Successful treatment of pregnant and postpartum women with severe COVID-19 associated acute respiratory distress syndrome with extracorporeal membrane oxygenation. ASAIO J 2021;67(2):132–6.

117. Li N, Han L, Peng M, et al. Maternal and neonatal outcomes of pregnant women with coronavirus disease 2019 (COVID-19) pneumonia: a case-control study. Clin Infect Dis 2020;71(16):2035–41.

118. Prabhu M, Cagino K, Matthews KC, et al. Pregnancy and postpartum outcomes in a universally tested population for SARS-CoV-2 in New York City: a prospective cohort study. BJOG 2020;127(12):1548–56.

119. Martin JA, Hamilton BE, Osterman MJK, et al. Births: final data for 2019. Natl Vital Stat Rep 2021;70(2):1–51.

120. Moore SA, Dietl CA, Coleman DM. Extracorporeal life support during pregnancy. J Thorac Cardiovasc Surg 2016;151(4):1154–60.

121. Pattinson KTS. Opioids and the control of respiration. Br J Anaesth 2008;100(6): 747–58.

122. Boom M, Niesters M, Sarton E, et al. Non-analgesic effects of opioids: opioid-induced respiratory depression. Curr Pharm Des 2012;18(37):5994–6004.

123. Lalley PM. Mu-opioid receptor agonist effects on medullary respiratory neurons in the cat: evidence for involvement in certain types of ventilatory disturbances. Am J Physiol Regul Integr Comp Physiol 2003;285(6):R1287–304.

124. Taylor S, Kirton OC, Staff I, et al. Postoperative day one: a high risk period for respiratory events. Am J Surg 2005;190(5):752–6.

125. Weingarten TN, Herasevich V, McGlinch MC, et al. Predictors of delayed postoperative respiratory depression assessed from naloxone administration. Anesth Analg 2015;121(2):422–9.

126. Ramachandran SK, Haider N, Saran KA, et al. Life-threatening critical respiratory events: a retrospective study of postoperative patients found unresponsive during analgesic therapy. J Clin Anesth 2011;23(3):207–13.

127. Gordon DB, Pellino TA. Incidence and characteristics of naloxone use in postoperative pain management: a critical examination of naloxone use as a potential quality measure. Pain Manag Nurs 2005;6(1):30–6.

128. Weingarten TN, Chong EY, Schroeder DR, et al. Predictors and outcomes following naloxone administration during Phase I anesthesia recovery. J Anesth 2016;30(1):116–22.

129. Ramachandran SK, Pandit J, Devine S, et al. Postoperative respiratory complications in patients at risk for obstructive sleep apnea: a single-institution cohort study. Anesth Analg 2017;125(1):272–9.

130. Toledano RD, Kodali BS, Camann WR. Anesthesia drugs in the obstetric and gynecologic practice. Rev Obstet Gynecol 2009;2(2):93–100.

131. Guglielminotti J, Landau R, Li G. Adverse events and factors associated with potentially avoidable use of general anesthesia in cesarean deliveries. Anesthesiology 2019;130(6):912–22.

132. Mhyre JM, Sultan P. General anesthesia for cesarean delivery: occasionally essential but best avoided. Anesthesiology 2019;130(6):864–6.

133. Carron M, Guzzinati S, Ori C. Simplified estimation of ideal and lean body weights in morbidly obese patients. Br J Anaesth 2012;109(5):829–30.

134. Gin T, Chan MT, Chan KL, et al. Prolonged neuromuscular block after rocuronium in postpartum patients. Anesth Analg 2002;94(3):686–9, table of contents.

135. Mercer BM, Merlino AA, Society for Maternal-Fetal M. Magnesium sulfate for preterm labor and preterm birth. Obstet Gynecol 2009;114(3):650–68.
136. Berdai MA, Labib S, Harandou M. Prolonged neuromuscular block in a pre-eclamptic patient induced by magnesium sulfate. Pan Afr Med J 2016;25:5.
137. Richardson MG, Raymond BL. Sugammadex administration in pregnant women and in women of reproductive potential: a narrative review. Anesth Analg 2020; 130(6):1628–37.
138. Society for Obstetric Anesthesia and Perinatology S. Statement on Sugammadex during pregnancy and lactation. 2019.

Preeclampsia in 2021— a Perioperative Medical Challenge for the Anesthesiologist

Dominique van Dyk, MBChB (UCT), FCA (SA)*,
Robert A. Dyer, MBChB (UCT), FCA (SA), PhD,
Nicole L. Fernandes, MBChB (UCT), MMed (UCT), FCA (SA)

KEYWORDS

- Preeclampsia • Eclampsia • Hemodynamic monitoring • Anesthesia
- Perioperative care

KEY POINTS

- Preeclampsia is a multisystem pregnancy disorder associated with endothelial dysfunction.
- In the case of preeclampsia with severe features, the anesthesiologist must be aware that there may be rapid deterioration in the clinical condition of the patient.
- Cardiovascular involvement is typified by elevated systemic vascular resistance and hypertension, left ventricular diastolic dysfunction, left ventricular hypertrophy, normal to increased cardiac output, and increased pericardial fluid.
- Point-of-care ultrasound has utility in quantifying disease severity, elucidating the cause of pulmonary edema, informing the anesthesia strategy, and guiding resuscitation in the case of hemorrhage or collapse.
- In the absence of epidural analgesia for labor, spinal anesthesia is the preferred option for cesarean delivery where there are no contraindications.

INTRODUCTION

A recent editorial calls for the prioritization of pregnant women by the discipline of perioperative medicine.[1] Nowhere is this more appropriate than in preeclampsia, where patients in low- and middle-income countries (LMICs) are often neglected and present late to the multidisciplinary team involved in feto-maternal care. Anesthesiologists have a

Department of Anaesthesia and Perioperative Medicine, University of Cape Town, D23 Department of Anaesthesia and Perioperative Medicine, Groote Schuur Hospital, Anzio Road, Observatory, 7925, Cape Town, South Africa
* Corresponding author.
E-mail address: d.vandyk@uct.ac.za

Anesthesiology Clin 39 (2021) 711–725
https://doi.org/10.1016/j.anclin.2021.08.005 **anesthesiology.theclinics.com**
1932-2275/21/© 2021 Elsevier Inc. All rights reserved.

prominent role to play. For effective practice, they need to understand the pathogenesis and cardiovascular pathophysiology, be able to assess the severity of cardiorespiratory disease and complications, make rational decisions on anesthesia technique, institute appropriate hemodynamic and respiratory monitoring, and be aware of long-term outcomes.

BACKGROUND

Preeclampsia is a multisystem disease of pregnancy, whose main feature is endothelial dysfunction. Maternal complications include abruptio placentae, pulmonary edema, acute renal failure, liver failure, and stroke. Neonatal complications include preterm delivery, fetal growth restriction, hypoxic-ischemic encephalopathy, and perinatal death.[2] The emergence of the severe acute respiratory syndrome coronavirus 2 (SARS-CoV-2) pandemic has added further complexity to the anesthesia management of patients with preeclampsia. SARS-CoV-2 illness in pregnancy has a strong independent association with preeclampsia, particularly in nulliparous women, and each condition is additive in its association with preterm delivery and adverse maternal outcomes.[3]

The International Society for the Study of Hypertension in Pregnancy has revised its definition of preeclampsia; in addition to the previous definition of new-onset hypertension after 20 weeks' gestation and proteinuria, we should also recognize the new onset of so-called severe features,[4] which include thrombocytopenia, renal insufficiency, impaired liver function, pulmonary edema, and cerebral or visual symptoms, and not necessarily proteinuria; this removes the categories "mild" and "severe" preeclampsia, which may be misleading when the disease severity may change so rapidly.

PATHOGENESIS

Anesthesia practice is based on an understanding of the relevant pathophysiology. Current theory suggests that in preeclampsia there is failure of the usual vascular remodeling of the spiral arteries by invasion by the cytotrophoblast. There is resultant activation of clotting pathways, release of cytokines and antiangiogenic proteins, endothelial dysfunction, vasoconstriction, and finally reduced organ perfusion, with its associated symptoms and signs.[5] It has also been postulated that the mechanisms of abnormal placentation may be different in early and late-onset disease.[6] Two recent reviews on the cardiovascular system in preeclampsia emphasize that clinical findings supporting the triad of inadequate placentation, placental insufficiency, and vascular reactivity are only found in a small proportion of cases.[7,8]

An alternative theory is that maternal systemic and uterine vascular impairment may predate placental maldevelopment. There is evidence of elevated systemic vascular resistance (SVR) and lower cardiac output before conception in at-risk women. Maladaptive responses to the increasing physiologic demands of pregnancy culminate in exaggerated concentric hypertrophy, increased left ventricular mass, and diastolic dysfunction characteristic of preeclampsia (**Fig. 1**). In support of a shared cardiovascular predisposition to preeclampsia and cardiovascular disease, current prophylaxis and management include aspirin, statins, metformin, and antihypertensive agents.

MORBIDITY AND MORTALITY

Mortality in preeclampsia is very different in low- and high-resource environments. For example, in the triennium 2012 to 2014 in the United Kingdom, there were 3 maternal

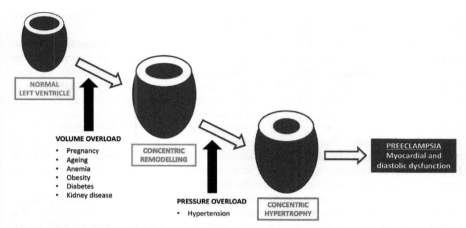

Fig. 1. Left ventricular remodeling induced by pregnancy and preeclampsia may progress to a maladaptive state with symptomatic cardiac failure. (*From* Ridder A, Giorgione V, Khalil A, Thilaganathan B. Preeclampsia: The Relationship between Uterine Artery Blood Flow and Trophoblast Function. Int J Mol Sci. 2019;20(13):3263; with permission.)

deaths (0.1 per 100,000 live births) due to preeclampsia, none of which had a cardiopulmonary cause[9]; this is in sharp contrast with the situation in South Africa, where in the triennium 2014 to 2016 there were 661 deaths, 34% of which had a cardiopulmonary cause.[10] The anesthesiologist therefore needs to have a keen understanding of cardiopulmonary function, as well as cerebrovascular dysfunction, in preeclampsia and eclampsia, and must be able to assess disease severity in order to predict, prevent, and treat life-threatening complications.

CARDIAC FUNCTION IN PREECLAMPSIA

The assessment of cardiac function in preeclampsia has been considerably advanced in recent years, with anesthesiologists playing a leading role in this field. Transthoracic echocardiography has been a major research tool in the elucidation of central hemodynamics and as a point-of-care tool for assessment of severity of cardiac dysfunction in preeclampsia. Dennis has depicted the disease as an "inovasoconstrictor state of pregnancy," with echocardiographic evidence of abnormal Doppler (left ventricular filling) and tissue Doppler (left ventricular movement) indices, increased left ventricular mass, increased inotropy with normal to increased cardiac output, an elevated SVR, and increased pericardial fluid.[11]

Sophisticated methodology has further characterized cardiac dysfunction. A comparison of cardiac function in early and late-onset preeclampsia used 3-dimensional (3D) speckle tracking echocardiography and showed that all strain indices correlated with gestational age. "Speckles" are generated by ultrasound–myocardial tissue interactions; this provides non-Doppler, less load-dependent information about global and segmental myocardial deformation or strain. Early onset disease was associated with a higher left ventricular mass index and lower (less negative) 3D derived strain values, different from late-onset preeclampsia.[12] In addition, a recent systematic review of 36 echocardiographic studies has shown that patients developing preeclampsia have lower prepregnancy cardiac output and higher SVR and that early onset disease is associated with more severe diastolic dysfunction, as well as more systolic dysfunction. The latter patients also have a lower cardiac output and higher SVR at 20 weeks' gestation.[13] It is important to appreciate that early and late-onset preeclampsia are different diseases from a cardiovascular point of view.

Can there be a progression to severe systolic dysfunction and low ejection fraction heart failure? Probably, yes. Firstly, there is recent evidence for shared genetic mutations in peripartum cardiomyopathy (PPCM) and preeclampsia.[14] Secondly, this diagram from a recent review on PPCM shows the potential interplay of pathways in the pathogenesis of PPCM, preeclampsia, and systolic heart failure (**Fig. 2**). Oxidative stress leads to the generation of a 16kDA prolactin fragment, which is thought to lead to endothelial dysfunction, followed by the generation of microRNA, which leads to cardiomyocyte death. The diagram also shows the generation of large amounts of circulating soluble FMS-like tyrosine kinase-1 (sFlt-1), which may occur both in PPCM and preeclampsia. sFlt-1 binds to endothelial growth factor and is antiangiogenic, and this may lead to severe systolic hypofunction.

Ultimately, management of cardiac dysfunction in complicated preeclampsia revolves around abnormalities of angiogenesis in pregnancy, which depends on the balance between pro- and antiangiogenic factors such as placental growth factor and sFlt-1.

PREDICTION OF SEVERITY OF CARDIORESPIRATORY DYSFUNCTION

Recent work on the prediction of severity of cardiorespiratory complications suggested that easily performed lung ultrasound may predict interstitial pulmonary edema

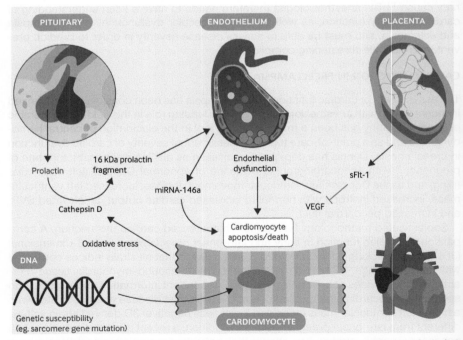

Fig. 2. Pathophysiology of peripartum cardiomyopathy. miRNA-146a, endothelial microRNA-146a; sFlt-1, soluble fms-like tyrosine kinase receptor 1; VEGF, vascular endothelial growth factor. (*From* Honigberg MC, Givertz MM. Peripartum cardiomyopathy. *BMJ*. 2019;364:k5287; with permission.)

(IPE), which is probably the precursor of life-threatening alveolar edema.[15] When the interlobular septa become edematous, there are multiple reverberations of the ultrasound beam, which give rise to "comet tails" or B lines. The density and width between the comets predict whether there is interstitial or alveolar edema. A positive B line pattern is defined as 3 to 6 per image, which, if they are less than 3 mm apart, implies alveolar edema.[16] Optic nerve sheath diameter (ONSD) may also be a predictor of raised intracranial pressure (ICP) and/or increased disease severity. In 20% of preeclamptic women ONSD reaches values compatible with ICP greater than 20 mm Hg.[17] A recent paper addresses the controversies related to the procedure and acquisition of the images in women with preeclampsia and the conclusions that can be drawn from these measurements.[18]

A recent study has attempted to elucidate the contributors to pulmonary edema in preeclampsia. The prevalence of point-of-care ultrasound (POCUS) abnormalities was established using transthoracic echocardiography, lung ultrasound, and ONSD in late-onset severe preeclampsia, as well as the association with serum albumin and brain natriuretic peptide (BNP).[19] The overall incidence of POCUS abnormalities was 59%, with nearly one-quarter exhibiting IPE (**Fig. 3**). There was no difference in serum albumin in patients with and without IPE. However, there were more cardiac abnormalities, and BNP was higher in patients with IPE, suggesting that cardiac dysfunction may be more important than colloid osmotic pressure in the generation of pulmonary edema. Indeed, the absence of IPE might exclude raised left ventricular end-diastolic pressure (LVEDP).

FLUID MANAGEMENT

Two systematic reviews have shown that there is insufficient evidence from randomized trials to favor a particular fluid management strategy to avoid pulmonary edema in preeclampsia.[20,21] Considerable variability in stroke volume responsiveness has been shown in observational studies.[22] Fluid restriction to less than 80 mL/h, as recommended by the Royal College of Obstetricians and Gynecologists (NICE guidelines),[23] seems safer in the absence of reliable measurement of stroke volume responsiveness in individual

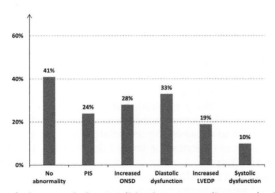

Fig. 3. Prevalence of ultrasound abnormalities in women diagnosed with late-onset preeclampsia and severe features. LVEDP, left ventricular end-diastolic pressure; ONSD, optic nerve sheath diameter; PIS, pulmonary interstitial syndrome. (*From* Ortner CM, Krishnamoorthy V, et al. Point-of-Care Ultrasound Abnormalities in Late-Onset Severe Preeclampsia: Prevalence and Association with Serum Albumin and Brain Natriuretic Peptide. Anesth Analg. 2019;128(6):1208-1216; with permission.)

cases. However, the incidence of chronic renal failure may be higher in women who have had preeclampsia than following a healthy pregnancy.[24] In patients with hemorrhage, resuscitation should proceed as in the healthy parturient, and there should be a low threshold for mechanical ventilation. In this situation, intra-arterial monitoring would allow for the assessment of stroke volume- and arterial pressure variability to guide fluid administration.

HEMODYNAMIC MONITORING IN CLINICAL PRACTICE

Initial management of preeclampsia with severe features includes urgent reduction of systolic blood pressure (SBP) to less than 160 mm Hg, to avoid stroke, followed by seizure prophylaxis using magnesium sulfate, usually a bolus of 4 g slowly intravenously (IV), followed by 1 g hourly. Therefore, accurate determination of blood pressure is crucial for diagnostic purposes. There are very few noninvasive blood pressure algorithms validated for accuracy in preeclampsia; most underestimate the SBP. The validated Microlife CRADLE Vital Signs Alert device, which incorporates the Microlife 3AS1-2 algorithm, is a hand-held, upper arm semi-automated device with a traffic light warning system.[25] This device has been used for early identification of preeclampsia in Africa and has been used in several clinical trials. For monitoring during anesthesia, many automated noninvasive monitors not validated for use in preeclampsia are available and seem to be adequate for the measurement of trends and changes in blood pressure.

There should be a low threshold for arterial line placement in preeclampsia, particularly in the setting of poorly controlled hypertension, renal failure, hemorrhage, pulmonary edema, and mechanical ventilation. Transthoracic echocardiography is a useful point-of-care tool for assessment of intravascular volume status, ventricular function, and comorbidities such as valvular heart disease.[11] The latest Cochrane review on pulmonary artery catheterization in preeclampsia found no randomized trials on which to base recommendations,[26] and the indications for this monitor are the same as in the general population.

ANESTHESIA MANAGEMENT
Regional Anesthesia

Historically Newsome, using the pulmonary artery catheter, demonstrated that there was only mild afterload reduction during epidural analgesia for labor in women with severe preeclampsia and receiving magnesium sulfate.[27] Blood pressure and cardiac output were well preserved. From first principles, epidural anesthesia should therefore be initiated wherever possible in women with preeclampsia in active labor, because the analgesia forms part of blood pressure control.

In a purely experimental study in 1950, healthy pregnant women, nonpregnant volunteers, and preeclamptic women were given either ganglion blockers or spinal anesthesia (SA), in order to observe the associated hemodynamic changes.[28] This study was the first paper to describe the limited degree of spinal hypotension in patients with severe preeclampsia. A major advance in obstetric anesthesia practice in the past 25 years has been the establishment of the safety of SA for cesarean section (CS) in uncomplicated severe preeclampsia, in the absence of contraindications, even in the setting of a nonreassuring fetal heart tracing.[29]

Using minimally invasive cardiac output monitoring in severe preeclampsia, it has been shown that SA is associated with only mild afterload reduction and that preload is not the major concern in the absence of hemorrhage or other comorbidities.[30] Sympathetic blockade, and modest afterload reduction with only minor changes in preload, are textbook management for diastolic dysfunction, which is the hallmark of cardiovascular dysfunction in preeclampsia.

Also using minimally invasive cardiac output monitoring, a randomized trial in 42 women with severe early onset preeclampsia showed that spinal hypotension in 20 patients was associated with an increase in cardiac index of 0.6 L/min/m.[2] Phenylephrine (initial dose 50 μg, median [range] 50 [50–150 μg]), in comparison with ephedrine (7.5 mg, [7.5–37.5 mg]) was associated with a change in cardiac output of -12 (7.3) versus 2.6 (6) percent and in SVR of 22.3 (7.5) versus -1.9 (10.5) percent respectively, $P < .0001$ in each case.[22] In a further study on early neonatal outcome, comparing phenylephrine, 50 to 100 ug, with ephedrine, 7.5 mg, for spinal hypotension in patients with fetal compromise, there were no significant between-group differences in neonatal acid base status (umbilical arterial base deficit −6.0 [4.6] versus −4.8 [3.7] mmol/L, 95% confidence interval [CI] of the difference −1 to 3.3 mmol/L).[31] Thus, the vasopressor used should be based on maternal hemodynamic status. Phenylephrine is the first-line vasopressor if systolic function is preserved. A recent meta-analysis of 5 randomized controlled clinical trials, which included the aforementioned 2 papers, compared incidences of fetal acidosis when either phenylephrine or ephedrine was used to treat spinal hypotension in parturients undergoing high risk CS.[32] The investigators concluded that further research with adequate power is needed to clarify outcomes using the 2 vasopressors. However, the effect size was small, and the sample size required to demonstrate either a difference or an equivalence between proportions would be greater than 1000 women. It would be ethically unjustifiable and impracticable to expend the time and major clinical resources required to subject large numbers of such a vulnerable group of patients to further clinical trials for the sake of merely demonstrating statistical significance for an anticipated small effect size.

Two publications have described the use of noradrenaline during SA in preeclampsia.[33,34] In the authors' view, noradrenaline is contraindicated in the routine management of spinal hypotension in preeclampsia, because even minor dose errors using this potent vasoconstrictor could cause precipitous hypertension in these patients, with potential associated severe morbidity; this is especially true in underresourced environments, where anesthesia providers may be inexperienced, with little supervision.

There is no definitive literature on specific contraindications to SA in severe preeclampsia, other than the presence of hypovolemia and thrombocytopenia. Because of the high incidence of severe disease in LMICs, there is not infrequently further cardiac comorbidity, which requires careful titration of epidural or general anesthesia (GA) with appropriate monitoring, including echocardiography. Clinical experience in our high-risk referral unit (Groote Schuur Hospital, Cape Town, South Africa) has been that relative contraindications to single-shot SA include pulmonary edema with severe systolic hypofunction, or comorbidities such as clinically significant valvular heart disease, in particular mitral stenosis, complicated grown-up congenital heart disease, hypertrophic obstructive cardiomyopathy, or pericardial effusion.

Thrombocytopenia and the Risks of Regional Anesthesia

The lower limit of the platelet count for safe performance of regional anesthesia in preeclampsia remains controversial. In a recent large retrospective study of 1524 patients receiving obstetric neuraxial anesthesia with a platelet count less than 100×10^9/L, there were no cases of epidural hematoma, but the upper bounds of the 95% CI of the risk were high for the groups with low platelet counts, due to limited numbers of observations.[35] Most clinicians are still guided by an early study that showed that the maximum amplitude of the thromboelastograph tracing in women with preeclampsia decreased markedly when the platelet count decreased to less than 75×10^9/L.[36] A recent SOAP Task Force performed a systematic review and a Delphi process and concluded that the risk of spinal epidural hematoma associated with a platelet count $\geq$ 70×10^9/L would be low in hypertensive disorders of pregnancy; factors to be considered with relevance to preeclampsia include airway status, available equipment, and the risk of GA, which to some extent would be determined by the experience of the anesthesia provider.[37] All these factors should also be considered when deciding on the method of anesthesia in women with preeclampsia or eclampsia who have thrombocytopenia or when a platelet count is not available.

In HELLP syndrome (hemolysis, elevated liver enzymes, low platelets) thrombocytopenia occurs more frequently, and the platelet count may decrease precipitously to less than 75×10^9/L. In these parturients it is essential that one follows the trend in platelet counts closely.[38] In contrast with the SOAP consensus guidelines, the NICE guidelines do not recommend a specific platelet threshold that precludes neuraxial blockade. Instead, they suggest an individualized approach, where one takes into consideration the risk of bleeding and opportunity for correction, the use of anticoagulants, anticipated difficulty of the procedure, as well as the proposed method (epidural or SA).[39]

Current guidance recommends that pregnant women hospitalized with SARS-CoV-2 infection receive prophylactic anticoagulation, generally with low-molecular-weight heparins, in the absence of contraindications.[40] The choice of anticoagulant and its dosing in undelivered patients with preeclampsia and SARS-CoV-2 should take into consideration the likelihood of residual anticoagulation should a category 1 or 2 emergency CS become indicated. It is prudent to have a recent platelet count available, as each of the conditions and the heparin anticoagulants may be associated with thrombocytopenia.

General Anesthesia

Should GA be required, it is of great importance to obtund the hypertensive response to tracheal intubation, thus avoiding potential cerebrovascular complications. The most effective pharmacologic technique for this purpose remains controversial. In a narrative review, all aspects of the pharmacology of beta-blockers, vasodilators, opiates, and magnesium sulfate were discussed.[41] The authors recommend esmolol or nitroglycerine. However, most drugs considered have risks and benefits. For example, remifentanil causes neonatal respiratory depression, and hydralazine has a delayed onset and prolonged effect. Recent literature on dexmedetomidine as an adjunct to GA shows that maternal recovery may be prolonged.[42] Early randomized trials confirmed the effectiveness of IV bolus magnesium sulfate (30–45 mg/kg after administration of the IV induction agent), with minimal neonatal side effects. Discussion of these studies was included in correspondence, which summarized the evidence in favor of the use of this agent.[43]

Data from 402 patients receiving GA in obstetrics, in a recently established obstetric airway management registry at Groote Schuur Hospital, Cape Town, were compared in women with and without hypertensive disorders of pregnancy (HDP). It was shown that hypoxemia occurred in 19% with and 9% without hypertension (estimated risk difference 10%, 95% CI 2–17, $P = .005$).[44] It could be hypothesized that the presence of IPE could impair gas exchange and contribute to rapid desaturation during apnea. In addition, LVEDP may increase due to the hypertensive response to tracheal intubation in patients with severe preeclampsia and result in IPE. HDP and elevated body mass index were both associated with hypoxemia, and the effects were additive (**Fig. 4**); this is particularly relevant because obstructive sleep apnea in obese pregnant women is

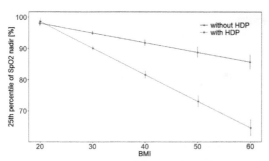

Fig. 4. Interaction plot of the combined effects of hypertensive disorders of pregnancy and body mass index on the 25th percentile (Q1) of SpO2 nadir. Vertical bars represent 95% confidence intervals. Blue and red lines represent predicted 25th percentiles for patient groups with and without HDP, respectively. HDP, hypertensive disorders of pregnancy; BMI, body mass index (kg/m^2). (*From* Smit MI, du Toit L, Dyer RA, et al. Hypoxaemia during tracheal intubation in patients with hypertensive disorders of pregnancy: analysis of data from an obstetric airway management registry. Int J Obstet Anesth. 2021;45:41-48; with permission.)

associated with more frequent preeclampsia, neonatal intensive care unit admissions, and CS.[45] Future studies could include the use of gentle mask ventilation after administration of muscle relaxant and the use of high flow nasal oxygen in order to prolong apneic oxygenation.

Intubation of the eclamptic patient with a bitten tongue poses a particular challenge for induction of GA. Logically, the worst of the lingual trauma and swelling is situated anterior in the buccal cavity, but the possibility of blood and edema deeper in the upper airway must be recognized. The use of a channeled video laryngoscope, such as the Airtraq, is likely to be of utility in viewing the glottis and advancing the endotracheal tube under continuous vision. There is no evidence in this scenario as to whether the use of suxamethonium has advantages over rocuronium; the latter's reversal by sugammadex is not impeded by prior magnesium sulfate administration.[46] If there is doubt about the ability to achieve an adequate view of the vocal cords after rapid sequence induction, an inhalational induction can be considered. Fiberoptic bronchoscopic intubation is usually impractical in this clinical context.

There are shared risk factors for the development of preeclampsia and severe SARS-CoV-2 disease. In general, patients are managed and delivered according to the status of their preeclampsia; however, earlier delivery may be indicated should there be respiratory compromise, particularly if prone ventilation or extracorporeal membrane oxygenation is required as part of SARS-CoV-2 therapy. Where the patient's respiratory status and coagulation status allow it, neuraxial anesthesia is strongly preferred.

The Use of Uterotonic Agents

Specific work on the effects of uterotonic agents in preeclampsia is especially relevant given the increased risk of postpartum hemorrhage. A slowly administered oxytocin bolus dose, in line with current international consensus recommendations, has been shown to cause similar short-lived vasodilatation and hypotension as in healthy parturients at CS,[47] although the hemodynamic response may be more variable in severe preeclampsia.[48] There are growing data suggesting that carbetocin is a safe and efficacious alternative oxytocic, even though its manufacturing license lists preeclampsia as a contraindication to its use.[49] Second-line uterotonic agents remain largely limited to prostaglandins such as misoprostol, because the ergot alkaloids may provoke a pronounced hypertensive response.

Postcesarean Analgesia

Adequate analgesia, as during labor, is not only a patient's right but also a crucial component of blood pressure management after CS. A multimodal approach is typically recommended, but there has been limited work done on postoperative analgesia in preeclamptic women. Dennis and colleagues demonstrated lower pain scores and analgesic requirements in the early postoperative period in preeclamptic women after SA for CS and postulated that this may be due to the effects of peripartum magnesium sulfate infusion and the higher neuraxial local anesthetic dose administered for the delivery of growth-restricted, preterm fetuses.[50] The use of nonsteroidal antiinflammatory drugs (NSAIDs) remains controversial, with concerns around the propensity of these drugs to impair renal and platelet function and control of hypertension in preeclamptic women. An adequately powered retrospective cohort study in women with preeclampsia and severe features has shown no association between the use of postdelivery NSAIDs and persistent postpartum hypertension.[51]

ECLAMPSIA

Eclampsia remains a major challenge for the anesthesiologist. In a cohort study examining maternal and fetal outcomes in preeclampsia in South Africa, young maternal age and low body mass index were significant predictors of eclampsia.[52] Progression to eclamptic seizures may be associated with cytotoxic edema and cerebral infarction and/or vasogenic edema, with loss of cerebral autoregulation and increased capillary permeability, placing the patient at risk of intracerebral hemorrhage.[53] In the latest Report on Confidential Enquiries into Maternal Deaths in South Africa, cerebral complications were the most common cause of death in patients with hypertensive disorders (357/661 [54%]).[10]

Current clinical opinion is that patients with eclampsia with a Glasgow Coma Scale score (GCS) < 14 and a high likelihood that there is elevated ICP should receive GA for CS with similar considerations as in neuroanaesthesia.[2] These include normoxia and normocarbia, control of blood pressure so that cerebral perfusion is maintained in the setting of elevated ICP, and postoperative ventilation with careful sedation until neurologic recovery is achieved, in an intensive care unit. In limited-resource environments, the capacity for postoperative ventilation is often not available. For example, 12/82 (15%) of women received mechanical ventilation in a recent report from Nigeria.[54]

In an early study comparing outcomes following GA versus neuraxial anesthesia for CS in conscious women with stable eclampsia, epidural anesthesia was favored over SA.[55] Patients were defined as "stable" if the blood pressure did not require acute management, GCS was ≥ 14, the fetal heart tracing was normal, platelet count was > 100 × 10⁹/L, magnesium therapy had been initiated, and central venous pressure was maintained at 4 to 6 cm H_2O. Epidural anesthesia was found to be associated with similar maternal and neonatal outcomes as GA, except for higher 1-minute Apgar scores in the epidural group. This study was conducted before the acceptance of SA as the method of choice in women with preeclampsia for CS in the absence of contraindications. A subsequent case series described good hemodynamic stability in a series of 12 women with stable eclampsia receiving SA for CS.[56]

A recent retrospective audit was performed of anesthesia for CS in eclampsia, in a high-risk referral unit in Cape Town, South Africa.[57] The primary outcome was the proportion of patients receiving SA or GA. An assessment was also performed of the rationale for the choice of anesthesia. Seven of eighty-nine (7.9%) patients received SA and 82/89 (92.1%) GA. Overall, 63/89 (70.8%) had a preoperative GCS < 14, and 26/89 (29.2%) patients had GCS ≥ 14. Seven of twenty-six patients with GCS ≥ 14 had SA, and the remaining 19/26 received GA. In many of these the audit showed that SA would likely have been safe. Median Apgar scores at 1 and 5 minutes in SA patients were significantly higher than those in GA patients with GCS $\geq$ 14 and < 14. Eclamptic women had minimal hemodynamic changes during SA; 3 patients required small doses of vasopressor. Seven of sixty-three patients with GCS < 14 had cerebral edema and 2 had a cerebral infarct. There were 2 maternal deaths.

In view of the undoubted risk associated with GA in women with eclampsia, careful consideration should be given to the use of SA in all women with a GCS $\geq$ 14. In patients who have had several seizures, focal neurologic signs, and/or HELLP syndrome, GA should be provided. Major audits of anesthesia practice in high- and low-income environments would be useful, so that one could plan optimal management depending on resources available.

LONG-TERM CARDIOVASCULAR RISK

Preeclampsia is now well recognized as a risk factor for long-term cardiovascular disease, which clearly affects anesthesia practice. Both diastolic and systolic dysfunction persist in early onset disease for at least 1 year. In the longer term, women who have had preeclampsia are at increased risk for coronary, cerebrovascular or peripheral vascular disease, stroke, thromboembolism,[58,59] white matter lesions post eclampsia,[60] as well as diabetes and end-stage renal disease.[24,61] Overall, 14% of women with preeclampsia develop chronic hypertension within 10 years if the first pregnancy was in their 20s, versus 4% who were normotensive in pregnancy, and 32% versus 11% if preeclampsia occurred when older than 40 years.[62] A history of hypertensive disorders of pregnancy has been found to be independently associated with impaired memory and verbal learning 15 years later.[63]

SUMMARY

Anesthesiologists have for many years been at the forefront of research whose goal has been the establishment of safe regional anesthesia in preeclampsia, both epidural anesthesia for labor and SA for CS. Advances in GA in this field include an understanding of the mechanisms of hypoxemia, and the introduction of sophisticated aids to tracheal intubation. More recently, anesthesiologists have become proficient in the use of echocardiography and other ultrasound modalities, which has led to research elucidating cardiac function, and point-of-care identification of many aspects of cardiac and pulmonary function. The close involvement of the anesthesiologist in the perioperative interdisciplinary team including nurses, obstetricians, physicians, and cardiologists has improved the prediction of severity of disease and will likely improve safety in patients with complicated preeclampsia with severe features.

CLINICS CARE POINTS

- Point-of-care lung ultrasound is useful to identify those patients with preeclampsia with IPE, who would benefit from judicious fluid restriction and afterload reduction, to avoid progression to life-threatening alveolar edema.

- Point-of-care transthoracic echocardiography is useful to delineate the cause of pulmonary edema and allows differentiation between diastolic dysfunction, systolic hypofunction, and preexisting valvular heart disease.

- In the absence of contraindications, SA is a well-tolerated technique for urgent CS, with less hypotension than in normotensive women.

- Induction of GA requires skilled administration of agents to control peri-induction hypertension and an awareness of the propensity for rapid desaturation and airway edema.
- Anesthesiologists should be aware of the long-term cardiovascular effects of preeclampsia, many of which influence the choice of technique and detailed practice of anesthesia.

DISCLOSURE

Dominique van Dyk, Nicole Fernandes, and Robert Dyer certify that they have no commercial or financial interests in the material contained in the article and have received no funding for its preparation.

REFERENCES

1. Dennis AT, Sheridan N. Sex, suffering and silence - why peri-operative medicine must prioritise pregnant women. Anaesthesia 2019;74(12):1504–8.
2. Chestnut D, Wong C, Tsen L, et al. Chestnut's obstetric anesthesia: principles and practice. 6th edition. Philadelphia, PA: Elsevier; 2020.
3. Papageorghiou AT, Deruelle P, Gunier RB, et al. Preeclampsia and COVID-19: results from the INTERCOVID prospective longitudinal study. Am J Obstet Gynecol 2021;S0002-9378(21):00561–5.
4. Hypertension in pregnancy. Report of the American College of Obstetricians and Gynecologists' Task Force on Hypertension in Pregnancy. Obstet Gynecol 2013; 122(5):1122–31.
5. Powe CE, Levine RJ, Karumanchi SA. Preeclampsia, a disease of the maternal endothelium: the role of antiangiogenic factors and implications for later cardiovascular disease. Circulation 2011;123(24):2856–69.
6. Redman CW, Sargent IL, Staff AC. IFPA Senior Award Lecture: making sense of pre-eclampsia - two placental causes of preeclampsia? Placenta 2014; 35(Suppl):S20–5.
7. Thilaganathan B, Kalafat E. Cardiovascular System in Preeclampsia and Beyond. Hypertension 2019;73(3):522–31.
8. Ridder A, Giorgione V, Khalil A, Thilaganathan B. Preeclampsia: The Relationship between Uterine Artery Blood Flow and Trophoblast Function. Int J Mol Sci 2019; 20(13):3263.
9. MBRRACE-UK - Saving Lives. Improving Mothers' care. 2016. https://www.npeu. ox.ac.uk/mbrrace-uk. [Accessed 5 June 2021]. Accessed.
10. Moodley J. Saving Mothers 2014-2016: Seventh triennial report on confidential enquiries into maternal deaths in South Africa, short report. Pretoria: Department of Health; 2018.
11. Dennis AT. Transthoracic echocardiography in women with preeclampsia. Curr Opin Anaesthesiol 2015;28(3):254–60.
12. Cong J, Fan T, Yang X, Shen J, Cheng G, Zhang Z. Maternal cardiac remodeling and dysfunction in preeclampsia: a three-dimensional speckle-tracking echocardiography study. Int J Cardiovasc Imaging 2015;31(7):1361–8.
13. Castleman JS, Ganapathy R, Taki F, Lip GY, Steeds RP, Kotecha D. Echocardiographic Structure and Function in Hypertensive Disorders of Pregnancy: A Systematic Review. Circ Cardiovasc Imaging 2016;9(9):e004888.
14. Gammill HS, Chettier R, Brewer A, et al. Cardiomyopathy and Preeclampsia. Circulation 2018;138(21):2359–66.

15. Zieleskiewicz L, Contargyris C, Brun C, et al. Lung ultrasound predicts interstitial syndrome and hemodynamic profile in parturients with severe preeclampsia. Anesthesiology 2014;120(4):906–14.

16. Volpicelli G, Elbarbary M, Blaivas M, et al. International evidence-based recommendations for point-of-care lung ultrasound. Intensive Care Med 2012;38(4): 577–91.

17. Dubost C, Le Gouez A, Jouffroy V, et al. Optic nerve sheath diameter used as ultrasonographic assessment of the incidence of raised intracranial pressure in preeclampsia: a pilot study. Anesthesiology 2012;116(5):1066–71.

18. Ortner CM, Macias P, Neethling E, et al. Ocular sonography in pre-eclampsia: a simple technique to detect raised intracranial pressure? Int J Obstet Anesth 2020;41:1–6. https://doi.org/10.1016/j.ijoa.2019.09.002.

19. Ortner CM, Krishnamoorthy V, Neethling E, et al. Point-of-Care Ultrasound Abnormalities in Late-Onset Severe Preeclampsia: Prevalence and Association With Serum Albumin and Brain Natriuretic Peptide. Anesth Analg 2019;128(6): 1208–16.

20. Duley L, Williams J, Henderson-Smart DJ. Plasma volume expansion for treatment of women with pre-eclampsia. Cochrane Database Syst Rev 2000;2: CD001805. https://doi.org/10.1002/14651858.CD001805.

21. Pretorius T, van Rensburg G, Dyer RA, Biccard BM. The influence of fluid management on outcomes in preeclampsia: a systematic review and meta-analysis. Int J Obstet Anesth 2018;34:85–95. https://doi.org/10.1016/j.ijoa.2017.12.004.

22. Dyer RA, Daniels A, Vorster A, et al. Maternal cardiac output response to colloid preload and vasopressor therapy during spinal anaesthesia for CS in patients with severe pre-eclampsia: a randomised, controlled trial. Anaesthesia 2018; 73(1):23–31.

23. NICE. Hypertension in pregnancy : diagnosis and management. 2020. Available at: https://www.nice.org.uk/guidance/ng133. Accessed 4 June 2021.

24. Vikse BE. Pre-eclampsia and the risk of kidney disease. Lancet 2013;382(9887): 104–6.

25. Nathan HL, de Greeff A, Hezelgrave NL, Chappell LC, Shennan AH. An accurate semiautomated oscillometric blood pressure device for use in pregnancy (including pre-eclampsia) in a low-income and middle-income country population: the Microlife 3AS1-2. Blood Press Monit 2015;20(1):52–5.

26. Li YH, Novikova N. Pulmonary artery flow catheters for directing management in pre-eclampsia. Cochrane Database Syst Rev 2012;6:CD008882. 10.1002/ 14651858.

27. Newsome LR, Bramwell RS, Curling PE. Severe preeclampsia: hemodynamic effects of lumbar epidural anesthesia. Anesth Analg 1986;65(1):31–6.

28. Assali NS, Prystowsky H. Studies on autonomic blockade. I. Comparison between the effects of tetraethylammonium chloride (TEAC) and high selective spinal anesthesia on blood pressure of normal and toxemic pregnancy. J Clin Invest 1950;29(10):1354–66.

29. Henke VG, Bateman BT, Leffert LR. Focused review: spinal anesthesia in severe preeclampsia. Anesth Analg 2013;117(3):686–93.

30. Dyer RA, Piercy JL, Reed AR, Lombard CJ, Schoeman LK, James MF. Hemodynamic changes associated with spinal anesthesia for cesarean delivery in severe preeclampsia. Anesthesiology 2008;108(5):802–11.

31. Dyer RA, Emmanuel A, Adams SC, et al. A randomised comparison of bolus phenylephrine and ephedrine for the management of spinal hypotension in

patients with severe preeclampsia and fetal compromise. Int J Obstet Anesth 2018;33:23–31. https://doi.org/10.1016/j.ijoa.2017.08.001.

32. Heesen M, Rijs K, Hilber N, et al. Ephedrine versus phenylephrine as a vasopressor for spinal anaesthesia-induced hypotension in parturients undergoing high-risk CS: meta-analysis, meta-regression and trial sequential analysis. Int J Obstet Anesth 2019;37:16–28. https://doi.org/10.1016/j.ijoa.2018.10.006.

33. Wang X, Mao M, Liu S, Xu S, Yang J. A Comparative Study of Bolus Norepinephrine, Phenylephrine, and Ephedrine for the Treatment of Maternal Hypotension in Parturients with Preeclampsia During Cesarean Delivery Under Spinal Anesthesia. Med Sci Monit 2019;25:1093–101. https://doi.org/10.12659/MSM.914143.

34. Wei C, Qian J, Zhang Y, Chang X, Hu H, Xiao F. Norepinephrine for the prevention of spinal-induced hypotension during caesarean delivery under combined spinal-epidural anaesthesia: Randomised, double-blind, dose-finding study. Eur J Anaesthesiol 2020;37(4):309–15.

35. Lee LO, Bateman BT, Kheterpal S, et al. Multicenter Perioperative Outcomes Group Investigators. Risk of Epidural Hematoma after Neuraxial Techniques in Thrombocytopenic Parturients: A Report from the Multicenter Perioperative Outcomes Group. Anesthesiology 2017;126(6):1053–63.

36. Sharma SK, Philip J, Whitten CW, Padakandla UB, Landers DF. Assessment of changes in coagulation in parturients with preeclampsia using thromboelastography. Anesthesiology 1999;90(2):385–90.

37. Bauer ME, Arendt K, Beilin Y, et al. The Society for Obstetric Anesthesia and Perinatology Interdisciplinary Consensus Statement on Neuraxial Procedures in Obstetric Patients With Thrombocytopenia. Anesth Analg 2021;132(6):1531–44.

38. Russell R. Preeclampsia and the anaesthesiologist: current management. Curr Opin Anaesthesiol 2020;33(3):305–10.

39. NICE. Intrapartum care for women with existing medical conditions or obstetric complications and their babies. 2020. Available at: https://www.nice.org.uk/guidance/ng121. Accessed 6 June 2021.

40. COVID-19 Treatment Guidelines Panel. Coronavirus disease 2019 (COVID-19) Treatment guidelines. National Institutes of Health. Available at: https://www.covid19treatmentguidelines.nih.gov/. Accessed 12 August 2021.

41. Pant M, Fong R, Scavone B. Prevention of peri-induction hypertension in preeclamptic patients: a focused review. Anesth Analg 2014;119(6):1350–6.

42. Brogly N, Guasch E. Hypertension control during CS in patients with preeclampsia: is dexmedetomidine an option? Minerva Anestesiol 2018;84(12):1329–31.

43. James MF, Dyer RA. Prevention of Peri-Induction Hypertension in Pre-Eclamptic Patients. Anesth Analg 2015;121(6):1678–9.

44. Smit MI, du Toit L, Dyer RA, et al. Hypoxaemia during tracheal intubation in patients with hypertensive disorders of pregnancy: analysis of data from an obstetric airway management registry. Int J Obstet Anesth 2021;45:41–8. https://doi.org/10.1016/j.ijoa.2020.10.012.

45. Louis J, Auckley D, Miladinovic B, et al. Perinatal outcomes associated with obstructive sleep apnea in obese pregnant women. Obstet Gynecol 2012;120(5):1085–92.

46. Grandjean B, Guerci P, Vial F, et al. Sugammadex and profound rocuronium neuromuscular blockade induced by magnesium sulphate. Ann Fr Anesth Reanim 2013;32(5):378–9.

47. Heesen M, Carvalho B, Carvalho JCA, et al. International consensus statement on the use of uterotonic agents during CS. Anaesthesia 2019;74(10):1305–19.

48. Langesæter E, Rosseland LA, Stubhaug A. Haemodynamic effects of oxytocin in women with severe preeclampsia. Int J Obstet Anesth 2011;20(1):26–9.
49. Nucci B, Aya AGM, Aubry E, Ripart J. Carbetocin for prevention of postcesarean hemorrhage in women with severe preeclampsia: a before-after cohort comparison with oxytocin. J Clin Anesth 2016;35:321–5. https://doi.org/10.1016/j.jclinane.2016.08.017.
50. Dennis AT, Mulligan SM. Analgesic requirements and pain experience after CS under neuraxial anesthesia in women with preeclampsia. Hypertens Pregnancy 2016;35(4):520–8.
51. Viteri OA, England JA, Alrais MA, et al. Association of Nonsteroidal Antiinflammatory Drugs and Postpartum Hypertension in Women With Preeclampsia With Severe Features. Obstet Gynecol 2017;130(4):830–5.
52. Nathan HL, Seed PT, Hezelgrave NL, et al. Maternal and perinatal adverse outcomes in women with pre-eclampsia cared for at facility-level in South Africa: a prospective cohort study. J Glob Health 2018;8(2):020401.
53. Zeeman GG, Fleckenstein JL, Twickler DM, Cunningham FG. Cerebral infarction in eclampsia. Am J Obstet Gynecol 2004;190(3):714–20.
54. Afolayan JM, Nwachukwu CE, Esangbedo ES, Omu PO, Amadasun FE, Fadare JO. Evolving pattern of spinal anaesthesia in stable eclamptic patients undergoing CS at University of Benin Teaching Hospital, Benin, Nigeria. Niger J Med 2014;23(4):288–95.
55. Moodley J, Jjuuko G, Rout C. Epidural compared with general anaesthesia for caesarean delivery in conscious women with eclampsia. BJOG 2001;108(4):378–82.
56. Singh R, Kumar N, Jain A, Chakraborty M. Spinal anesthesia for lower segment Cesarean section in patients with stable eclampsia. J Clin Anesth 2011;23(3):202–6.
57. Jordaan M, Reed AR, Cloete E, Dyer RA. A retrospective audit of anaesthesia for CS in parturients with eclampsia at a tertiary referral hospital in Cape Town. South Afr J Anaesth Analg 2020;26(4):192–7.
58. Ahmed R, Dunford J, Mehran R, Robson S, Kunadian V. Pre-eclampsia and future cardiovascular risk among women: a review. J Am Coll Cardiol 2014;63(18):1815–22.
59. Melchiorre K, Thilaganathan B, Giorgione V, Ridder A, Memmo A, Khalil A. Hypertensive Disorders of Pregnancy and Future Cardiovascular Health. Front Cardiovasc Med 2020;15(7):59. https://doi.org/10.3389/fcvm.2020.00059.
60. Wiegman MJ, Zeeman GG, Aukes AM, et al. Regional distribution of cerebral white matter lesions years after preeclampsia and eclampsia. Obstet Gynecol 2014;123(4):790–5.
61. Luyckx VA, Perico N, Somaschini M, et al. writing group of the Low Birth Weight and Nephron Number Working Group. A developmental approach to the prevention of hypertension and kidney disease: a report from the Low Birth Weight and Nephron Number Working Group. Lancet 2017;390(10092):424–8.
62. Behrens I, Basit S, Melbye M, et al. Risk of post-pregnancy hypertension in women with a history of hypertensive disorders of pregnancy: nationwide cohort study. BMJ 2017;358:j3078. https://doi.org/10.1136/bmj.j3078.
63. Adank MC, Hussainali RF, Oosterveer LC, et al. Hypertensive Disorders of Pregnancy and Cognitive Impairment: A Prospective Cohort Study. Neurology 2021;96(5):e709–18.

Neuraxial Techniques for Parturients with Thromboprophylaxis or Thrombocytopenia

Jacqueline M. Galvan, MD*, Heather C. Nixon, MD

KEYWORDS

- Thrombocytopenia • Thromboprophylaxis • Neuraxial anesthesia
- Spinal epidural hematoma

KEY POINTS

- Hypocoagulable states will be encountered in the parturient, including pharmacologic thromboprophylaxis against venous thromboembolism (VTE) and thrombocytopenia. Hypocoagulable states complicate the placement of neuraxial anesthesia, which is a cornerstone of obstetric anesthesia care.
- Risk factors for the development of VTE in pregnancy are increased, specifically obesity, smoking, preeclampsia, postpartum hemorrhage, and advanced maternal age.
- Risk of spinal epidural hematoma (SEH) is low in parturients after following minimum time requirements for prophylactic doses of unfractionated heparin or low-molecular-weight heparin in the obstetric population.
- Risk of SEH in parturients with thrombocytopenia due to gestational hypertension, hypertensive disease, or thrombocytopenia (ITP) is low. An acceptable low platelet count, in the absence of other concerning risk factors, is $> 70,000 \times 10^6$/L.
- The risk of an alternative anesthetic, typically general anesthesia, must be weighed against the risk of complications associated with neuraxial anesthesia in patient with alterations in coagulation status.

INTRODUCTION AND DEFINITIONS
Physiologic changes in anticoagulant activity and platelets in pregnancy

In general, pregnancy is a hypercoagulable state characterized by physiologic changes which serve as a protective mechanism against hemorrhage for mom and baby. In healthy pregnancy, there exists a delicate balance between uterine implantation, proliferation of spiral arteries, but also hemostatic maintenance that prevents

Department of Anesthesiology, University of Illinois at Chicago, 1740 West Taylor Street MW 3200W, Chicago, IL 60612, USA
* Corresponding author.
E-mail address: jackiemgalvan@gmail.com

Anesthesiology Clin 39 (2021) 727–742
https://doi.org/10.1016/j.anclin.2021.08.011
1932-2275/21/© 2021 Elsevier Inc. All rights reserved.

maternal hemorrhage after delivery. Pregnancy is characterized by an increase in blood clotting, with decreased anticoagulant, and fibrinolytic activity. An increase in endogenous procoagulant factors II, VII, VIII, IX, X, XII, XIII is accompanied by a concurrent increase in fibrinogen well above levels in the nonpregnant state.[1,2]

Similarly, increases in platelet activation and aggregation are also seen during pregnancy. Several studies of healthy pregnant women suggest an overall increase in platelet aggregation in pregnancy when exposed to factors that promote thrombosis, including collagen and arachidonic acid.[3,4] Currently, it is commonly accepted that physiologic changes in maternal blood volume and circulation contribute to an overall decrease in platelet numbers during pregnancy. A quantitative decrease in platelets during normal pregnancies can be due to dilutional factors and placental sequestration. Plasma volume can increase to 34% to 70% above baseline, representing plasma volumes ranging from 3200 L to 4200L at the end of pregnancy.[5]

Placental sequestration of platelets can also mirror normal splenic sequestration in nonpregnant healthy adult women. Increased splenic sequestration or "pooling" of radioactively tagged platelets in splenomegalic subjects compared to those with normal spleens is one apparent mechanism of lower platelets counts. An increase in spleen size, which is a low-resistance vascular system, can promote platelet pooling and therefore lower platelet numbers. In pregnancy not only is there an increase in spleen size, but there are additional low-resistance spaces for platelet sequestration: the placental intervillous spaces. This is supported by data that demonstrate lower platelet counts in twin pregnancies versus singleton pregnancies. The former may have larger placentas or 2 placentas, resulting in increased sequestration and lower platelet counts.[6,7]

Recent studies have shed some light on the course of platelets during pregnancy. A 2017 systematic review of a multinational assortment of 13 longitudinal and 33 cross-section studies aimed to describe the normal course of platelet counts during pregnancy. Individual studies of varying methodology had conflicting results. Some data suggested there was an increase, decrease, or no change in platelets during pregnancy. However, the overall results of the study suggested a gradual decrease in platelets from a mean of $250,000 \times 10^6$/L in the first trimester to $224,000 \times 10^6$/L in the third trimester. Similarly, a 2018 retrospective, United States (US)-based single-center study of 7000 pregnant women investigated platelet counts during pregnancy in uncomplicated and complicated pregnancies compared to nonpregnant controls. The data suggested a normally distributed decrease in platelet counts in all included healthy pregnant women than nonpregnant controls. In this cohort, platelet counts dropped during pregnancy from the first through the third trimester. The mean platelet value was $225,00 \times 10^6$/L in the third trimester.[8,9]

Abnormalities in these physiologic changes in pregnancy can precipitate hyper- or hypocoaguable states of pregnancy which represents unique challenges to the anesthesiologist. This is particularly salient when the decision to perform or withhold neuraxial anesthesia is in question. The risk of an alternative anesthetic, typically general anesthesia, must be weighed against the risk of complications associated with neuraxial anesthesia in patient with altered coagulation status.

NATURE OF THE PROBLEM: VENOUS THROMBOEMBOLISM IN PREGNANCY

According to the 2016 National Partnership for Maternal Safety Consensus Bundle on Venous Thromboembolism, obstetric venous thromboembolism (VTE) is a leading cause of maternal morbidity and mortality. Even in high-resource countries such as the US, United Kingdom, and Australia, VTE can account for anywhere from 14% to

30% of maternal deaths. VTEs that precipitate maternal morbidity, which include deep venous thrombosis (DVTs) and pulmonary embolisms (PEs), are likely multifactorial in etiology. The hypercoagulable state of pregnancy, venous stasis due to uterine mechanical obstruction, and decreased mobility are some of the notable causes of pregnancy-related VTE. The incidence of VTE events is greatly elevated (a 4-fold increase) in pregnancy than in nonpregnant patients.[10]

However, there is an alarming trend in the US suggesting an increasing prevalence of VTE.

Data from the National Inpatient Sample from 1994 to 1997 and 2006 to 2009 reviewed 118,000 pregnancy-related VTE-associated hospitalizations. Overall, the rate of VTE-associated hospitalization increased by 14% between 1994 to 1997 and 2006 to 2009 (1.74–1.99 per 1000 deliveries). The rate of VTE hospital admission attributed to PE (which can have devastating consequences if not diagnosed and treated quickly) increased by 128% over this same time period (0.32–0.73 per 1000 deliveries). This study noted that 50% of pregnancy-related VTE-associated hospitalizations were among women ages 25 to 35 years old. There was also a trend toward increased VTE-related antepartum and postpartum hospitalizations in urban areas. Another study analyzed the VTE incidence and use of VTE prophylaxis during vaginal delivery hospitalizations in the US between 2006 and 2012. These results again demonstrated an increased incidence of VTE hospitalizations from 15.6/100,000 to 29.8/100,000.[11,12]

Concomitant increases in maternal comorbid conditions associated with VTE can contribute to this alarming trend. These include rising rates of obesity, smoking, preeclampsia, postpartum hemorrhage, and advanced maternal age, to name a few. Consensus statements and safety bundles from the Society from Obstetric Anesthesia, National Partnership for Maternal Safety, and the California Maternal Quality Care Collaborative have highlighted the recognition and treatment of VTE in pregnancy as an opportunity to mitigate harm in these patients.[10,13]

Although mechanical thromboprophylaxis is generally a low-risk option, the use of pharmacologic therapies is gaining traction as a means for prophylaxis against VTE. However, this acquired hypocoagulable state may be in direct conflict with providing neuraxial anesthesia.

NATURE OF THE PROBLEM: THROMBOCYTOPENIA IN PREGNANCY

Identifying a normal range of platelets in pregnancy can distinguish between physiologic and pathologic states, which in turn can help define the management of obstetric patients. Specifically, thrombocytopenia (TCP) in pregnancy can influence the use of neuraxial anesthesia. Up to 12% of obstetric patients meet the criteria for TPC in pregnancy, with 1% experiencing moderate to severe disease (platelets $< 100,000 \times 10^6/$L). The ACOG (American College of Obstetrics and Gynecology) practice bulletin No. 207 defines thrombocytopenia as a platelet count less than $150,000 \times 10^6/$L, with moderate to severe thrombocytopenia being less than $100,000 \times 10^6/$L. However, the lower limit of normal platelet counts in otherwise healthy women is less well defined. Counts between $100,000 \times 10^6/$L and $150,000 \times 10^6/$L are not uncommon, and the clinical implications are unknown. Evaluation of maternal comorbid conditions, laboratory values and trends, gestational and obstetric history can help providers distinguish between the common etiologies of thrombocytopenia in pregnancy. Main etiologies of thrombocytopenia in pregnancy include gestational thrombocytopenia (GTCP), immune thrombocytopenia (ITP), thrombocytopenia associated with hypertensive disease of pregnancy and pseudothrombocytopenia.[14,15]

Differential diagnosis of thrombocytopenia by trimester

†First trimester or outside of pregnancy: immune thrombocytopenia

As the name suggests, ITP is antibody-induced destruction of platelets occurring in less than 1% of pregnancies. ITP often presents with moderately to severely low platelets (80–100,000 × 10^6/L), and often presents without any accompanying symptoms. It can occur anytime during pregnancy, and the patient may have thrombocytopenia outside of pregnancy. The effect of pregnancy on ITP (and vice versa) is ill-defined as most information comes from retrospective or observational data. A retrospective chart review of 92 women with ITP found that 77% experienced no or mild symptoms of thrombocytopenia. Only 3% (4 subjects) experienced severe bleeding symptoms, but none were hospitalized due to bleeding. Bleeding risk seemed to correlate with platelets levels less than 100,000 × 10^6/L.[16]

Second and third trimesters: gestational thrombocytopenia

GTCP is the most common cause of TCP in pregnancy, occurring in up to 5% to 11% of pregnancies. It is often idiopathic in nature and is a diagnosis of exclusion. Common presentation occurs during the late second into the third trimester, with platelet counts often greater than 75,000 × 10^6/L and otherwise asymptomatic from a bleeding perspective. Pregnant persons with GTCP have no TCP or bleeding history outside of pregnancy. Platelet levels return to normal after pregnancy. The etiology of GTCP is unknown, but probably related to dilutional or clearance processes. Interestingly, because mean platelets counts trend downwards throughout pregnancy, an estimated 17% decrease, pregnant persons at the low end of platelet counts at baseline will likely be in the thrombocytopenic range during pregnancy. Therefore, the risk of recurrent GTCP may be increased up to 14 times among pregnant people with a history of GTCP.[8,17]

Second and third trimesters: thrombocytopenia and hypertensive disorders

Thrombocytopenia manifests with hypertensive disorders, including preeclampsia, in 5% to 21% of pregnancies. In fact, hypertension and platelet count less than 100,000 × 10^6/L are diagnostic criteria for preeclampsia even in the absence of significant proteinuria according to recent ACOG guidelines. Unlike GTCP and ITP, women with hypertensive disorders of pregnancy and TCP often exhibit other clinical symptomatology including elevated systolic and diastolic blood pressures after 20 weeks of gestation, CNS disturbances, or impaired liver or kidney dysfunction. Thrombocytopenia associated with preeclampsia has been attributed to increased platelet activation, size, and consumption and reduced platelet lifespan. The relative imbalance between the placental production of thromboxane A2 and prostacyclin can contribute to increased vasoconstriction and platelet aggregation seen in preeclamptic women.[14,17]

A significant consideration is the platelet trends in women with preeclampsia. An impending coagulation disorder marked by TCP may affect anesthetic management. In a retrospective analysis of 984 women with preeclampsia, 6.5% had platelets less than 100,000 × 10^6/L, 2.1% less than 70,000 × 10^6/L, and 0.5% less than 50,000 × 10^6/L, respectively. They also found that within 72 hours surrounding delivery platelet counts were unlikely to change significantly. Progression to HELLP (hemolysis, elevated liver enzymes, low platelets) was associated with more precipitous decreases in platelets to levels less than 50,000 × 10^6/L. HELLP can be distinguished from other types of pregnancy-related hypertensive disease via laboratory tests. Commonly, but not reliably, substantially elevated aspartate aminotransferase (AST), alanine aminotransferase (ALT), and or lactate dehydrogenase (LDH) are present and can aid in the diagnosis of HELLP. Although the inclusion criteria for preeclampsia have changed over time, similar studies demonstrate the minority of preeclamptic women will have platelet counts less than $100,000 \times 10^6/L$. Clinically significant coagulopathy or hemorrhage in preeclamptic women is rare unless there is progression to HELLP or disseminated intravascular coagulopathy (DIC).[14,18,19]

All three trimesters: laboratory error/clumping/pseudothrombocytopenia
Sometimes laboratory artifacts can result in an erroneous diagnosis of TCP. Pseudothrombocytopenia, or platelet clumping, has a reported incidence of 0.1% in the general population. This occurs as a result of platelet activation in the presence of Ethylenediaminetetraacetic acid (EDTA), a widely used anticoagulant in laboratory medicine. EDTA-platelet complexes can trigger a cascade which ultimately leads to platelet clumping and therefore spuriously decreased counts. An expectedly low platelet count in the absence of other concerning clinical indicators of TCP may lead the clinician to suspect pseudothrombocytopenia. Obtaining a manual platelet count or recollecting the patient's blood sample (eg, using citrated platelets instead) can confirm a diagnosis of pseudothrombocytopenia.[20]

All three trimesters: other etiologies of thrombocytopenia in pregnancy
Pregnant patients may be thrombocytopenic for other reasons. Alternative etiologies include systemic dysfunction such as sepsis and DIC, immune-mediated disorders such as thrombotic thrombocytopenic purpura and hemolytic uremic syndromes, and nutritional disorders to name a few. A full discussion of these disorders is beyond the scope of this paper.

PHARMACOLOGIC THROMBOPROPHYLAXIS AGAINST VENOUS THROMBOEMBOLISM IN PREGNANCY
Anticoagulation during pregnancy

As previously stated, VTE is a leading cause of preventable maternal morbidity and mortality in the US. The reported incidence during pregnancy is 0.61–1.72 per 1000 deliveries. Pregnancy fosters the formation of VTE due to elements that are consistent with Virchow's triad: (1) stasis, (2) hypercoagulability, and (3) vascular trauma (ie, operative delivery). Acquired and inherited complications of pregnancy serve as clinical risk factors which contribute to the rising rates of VTE. Risk factors such as antiphospholipid antibody syndrome, diabetes, BMI greater than 25 with antepartum immobility, and hemorrhage with surgery carry odds ratios of VTE of 15.8, 2, 62, and 12, respectively.[21] Institution-specific protocols and safety bundles call for standardized screening, education, dosing, and communication strategies for pregnant patients at risk for VTE. Anticoagulation is a crucial component of VTE treatment and prevention to reduce maternal morbidity and mortality.[10,22]

A United Kingdom study demonstrated a reduction in VTE-related maternal deaths in women treated with low-molecular-weight heparin (LMWH). Maternal morbidity decreased from 1.26/100,000 births in 2009 to 2011 to 0.85/100,000 births in 2012 to 2014. It is clear that with implementing anticoagulation protocols for parturients at high risk for VTE, obstetric anesthesiologists will encounter these patients at or near the time a request for neuraxial anesthesia is made.

As mentioned, there are various safety bundles and consensus statements regarding VTE prophylaxis and treatment in pregnancy. This includes the National Partnership for Maternal Safety (NPMS), California Maternal Quality Care Collaborative, ACOG, American College of Chest Physicians (ACCP), and Royal College of Obstetricians and Gynecologists. Although no one guideline has demonstrated clear superiority in all situations, adoption, and adaptation of an institution-specific bundle to reduce maternal morbidity from VTE are the overarching goal.[10,14,22,23]

Unfractionated heparin and low-molecular-weight heparins

Heparins are an ideal choice for pregnancy as they do not cross the placenta and are accepted as safe for the fetus. Heparins reduce the risk of VTE by binding to and causing a conformational change in antithrombin III (AT III). ATIII inactivates thrombin and factor Xa, which is important in clot formation and stability. UFH pharmacokinetics in pregnancy are somewhat unpredictable and therefore clinical response varies. Data suggest that, compared to nonpregnant peers, single doses of UFH in pregnant patients produce lower serum heparin levels with little to no effect on activated partial thromboplastin time (aPTT). It is postulated that increased nonspecific heparin neutralizing proteins and/or increased factor VIII and fibrinogen may be the cause of relative heparin resistance in pregnancy. Furthermore, there also may be increased requirements in pregnancy and as gestational age advances, but the relationship is unclear. Dosing strategies are discussed later in this article. Important side effects include heparin-induced thrombocytopenia (HIT) and osteoporosis.[13,21]

LMWH is the preferred pharmacologic agent to prevent VTE in pregnancy due to better bioavailability, safety profile, and more predictable dosing. Enoxaparin, dalteparin, and tinzaparin are commonly used LMWHs during pregnancy. Reduced peripheral protein binding may aid in better bioavailability in the subcutaneous tissue. Longer serum half-life allows once to twice daily dosing strategies.[13,21]

CRUX OF THE PROBLEM: INCIDENCE AND RISK FACTORS FOR SPINAL EPIDURAL HEMATOMA IN PREGNANCY

Spinal epidural hematoma in pregnancy

Hypocoagulable states of pregnancy, either through the iatrogenic administration of anticoagulants or acquired thrombocytopenia, complicate anesthetic management for the patient and obstetric anesthesiologist. Both conditions require coordinated care due to the risks of neuraxial placement. The most feared risk is spinal epidural hematoma (SEH). The overall incidence of SEH, and therefore, neurologic sequelae is low in the obstetric population (1:200,000) compared to the elderly orthopedic population (1:3600).[24] The latter may be more prone to SEH after neuraxial blockade due to age-induced changes in the vasculature, spine, and medication clearance. Obstetric populations tend to be younger and healthy. When a parturient is presumed to be hypocoagulable due to thromboprophylaxis or TCP and requires neuraxial anesthesia, carefully evaluation with evidence-based guidelines of these apparent contraindications is paramount to a successful outcome.[24,25]

Spinal epidural hematoma and pharmacologic thromboprophylaxis

Expert guidelines from national anesthesiology societies recommend prophylactic anticoagulation for parturients at the risk of developing VTE. Anticoagulation is carefully weighed when deciding to perform a neuraxial anesthetic should it be requested or required for delivery. Avoiding inadvertent SEH, due to neuraxial placement or removal of a catheter in the presence of anticoagulation, is key. A large systematic review of published literature of parturients receiving pharmacologic thromboprophylaxis between 1952 and 2016, and the Anesthesia Close Claims Project Database (1950–2013), found no cases of SEH associated with neuraxial blockade.[25] Thromboprophylactic doses of UFH and LMWH were considered to be 5000 to 10,000 units subcutaneous (U SQ) given once to three times daily. LMWH dosing was variable and included weight-based and nonweight-based strategies: (0.5–1.0 mg/kg, SQ daily) and (30–60 mg, SQ daily or 20–30 mg SQ, twice daily). Of the 2 case reports found which described SEH in obstetric patients, 1 case of SEH occurred before the administration of a prophylactic dose of LMWH. In the other case, SEH was temporally related to a continuous spinal anesthetic with therapeutically dosed LMWH. Although there are inherent limitations of retrospective systematic reviews, multiple published data further support the hypothesis that SEH in obstetric patients receiving prophylactic doses of LMWH and UFH is desirably low if established guidelines are followed.[25–27]

Spinal epidural hematoma and thrombocytopenia

As previously stated, TCP will complicate up to 12% of pregnancies with less than 1% presenting with platelet counts less than 100,000 $\times$ 10^6/L. Similar to parturients on anticoagulation, parturients with moderate to severe thrombocytopenia may be denied neuraxial anesthesia to avoid the risk of SEH. There is currently not a universally accepted lower limit for platelet levels in obstetric patients for which the risk of SEH secondary to neuraxial placement is considered to be reliably safe. Although the overall incidence of SEH in the obstetric population has been described, the incidence specifically associated with TCP less than 100,00 $\times$ 10^6/L is unknown. A systematic review of 7476 published reports between 1947 and 2018 was reviewed for the incidence of SEH in thrombocytopenic patients (<100,000 $\times$ 10^6/L) who received a neuraxial anesthetic. The study population was heterogeneous and included both obstetric and nonobstetrical subjects. Neuraxial procedures included lumbar punctures, spinal, epidurals, combined spinal epidurals, and catheter removals. Of the 7509 lumbar neuraxial procedures, 33 cases of SEH were found. SEH was frequently associated with lumbar puncture procedures (n = 25) with platelet counts less than 50,000 $\times$ 10^6 L (n = 20). Five obstetric patients were affected by SEH: 2 after epidural and 3 after spinal. One had an arteriovenous malformation, 1 was coagulopathic during catheter removal, 2 patients had HELLP syndrome, and 1 had eclampsia. Overall, the number of SEH stratified by platelet count was described as: 1 to 25,000 $\times$ 10^6/L (n = 14), 26 to 50,000 $\times$ 10^6/L (n = 6), 51 to 75,000 $\times$ 10^6/L (n = 9), and 76 to 99,000 $\times$ 10^6/L (n = 4). A nonspecific inflection point around a platelet count of 75,000 $\times$ 10^6/L reflects a lower limit threshold whereby the risk of SEH is believed to be low enough that neuraxial anesthesia can be considered in some patients with thrombocytopenia. An observational single-center study of 984 women evaluated parturients with preeclampsia and catheter-based analgesic use. Although the primary aim was not to determine the incidence of SEH, neuraxial anesthesia was used in 40 of 64 patients with platelet counts of less than 100,000 $\times$ 10^6/L with no cases of SEH.[28,29]

Other large-scale retrospective data including the SCORE project (Serious Complications Related to Obstetric Anesthesia) support the conclusion that the risk of SEH in the obstetric population is low. These studies did not address the risk of SEH in the setting of TCP specifically, but they add to knowledge in contemporary practice.[26,27]

To further stratify a platelet threshold whereby the benefit of neuraxial anesthesia outweighs the risk of SEH, a 2017 study analyzed 573 thrombocytopenic patients (platelets < 100,000 $\times$ 10^6/L) who received neuraxial anesthesia. Another retrospective analysis of 417 thrombocytopenic parturients stratified patients by platelets levels for the risk of SEH in the setting of neuraxial anesthesia. Combined results indicated lower platelet counts correlated with increased risk of SEH; 9% (0–49,000 $\times$ 10^6/L), 2.6% (50,000–69,000 $\times$ 10^6/L), and 0.19% (70,000–100,000 $\times$ 10^6/L) with 95% confidence intervals.[30,31]

The 2020 Society for Obstetric Anesthesia and Perinatology (SOAP) Interdisciplinary Consensus statement on neuraxial anesthesia in obstetric patients with TCP concluded that the risk of SEH is reasonably low in obstetric patients with platelet counts greater than $70,000 \times 10^6$/L in the absence of other concerning coagulopathies receiving neuraxial anesthesia.[28]

RISK AND BENEFITS DISCUSSION: AVOIDING SPINAL EPIDURAL HEMATOMA VERSUS THE RISK OF GENERAL ANESTHESIA
Benefits of neuraxial anesthesia in obstetric care

Hypocoagulable states in the parturient due to VTE thromboprophylaxis or TCP will be encountered in contemporary obstetric anesthesia practice. These 2 states may complicate placement of neuraxial anesthetics for delivery, postpartum pain management, or noncesarean delivery (CD) procedures. Catheter-based techniques are the cornerstone of obstetric anesthesia practice because of their many well-described maternal, and by extension fetal, benefits. Although the decision to provide neuraxial analgesia or anesthesia should be individualized, providing neuraxial anesthesia, particularly in high-risk pregnancies, is a practice supported by the American Society of Anesthesiologists (ASA) and SOAP. In situ labor epidural catheters not only provide targeted analgesic management, but can facilitate a rapid conversion to surgical anesthesia in the setting of maternal or fetal distress during labor. This allows the mother to maintain consciousness and participate in the birth of her child should urgent or emergent CD become indicated.

Neuraxial procedures for CD similarly have demonstrated benefits over alternative anesthetics, namely general anesthesia. Neuraxial procedures for CD allow maternal participation in the birth process, avoid systemic and fetal exposure to anesthetic medications and facilitate administration of neuraxial morphine, which is the gold standard for CD pain.[32,33]

Risks of general anesthesia in obstetric care

Occasionally, neuraxial anesthesia is relatively or absolutely contraindicated when there is concern about maternal coagulation status. Hypocoagulable states (as discussed in this article), sepsis, umbilical cord prolapse, placental abruption, or uterine rupture may preclude the use of neuraxial anesthesia or make it clinically impossible due to time constraints. As such, when general anesthesia is used, providers need to be prepared for complications such as failed intubation, intraoperative awareness, and gastric content aspiration. Luckily, these are rare events. Data regarding anesthetic-related maternal mortality due to general anesthesia are encouraging. Data suggest a decrease in anesthetic-related maternal mortality from the use of general anesthesia; from 16.8 per million to 6.5 per million from the time period 1991% to 1996% to 1997% to 200,260% from 1991 to 2002.[34] Two-thirds of deaths associated with general anesthesia were caused by intubation failure or induction problems, speaking to the known incidence of difficult airway in parturients or anesthesiology provider unfamiliarity with the obstetric airway due to possible overreliance on catheter-based techniques. Additional complications are more common with general anesthesia than neuraxial techniques including higher postoperative pain scores, delayed mobilization, and impaired breastfeeding scores. It is often impossible to distinguish between the harm associated with general anesthesia during CD from the clinical circumstances which precipitate its use.

Not only does general anesthesia in obstetric care potentially increase the risk of death but can also precipitate lasting maternal harm. In a 2019 retrospective study analyzing outcomes associated with maternal adverse events and general anesthesia for CD, they found a 14% reduction of "potentially avoidable general anesthetics" over the study period (2003–2004 vs 2013–2014). "Avoidable general anesthetics" were those subjects lacking a code for a clear indication for general anesthesia such as fetal distress, severe postpartum hemorrhage, and placental abruption to name a few. The authors found that amongst those with avoidable general anesthetics, there was a significant increase in risk for anesthetic complications, severe complications, surgical site infections, and VTE. Therefore, thoughtful and careful use of neuraxial procedures in obstetric patients with pharmacologic thromboprophylaxis or thrombocytopenia may contribute to reducing the harm associated with unwarranted general anesthesia.[35] The risks of general anesthesia for CD, an alternative to neuraxial anesthesia, should be weighed carefully against the perceived risk of SEH in obstetric patients.

EVALUATING COAGULATION STATUS AND SUITABILITY FOR NEURAXIAL ANESTHESIA: WHAT TO DO WHEN FACED WITH THROMBOPROPHYLAXIS AND TCP

Thromboprophylaxis: history and physical examination

A thorough assessment of the patient's medical and obstetric history is a solid starting point to assess the suitability for neuraxial anesthesia in the setting of thromboprophylaxis. A global assessment for obvious clinical or hemodynamically significant bleeding can rapidly rule out a patient's suitability for neuraxial anesthesia. Indications for thromboprophylaxis, dosing, timing, and side effects are key components for making an informed decision on neuraxial anesthesia timing relative to the avoidance of SEH in the setting of thromboprophylaxis. Commonly used dosing of UFH SQ for thromboprophylaxis includes a <5000 U single dose twice daily or 3 times daily and ≤15,000 U in 24 hours for low dose. Doses greater than 5000 U and less than 10,000 U as a single dose or greater than 15,000 U in 24 hours are considered a high dose. In the LMWH category, dalteparin 5000 U once daily, enoxaparin 30 mg BID, and enoxaparin 40 mg once daily are all considered prophylactic dosing. According to the SOAP consensus statement and American Society of Regional Anesthesia (ASRA) guidelines, any amount greater than prophylactic dosing is considered therapeutic, the discussion of which is beyond the scope of this article in regards to neuraxial anesthetic techniques.[13]

Laboratory testing: prophylactic unfractionated heparin and low-molecular-weight heparins

In pregnancy, the altered volume of distribution, renal clearance, and coagulation status render interpretation of traditional coagulation markers a challenge. As discussed previously, UFH has a variable response between patients. A combination of time intervals (for metabolism) and assessment of coagulation laboratories are recommended. Activated partial prothrombin time (aPTT) is often used to evaluate the coagulation status of those patients on UFH. aPTT measures the speed of clot formation along the intrinsic and common coagulation pathways. Supratherapeutic levels of UFH, which can cause SEH, can be reflected in elevated aPTT levels. Although aPTT is widely available and easy to obtain in the US, there is no specific cut-off in obstetric patients to determine if the risk of SEH is reasonably low. In pregnant patients receiving UFH for greater than 4 days, the recommendation is to check a platelet count to rule out the possibility of HIT.

Clinical responsiveness to LMWHs is more predictable. Similar to UFH, most professional anesthesiology societies recommend time intervals specific for prophylactic and therapeutic dosing before proceeding with neuraxial anesthesia to avoid SEH. Factor Xa has been used in obstetric and nonobstetrical populations to describe the levels of anticoagulation in the setting of prophylactic LMWH, although the threshold for safe neuraxial anesthesia in the obstetric population is unknown. Factor Xa levels may not be readily available in some institutions.[13]

Thrombocytopenia

History and physical examination

Assessing underlying conditions that contribute to bleeding risk can help guide the decision to perform neuraxial anesthesia in parturients with thrombocytopenia. Anesthesia providers can ask about heavy menstrual bleeding, severe epistaxis, or easy bruising outside of pregnancy. Bleeding into major anatomic spaces, such as hemarthrosis or gastrointestinal bleeding, is also concerning for more severe disease. Positive findings may suggest inherited bleeding disorders which warrant further investigation. Excessive hemorrhage, or bleeding into mucous membranes, or IV sites might suggest an acute process and also require a pause to determine if neuraxial anesthesia is appropriate. Should TCP be discovered on the initial laboratory testing, platelet levels, trends, and blood pressures should be investigated to help determine an etiology.[15]

Laboratory testing

The 2016 ASA practice guidelines for Obstetric Anesthesia do not recommend intrapartum platelet count as a routine for healthy patients.[32] However, in the setting of comorbid conditions such as hypertensive disease, it is unknown at what regular intervals complete blood count (CBC) or platelet count should be drawn. Clinical practice varies, but published recommendations suggest a range of 6 to 12 hours for rechecking laboratories in conditions whereby platelets are likely to decline. The frequency of platelet counts is impacted by the labor course, fetal status, severity of thrombocytopenia, intended anesthetic, and maternal comorbid conditions. Unfortunately, platelet counts do not necessarily provide information on platelet function and therefore, may not provide enough information about SEH risk from qualitative deficits. aPTT and prothrombin time (PT) both test for acquired or inherited factor deficiencies and are not useful to determine platelet function.[15,32,36]

Viscoelastic testing: thrombocytopenia

There are very limited data to support the use of thromboelastography (TEG) before neuraxial anesthesia in parturients with thrombocytopenia. TEG is a point of care test which measures whole blood clotting and provides information about all phases of coagulation, fibrinolysis, and platelet function.[37] Small studies with healthy parturients, those with preeclampsia, and case reports suggest TEG is a useful adjunctive tool in addition to history, physical examination, and traditional measures of coagulation. In a study of 172 healthy term pregnancies (18 of whom had platelets <100,000 × 10^6/L), there was a positive correlation between TEG-derived maximum amplitude (MA) and platelet counts.[37] An MA cutoff of 53 mm has been suggested as a lower limit for pregnancy that is a surrogate marker for adequate hemostasis.

Additional TEG studies demonstrate a trend toward alterations in the hypercoagulable state in preeclamptic women. The same MA of less than 53 mm correlated with severe preeclampsia and platelets less than 75,000 × 10^6/L. The clinical correlation between these findings and the risk of SEH is unclear. Although the addition of TEG is useful in evaluating parturients with thrombocytopenia, identified parameters do not yet exist that suggest a reduced risk of SEH.[38–40]

RECOMMENDATIONS

Hypocoagulable states as suggested by pharmacologic thromboprophylaxis or thrombocytopenia in the parturient present unique challenges in obstetric management for the anesthesiologist, specifically regarding who is "safe" for neuraxial anesthesia given the numerous benefits when compared with general anesthesia. A quick but thorough and evidence-based application of these guidelines can help clinicians and patients make informed decisions about when to proceed with neuraxial anesthesia in parturients with thromboprophylaxis or TCP, especially when time is of the essence. Careful coordination with the obstetric team, nursing staff, and the patient is paramount to a successful outcome. Relevant metrics to consider are maternal comorbidities, obstetric concerns, fetal well-being, delivery plan, risks of difficult airway, risks of general anesthesia, rescue equipment and personnel availability, and patient preference.

Steps to assess a patient with thrombocytopenia

Step 1: Assess whether the patient may have a life-threatening condition (DIC) or suspected underlying coagulation disorder due to thrombocytopenia. If yes, it may be unsafe to proceed with neuraxial anesthesia. If the patient's thrombocytopenia is due to gestational TCP, hypertensive disorders, or ITP, proceed to Step 2.

Step 2: Assess platelet values and trends. In the absence of additional concerning risk factors:

- greater than $100,000 \times 10^6$/L: risk of SEH is reasonably low. OK to proceed with neuraxial anesthesia
- 70 to $100,000 \times 10^6$/L: risk of SEH is reasonably low. OK to proceed with neuraxial anesthesia
- 50 to $70,000 \times 10^6$/L: certain high-risk circumstances may warrant the use of neuraxial anesthesia in favor of the risks of general anesthesia. Multidisciplinary discussion is needed.
- less than $50,000 \times 10^6$/L: risk of SEH may be clinically significant and avoiding neuraxial anesthesia is reasonable.

Special circumstances

- HELLP syndrome: HELLP is a recognized complication of preeclampsia. Identifying those with HELLP may be challenging due to the lack of hypertension in up to 15% of these patients. As discussed earlier, elevations in LDH, AST, and ALT and severe TCP may suggest the diagnosis. Due to unpredictable drop in platelets in this subset, and the demonstrated benefits of in situ neuraxial anesthesia, anesthesia providers may consider prioritizing placement of early neuraxial anesthesia when the platelets are within a safe range, usually within 6 hours of last laboratory values.
- High-risk delivery providers should consider maternal comorbidities, obstetric complications or concerns, airway examination, and the possible need for urgent or emergent general anesthesia.
- Risk of SEH in a patient with an unknown diagnosis for thrombocytopenia less than $70,000 \times 10^6$/L is not clear. This situation may require further laboratory and clinical assessment.[15,41]

Pharmacologic thromboprophylaxis

Ideally, the labor unit should have a tailored protocol for how to navigate low, intermediate, and high-dose UFH and LMWH in elective and urgent procedures for parturients on pharmacologic thromboprophylaxis. Elective procedures may include induction of labor and planned CD. Obstetricians, nurses, patients, and anesthesiologists should all be involved in the decision making regarding the risk of SEH than the benefits of neuraxial techniques, particularly for vaginal and CD.

Consider the following framework for deciding suitability for neuraxial anesthetic techniques, based on the type of heparin, dose and timing, and urgency of the procedure.

For prophylactic low-dose UFH dosing and elective procedures: 5000 U twice daily or 3 times daily
- greater than 4 hrs since the last dose: can proceed with neuraxial
- less than 4 hours since the last dose AND aPTT levels available: can proceed with neuraxial

For prophylactic low-dose UFH dosing and urgent procedures: 5000 U twice daily or three times daily
- greater than 4 hrs since the last dose: can proceed with neuraxial
- less than 4 hours since the last dose: risk/benefit assessment of general anesthesia versus SEH. In select circumstances, it may be OK to proceed with neuraxial anesthesia.

For prophylactic intermediate-dose UFH and elective procedures: 7000 to 10,000 twice daily (<20,000 U per day)
- greater than 12 hours from the last dose: OK to proceed with neuraxial anesthesia
- less than 12 hours from the last dose AND normal aPTT: assess risk/benefit assessment of general anesthesia versus SEH. In select circumstances, it may be OK to proceed with neuraxial anesthesia.

For prophylactic intermediate-dose UFH and urgent procedures: 7000 to 10,000 twice daily (<20,000 U per day)
- less than 12 hours from the last dose: obtain aPTT and perform risk/benefit assessment of general anesthesia versus SEH. In select circumstances, it may be OK to proceed with neuraxial anesthesia.

For prophylactic high-dose UFH and elective procedures: Individual dose greater than 10,000 U per dose or total daily dose greater than 20,000 U
- greater than 24 hours since the last dose AND normal aPTT: OK to proceed with neuraxial
- less than 24 hours since the last dose: minimal data to describe the risk of SEH. It may be reasonable to avoid neuraxial anesthesia.

For prophylactic high-dose UFH and urgent procedures: Individual dose greater than 10,000 U per dose or total daily dose greater than 20,000 U
- less than 24 hours since the last dose: minimal data to describe the risk of SEH. It may be reasonable to avoid neuraxial anesthesia.

For prophylactic low-dose LMWH and elective procedures: Enoxaparin less than 40 mg SQ Daily or 30 mg SQ BID or dalteparin 5000 U SQ once daily
- greater than 12 hours since the last dose: Ok to proceed with neuraxial anesthesia
- less than 12 hours since the last dose: risk of SEH may be increased with neuraxial anesthesia.

For prophylactic low-dose LMWH and urgent procedures:
Enoxaparin less than 40 mg SQ Daily or 30 mg SQ BID or dalteparin 5000 U SQ once daily
- less than 12 hours since the last dose: insufficient data to guide management. Perform risk/benefit assessment of general anesthesia versus SEH. In select circumstances, it may be OK to proceed with neuraxial anesthesia.

For prophylactic intermediate-dose LMWH and elective or urgent procedures:
Enoxaparin: greater than 40 mg SQ daily, greater than 30 mg BID, less than 1 mg/kg SQ BID, or 1.5 mg/kg SQ daily
Dalteparin greater than 5000 U SQ daily
- Not enough evidence to suggest an appropriate time interval between 12 and 24 hours to wait before proceeding with neuraxial.
- In elective procedures may defer for 24 hours
- In urgent procedures, must weigh risks, and benefits of procedure between 12 and 24 hours

For high-dose LMWH and elective or urgent procedures:
Enoxaparin 1 mg/kg SQ twice daily or 1.5 mg/kg SQ daily
Dalteparin 120 U/kg SQ twice daily or 200 U/kg twice daily
- greater than 24 hours since the last dose: OK to proceed with neuraxial anesthesia
- less than 24 hours: risk of SEH may be increased with neuraxial anesthesia.[13]

SUMMARY

Neuraxial anesthesia has numerous benefits in obstetric patients than general anesthesia. Avoidance of maternal airway, minimizing the risk of anesthetic complications due to general anesthesia, and optimizing delivery outcomes are some of the known benefits. Occasionally, obstetric anesthesiology clinicians will encounter parturients who have relative contraindications to neuraxial anesthesia. These include those on pharmacologic thromboprophylaxis to VTE or those who have thrombocytopenia. Pharmacologic thromboprophylaxis and thrombocytopenia are risk factors for SEH. Maternal physiologic adaptations in coagulation status alter responses to anticoagulation and lower platelet counts in pregnancy than nonpregnant peers. In urgent, high-risk patient care scenarios, timely assessment of pharmacologic thromboprophylaxis for VTE or etiology and extent of thrombocytopenia can allow safe placement of neuraxial anesthesia in select obstetric patients who would otherwise have a perceived elevated risk of SEH.

CLINICS CARE POINTS

- In parturients with thrombocytopenia or thromboprophylaxis, consider following the SOAP guidelines when evaluating patients for neuraxial anesthetic techniques.
- Evaluate whether there is a dynamic underlying cause to a patient's unexplained thrombocytopenia that may worsen over time.
- Advanced hemostatic techniques (such as TEG) can augment standard laboratory evaluation of possible hypocoagulable states.

DISCLOSURE

The authors have nothing to disclose.

REFERENCES

1. Brenner B. Haemostatic changes in pregnancy. Thromb Res 2004;114:409–14.
2. American College of Obstetricians and Gynecologists' Committee on Practice Bulletins–Obstetrics. ACOG practice bulletin no. 197: inherited thrombophilias in pregnancy. Obstet Gynecol 2018;132(1):e18–34.
3. Burke N, Flood K, Murray A, et al. Platelet reactivity changes significantly throughout all trimesters of pregnancy compared with the nonpregnant state: a prospective study. BJOG 2013;120(13):1599–604.
4. Norris LA, Gleeson N, Sheppard BL, et al. Whole blood platelet aggregation in moderate and severe pre-eclampsia. Br J Obstet Gynaecol 1993;100:684–8.
5. Abduljalil K, Furness P, Johnson TN, et al. Anatomical, physiological and metabolic changes with gestational age during normal pregnancy. Clin Pharmacokinet 2012;51:365–96.
6. Aster RH. Pooling of platelets in the spleen: role in the pathogenesis of "hypersplenic" thrombocytopenia. J Clin Invest 1966;45(5):645–57.
7. Almog B, Shehata F, Aljabri S, et al. Placenta weight percentile curves for singleton and twins deliveries. Placenta 2011;32:58–62.
8. Reese JA, Peck JD, Deschamps DR, et al. Platelet counts during pregnancy. N Engl J Med 2018;379(1):32–43.
9. Reese JA, Peck JD, McIntosh JJ, et al. Platelet counts in women with normal pregnancies: A systematic review. Am J Hematol 2017;92(11):1224–32.
10. D'Alton ME, Friedman AM, Smiley RM, et al. National Partnership for maternal safety: consensus bundle on venous thromboembolism. Obstet Gynecol 2016;128(4):688–98.
11. Ghaji N, Boulet SL, Tepper N, et al. Trends in venous thromboembolism among pregnancy-related hospitalizations, United States, 1994-2009. Am J Obstet Gynecol 2013;209(5):433.e1–8.
12. Friedman AM, Ananth CV, Prendergast E, et al. Thromboembolism incidence and prophylaxis during vaginal delivery hospitalizations. Am J Obstet Gynecol 2015;212(2):221.e1-12.
13. Leffert L, Butwick A, Carvalho B, et al. The society for obstetric anesthesia and perinatology consensus statement on the anesthetic management of pregnant and postpartum women receiving thromboprophylaxis or higher dose anticoagulants. Anesth Analg 2018;126(3):928–44.
14. ACOG practice bulletin no. 207: thrombocytopenia in pregnancy. Obstet Gynecol 2019;133(3):e181–93.
15. Bauer ME, Arendt K, Beilin Y, et al. The society for obstetric anesthesia and perinatology interdisciplinary consensus statement on neuraxial procedures in obstetric patients with thrombocytopenia. Anesth Analg 2021;132(6):1531–44.
16. Webert KE, Mittal R, Sigouin C, et al. A retrospective 11-year analysis of obstetric patients with idiopathic thrombocytopenic purpura. Blood 2003;102(13):4306–11.
17. Chaiworapongsa T, Chaemsaithong P, Yeo L, et al. Pre-eclampsia part 1: current understanding of its pathophysiology. Nat Rev Nephrol 2014;10(8):466–80.
18. Beilin Y, Katz DJ. Analgesia use among 984 women with preeclampsia: a retrospective observational single-center study. J Clin Anesth 2020;62:109741.

19. Romero R, Mazor M, Lockwood CJ, et al. Clinical significance, prevalence, and natural history of thrombocytopenia in pregnancy-induced hypertension. Am J Perinatol 1989;6(1):32–8.
20. Lippi G, Plebani M. EDTA-dependent pseudothrombocytopenia: further insights and recommendations for prevention of a clinically threatening artifact. Clin Chem Lab Med 2012;50(8):1281–5.
21. Davis SM, Branch DW. Thromboprophylaxis in pregnancy: who and how? Obstet Gynecol Clin North Am 2010;37(2):333–43.
22. Improving health care response to maternal venous thromboembolism (California Maternal Quality Care Collaborative Toolkit to transform maternity care) Developed under contract #11-10006 with the California Department of Public Health; Maternal, Child and Adolescent Health Division; To be published by the California Maternal Quality Care Collaborative; Personal Correspondence with Doug Montgomery. Available at: https://www.cmqcc.org/resources-tool-kits/toolkits. Accessed September 29, 2021.
23. Bates SM, Greer IA, Middeldorp S, et al. VTE, thrombophilia, antithrombotic therapy, and pregnancy: antithrombotic therapy and prevention of thrombosis, 9th ed: American College of Chest Physicians Evidence-Based Clinical Practice Guidelines. Chest 2012;141:e691S–736S.
24. Moen V, Dahlgren N, Irestedt L. Severe neurological complications after central neuraxial blockades in Sweden 1990-1999. Anesthesiology 2004;101(4):950–9.
25. Leffert LR, Dubois HM, Butwick AJ, et al. Neuraxial anesthesia in obstetric patients receiving thromboprophylaxis with unfractionated or low-molecular-weight heparin: a systematic review of spinal epidural hematoma. Anesth Analg 2017; 125(1):223–31.
26. D'Angelo R, Smiley RM, Riley ET, et al. Serious complications related to obstetric anesthesia: the serious complication repository project of the society for obstetric anesthesia and perinatology. Anesthesiology 2014;120:1505–12.
27. Bateman BT, Mhyre JM, Ehrenfeld J, et al. The risk and outcomes of epidural hematomas after perioperative and obstetric epidural catheterization: a report from the multicenter perioperative outcomes group research consortium. Anesth Analg 2013;116:1380–5.
28. Bauer ME, Toledano RD, Houle T, et al. Lumbar neuraxial procedures in thrombocytopenic patients across populations: A systematic review and meta-analysis. J Clin Anesth 2020;61:109666.
29. Beilin Y, Katz DJ. Analgesia use among 984 women with preeclampsia: a retrospective observational single-center study. J Clin Anesth 2020;62:109741.
30. Lee LO, Bateman BT, Kheterpal S, et al. Risk of epidural hematoma after neuraxial techniques in thrombocytopenic parturients: a report from the multicenter perioperative outcomes group. Anesthesiology 2017;126(6):1053–63.
31. Levy N, Goren O, Cattan A, et al. Neuraxial block for delivery among women with low platelet counts: a retrospective analysis. Int J Obstet Anesth 2018;35:4–9.
32. Practice guidelines for obstetric anesthesia: an updated report by the american society of anesthesiologists task force on obstetric anesthesia and the society for obstetric anesthesia and perinatology. Anesthesiology 2016;124(2):270–300.
33. Mhyre JM, Sultan P. General anesthesia for cesarean delivery: occasionally essential but best avoided. Anesthesiology 2019;130(6):864–6.
34. Hawkins JL, Chang J, Palmer SK, et al. Anesthesia-related maternal mortality in the United States: 1979-2002. Obstet Gynecol 2011;117(1):69–74.

35. Guglielminotti J, Landau R, Li G. Adverse events and factors associated with potentially avoidable use of general anesthesia in cesarean deliveries. Anesthesiology 2019;130(6):912–22.

36. Working Party, Association of Anaesthetists of Great Britain & Ireland, Obstetric Anaesthetists' Association, Regional Anaesthesia UK. Regional anaesthesia and patients with abnormalities of coagulation: the Association of Anaesthetists of Great Britain & Ireland The Obstetric Anaesthetists' Association Regional Anaesthesia UK [published correction appears in Anaesthesia. 2016 Mar;71(3):352]. Anaesthesia 2013;68(9):966–72.

37. Beilin Y, Arnold I, Hossain S. Evaluation of the platelet function analyzer (PFA-100) vs. the thromboelastogram (TEG) in the parturient. Int J Obstet Anesth 2006; 15(1):7–12.

38. Orlikowski CE, Rocke DA, Murray WB, et al. Thrombelastography changes in pre-eclampsia and eclampsia. Br J Anaesth 1996;77(2):157–61.

39. Sharma SK, Philip J, Whitten CW, et al. Assessment of changes in coagulation in parturients with preeclampsia using thromboelastography. Anesthesiology 1999; 90(2):385–90.

40. Huang J, McKenna N, Babins N. Utility of thromboelastography during neuraxial blockade in the parturient with thrombocytopenia. AANA J 2014;82(2):127–30.

41. Sibai BM. Diagnosis, controversies, and management of the syndrome of hemolysis, elevated liver enzymes, and low platelet count. Obstet Gynecol 2004;103(5 Pt 1):981–91.

Enhanced Recovery after Surgery: Cesarean Delivery

Laura L. Sorabella, MD*, Jeanette R. Bauchat, MD, MS

KEYWORDS

- Cesarean delivery • Enhanced recovery after surgery • Enhanced recovery pathway
- Cesarean section

KEY POINTS

- Implementation of enhanced recovery after surgery (ERAS) protocols for cesarean deliveries (CDs) can have a large impact on population-based patient outcomes and medical resource consumption.
- ERAS for CD (ERAC) protocols have similar elements to ERAS protocols in the nonobstetric surgical population but also include unique elements to the peripartum period.
- ERAC requires multidisciplinary collaboration with multiple stakeholders including the patients, nursing staff, lactation consultants, obstetricians, anesthesiologists, and neonatologists.
- Anesthesiologists are critical members to ensure anesthesia-specific evidence-based practices and guidelines are incorporated into individual institutional ERAC protocols.

INTRODUCTION: PRINCIPLES OF ENHANCED RECOVERY AFTER SURGERY

Enhanced recovery after surgery (ERAS) is a perioperative management strategy that aims to improve the care of surgical patients from preoperative planning through their postoperative recovery. ERAS protocols are designed to minimize the physiologic stress of surgery and accelerate the return to normal function. When implemented successfully, ERAS protocols improve patient outcomes and satisfaction scores.[1] Institutions implementing ERAS protocols see improved efficiency with reduced lengths of stay and lower complications and costs.[1,2] ERAS protocol origins came from colorectal surgery but was adapted to almost every surgical subspecialty and procedure and now for CD.

Although ERAS protocols vary by specialty surgery, common themes include patient education/participation and standardized preoperative, intraoperative, and postoperative elements. ERAS protocols include common elements such as hemoglobin

Vanderbilt University Medical Center, 1211 Medical Center Drive, VUH 4202, Nashville, TN 37232, USA
* Corresponding author.
E-mail address: Laura.l.sorabella@vumc.org
Twitter: @jrbcpyw (J.R.B.)

Anesthesiology Clin 39 (2021) 743–760
https://doi.org/10.1016/j.anclin.2021.08.012   anesthesiology.theclinics.com
1932-2275/21/© 2021 Elsevier Inc. All rights reserved.

optimization, fluid and nutritional management, prevention of intraoperative and post-operative nausea and vomiting, infection prevention, multimodal analgesia, venous thromboembolism prophylaxis, promotion of early mobility, removal of urinary catheters, return of bowel function, and discharge planning. Individual ERAS protocols include unique elements based on scientific evidence for that particular subspecialty surgery. In ERAS for CD, uterotonic administration, delayed umbilical cord clamping, promotion of maternal rest, and breastfeeding support are unique additions.

WHY IS ENHANCED RECOVERY AFTER SURGERY FOR CESAREAN DELIVERY (ENHANCED RECOVERY AFTER CESAREAN) IMPORTANT?

CD is the most common major surgery worldwide, encompassing nearly 18.5 million births annually.[3] Approximately 1 in 3 women in the United States will deliver via cesarean. Unlike other major abdominal surgeries, cesarean deliveries (CDs) are unique in their expectation for rapid and complete maternal functional recovery. Within 72 hours, a woman is expected to be able to care for herself, a newborn, and return to activities of daily living.

Implemented successfully, enhanced recovery after cesarean (ERAC) protocols will have a broad and meaningful impact worldwide. Cesarean rates and maternal morbidity and mortality continue to climb and standardization using the best-available scientific evidence is critical to ensure high quality and safe outcomes. ERAC protocols should provide a continuum of care that starts in preconception outreach and continues through postpartum care. ERAC protocols can reduce variation and bias in practice by individual providers and health care systems, reducing health care disparities and promoting equity across broad populations of mothers worldwide.[4] The United States has the highest financial costs for CDs and the potential financial benefits of lower complication rates using enhanced recovery pathways are staggering.[4–6]

This review highlights evidence-based perioperative elements for inclusion in an ERAS for CD protocol. There is a multitude of ERAS protocols for CD; however, for this review, we use the Society of Obstetric Anesthesiology and Perinatology (SOAP) Consensus Statement and Recommendations for ERAC to guide our discussion. **Table 1**[7]

ENHANCED RECOVERY AFTER CESAREAN PATHWAY ELEMENTS
Hemoglobin Optimization

The prevalence of anemia during pregnancy ranges from 17% to 31% with 20% of women having a Hgb less than 8 at delivery.[8] Iron deficiency is the most common cause of anemia[8,9] and is defined as Hgb 11.0 g/dL in the first and third trimesters, and 10.5 g/dL in the second trimester.[10] Maternal effects of anemia include fatigue, depression, decreased mental and physical performance, cardiovascular symptoms, increased risk for transfusion, insufficient milk production, poor temperature regulation, and increased risk of surgical site infection (SSI). Neonatal consequences can be significant including small for gestational age, intrauterine growth restriction, death in utero, doubled risk of preterm delivery, neonatal intensive care unit admission, infection, and increased risk of neurocognitive impairment.

The American College of Obstetricians and Gynecologists (ACOG) recommends that all pregnant women be screened for anemia, and that those with iron deficiency anemia are treated with supplemental iron.[10] Oral iron therapy is the recommended treatment of iron deficiency anemia, but requires 4 weeks of therapy for correction. Intravenous iron therapy is safe in pregnancy, and provides faster correction of anemia

Table 1
Summary of enhanced recovery after cesarean delivery elements

ERAS Element	Recommendation	Future Studies
Preoperative ERAS Cesarean delivery pathway elements		
1. Limit Fasting Interval	• No solids 8 h before surgery • Clear fluids up until 2 h before surgery	Unscheduled CD fasting recommendations and gastric ultrasound
2. Nonparticulate liquid carbohydrate loading	• Nonparticulate carbohydrate drinks 2 h before surgery in nondiabetics	Gestational diabetic population and carbohydrate loading practices
3. Patient education	• Create/disseminate educational materials with predelivery instructions, expectations, and enhanced recovery information before admission • Inform patients about ERAS for CD goals and the personalization of their care	Patient feedback on utility and improvement of educational materials
4. Lactation/breastfeeding preparation and education	Create handout or educational tool with information about breastfeeding, common obstacles and complications, resources, and support structures	ERAS effects on breastfeeding success
5. Hemoglobin optimization	Screen all pregnant women per ACOG guidelines for anemia; evaluate and treat as indicated (PO or IV iron)	• Most effective PO iron regimen • Use of IV iron therapy in preterm labor • Best tests for guiding iron therapy in pregnancy
Intraoperative ERAS Cesarean Delivery Pathway Elements		
1. Prevent spinal anesthesia-induced hypotension	• Maintain normotension • Use prophylactic vasopressor infusion	Vasopressor type and optimal dose and duration
2. Maintain normothermia	• Active warming • Warm IV fluids • OR Temperature to 25° Celsius	WHO recommended OR temperature effects on maternal and neonatal outcomes
3. Optimal uterotonic administration	• Use lowest effective dose of uterotonic to achieve adequate uterine tone	Novel uterotonics with less side effects

(*continued on next page*)

Table 1
(continued)

ERAS Element	Recommendation	Future Studies
4. Antibiotic prophylaxis	• Preincision antibiotics • Redose after 1500 mL blood loss and/or 4 h	Antibiotic type and frequency guidance of redosing with PPH
5. IONV/PONV prophylaxis	• Use prophylactic vasopressor infusion • Consider skipping uterine exteriorization • Use 2 or more prophylactic IV antiemetic medications	• Optimal antiemetic drug combinations for CD • Risk stratification tool validated in the obstetric population

6. Initiate multimodal analgesia	• Neuraxial low-dose, long-acting opioid
	• Start nonopioid analgesia preop or in OR when possible
	  ○ IV NSAID
	  ○ Acetaminophen
	  ○ Local anesthetic blocks as indicated
		• Optimal timing of scheduled nonopioid analgesic medications
		• Regional blocks as rescue analgesia
		• Analgesic regimen in women with opioid use disorder

7. Promote breastfeeding and maternal–infant bonding	Skin-to-skin contact between mother and infant as soon as possible	Impact of intraoperative skin to skin on breastfeeding and neonatal hypothermia outcomes
8. Intravenous fluid optimization	Limit IV fluids to < 3L	Optimal fluid administration for unscheduled CD
9. Delayed umbilical cord clamping	Delay cord clamping $\geq$60 s in vigorous infants	Comparisons of cord milking practices vs delayed cord clamping practices
Postoperative ERAS Cesarean Delivery Pathway Elements		
1. Early oral intake	• Ice chips or water within 60 min in PACU • Lock IV as soon as taking orals and infusions complete • Advance to regular diet 4 h postpartum	• Optimal early oral intake regimen studies • Standardize recommendations across professional society guidelines
2. Early mobilization	• Ambulate when motor function returned • Increase frequency throughout stay	Optimal amount of mobility to promote recovery
3. Promote maternal rest	Optimize environment for sleep and recovery by clustering visits, interventions, and disturbances	Patient-centered outcomes with cluster visits

(continued on next page)

Table 1
(continued)

ERAS Element	Recommendation	Future Studies
4. Early urinary catheter removal	• Urinary catheter removed by 6–12 h • Establish protocol to manage urinary retention after removal	Evaluate urinary tract infection rates following ERAS protocol implementation
5. Venous thromboembolism prophylaxis	• Follow ACOG and ACCP guidelines to create institutional practice	Standardize recommendations across professional society guidelines for thromboprophylaxis
6. Facilitate early discharge	• Standardize and coordinate discharge planning which begins in the preadmission period • Personalize discharge analgesia plans including # opioid tablets • Use metrics to monitor for appropriate early discharges	• Patient understanding of discharge instructions • Patient-centered and safety outcomes with follow-up before traditional 6 wk
7. Anemia remediation	• Monitor for and treat anemia when indicated	Protocols for optimal transfusion thresholds in the postpartum period
8. Breastfeeding support	• Establish robust institutional lactation support protocols	See above

9. Multimodal analgesia	• Establish multimodal analgesia protocol to include
	  ○ Low-dose long-acting neuraxial opioid
	  ○ Scheduled acetaminophen and NSAID
	  ○ Local anesthetic techniques (TAP, QL) as indicated
		See above

10. Glycemic control	• Prioritize diabetics early in case order • Maintain normoglycemia using institutional protocol based on ACOG guideline	• Optimal glucose management in the postpartum period to prevent surgical site infection • Optimal blood glucose level during CD to prevent SSI and neonatal hypoglycemia • Pump settings for Type1 DM during CD

(continued on next page)

Table 1 (continued)		
ERAS Element	Recommendation	Future Studies
11. Promote return of bowel function	• Minimize systemic opioids • Encourage chewing gum and use of bowel medications • Encourage early mobility	• Optimal bowel regimens • Patient-centered outcomes and input in bowel regimens

Abbreviations: ACCP, American College of Chest Physicians; ACOG, American College of Obstetricians and Gynecologists; CD, cesarean delivery; ERAS, enhanced recovery after surgery; IV, intravenous; IONV/PONV, intraoperative/postoperative nausea vomiting; mg, milligram; L, liter; NSAID, nonsteroidal antiinflammatory drugs; PACU, postanesthesia care unit; PO, oral; QL, quadratus lumborum; TAP, transversus abdominus plane; WHO, World Health Organization.
Modified from Bollag L., Lim G., Sultan P. et al. Anesth Analg. 2021;132:1362 to 77.[7]

and repletion of iron stores but is more expensive.[11] The Network for the Advancement of Patient Blood Management, Haemostasis, and Thrombosis with the International Federation of Gynecology and Obstetrics (FIGO) and the European Board and College of Obstetrics and Gynecology recommend using intravenous iron therapy in women with Hgb less than 8 G/dL or if a woman cannot take or does not respond to oral iron therapy by an increase of 1 to 2 G/dL in 2 to 4 weeks.[12]

Perinatal anemia prevention is associated with transfusion avoidance and also quicker postpartum recovery and psychological benefits such as reduced postpartum depression and anxiety.[11,12] Identification and treatment of postpartum anemia should occur by postdelivery day 1 or 2, particularly in patients with postpartum hemorrhage (PPH) or preexisting anemia.[11] Treatment with either oral or intravenous iron formulations are acceptable, although intravenous formulations offer increased efficacy when compared with oral at 6 weeks postpartum visits.[11]

Fluid, Nutritional, and Digestive Optimization

Fluid optimization

Fluid optimization starts with appropriate institutional guidelines for fasting before the scheduled surgery. Most ERAS guidelines follow the American Society of Anesthesiologists (ASA) fasting guidelines to minimize the risk of aspiration during general anesthesia while also encouraging carbohydrate-containing liquids up to 2 hours before surgery to minimize dehydration and fasting ketosis.[13,14] **Box 1** These fasting guidelines apply to scheduled, healthy patients including those scheduled for CDs. These guidelines do not necessarily apply to CDs following labor or unscheduled CDs for fetal or maternal indications. Communication with the obstetric team must determine the urgency of the CD and this weighed against the risk of maternal aspiration.

Intraoperative fluid and vasopressor management strategies compensate for the expected hemodynamic changes from a regional sympathectomy, blood loss during CD, and vasodilation from uterotonic agent administration. A Cochrane review summarized the most effective methods to prevent hypotension under spinal anesthesia and demonstrated a coload of colloid or crystalloid with the spinal procedure to be more effective than preloading or no fluid administration.[15] Optimal intraoperative fluid management has been studied within the context of spinal sympathectomy in the obstetric population and is not as restrictive as in the colorectal surgical population whereby excessive fluids can lead to postoperative complications.[16] Prophylactic

Box 1	
American society of anesthesiologists perioperative fasting guidelines	
Liquid/Food Type	**Minimum Fasting Time**
Clear Liquids (ie, water, nonpulp fruit juice, black coffee)	2 h
Nonhuman milk	6 h
Light meal (ie, dry toast)	6 h
Fatty meal	8 h

Modified from the Practice Guidelines for Preoperative Fasting and the Use of Pharmacologic Agents to Reduce Risk of Pulmonary Aspiration.[14]

vasopressor medications should be used following a spinal anesthetic to prevent maternal hypotension, as fluids alone are ineffective.[17]

Nutritional and digestive optimization

To minimize time spent in a fasting state, meet nutritional needs, and promote the return of bowel function, ERAS protocols allow a general diet soon after surgery.[16] Early oral intake accelerates the return of bowel function while reducing postsurgical catabolism, the surgical stress response, and improving insulin sensitivity.[16] Resumption of a regular diet within 2 hours of CD is recommended by the ERAS Society.[18] The SOAP consensus statement recommends restarting clear liquids within 1 hour and a general diet at 4 hours following CD.[7] A systematic review and meta-analysis demonstrated that early feeding reduced thirst and hunger leading to improved patient satisfaction, earlier solid food intake, faster return of bowel function, and shorter lengths of stay.[19] Another meta-analysis evaluating early feeding (before 8 hours) after CD, found no increased risk of bowel complications such as nausea, vomiting, diarrhea, distension, or ileus.[20]

Adequate hydration, gum chewing, and minimized opioid consumption can expedite the return of normal bowel function. Post-CD order sets should include promotility agents (ie, docusate, polyethylene glycol, simethicone) and their use should be encouraged by providers[21] The postcesarean diet should include foods rich in fiber to prevent constipation and substantial enough in calories to aid in breastmilk production.

Prevention of Intraoperative and Postoperative Nausea and Vomiting

Prophylactic antiemetics

Per the Apfel risk scoring tool for postoperative nausea and vomiting, the obstetric population is a high-risk population, carrying a 40% to 80% risk of PONV.[22] Typical risk factors include, being female, undergoing a gynecologic surgery, receiving neuraxial opioid, nonsmoking, and having a history of PONV or motion sickness.[22] Risk stratification tools have been applied to the obstetric population, but have not been validated in this population. Women presenting for CD may have additional risk factors for experiencing IONV/PONV such as a history of hyperemesis gravidarum, presenting in active labor, not fasting before surgery, or supine hypotension of pregnancy.

These women have at least 2 risk factors for PONV and require 2 intravenous agents for antiemetic prophylaxis.[22] Many of the antiemetics used to treat general surgery patients are also effective for CD.[23] This patient population usually wants to avoid sedation to experience their birth and breastfeed as soon as possible. The preferred prophylactic antiemetic strategy should use and exhaust antiemetics without sedating properties before using those that cause sedation. (Clinical Care Point 1) After prophylactic antiemetics are administered, antiemetic medication from a different class should be used for rescue treatment.[22] Scopolamine is generally avoided due to concerns for reduced breast milk production.[24] Acupressure at PC6 may be a promising intervention for intraoperative nausea.[23]

Vasopressor Infusions

In addition to antiemetic medications, maintaining mean arterial pressure (MAP) at baseline using fluids and prophylactic vasopressor infusions prevents IONV associated with the sympathectomy from spinal anesthesia.[17] Combining a coload of crystalloid or colloid with a prophylactic vasopressor infusion (phenylephrine or norepinephrine), is the most effective way to prevent nausea and vomiting associated with the hemodynamic instability of spinal anesthesia.[15,17] Preventing uterine exteriorization has been recommended to reduce the risk of IONV[7]; although a recent meta-analysis showed no reduction in IONV, in situ uterine repair was associated with reduced blood loss and faster return of bowel function.[25]

Clinical Care Point 1: optimal strategies to minimize IONV and PONV

Preoperative	Intraoperative	Postoperative
Nonsedating Prophylactic Antiemetics (2 of 3)	Maintain MAP at baseline using fluids and prophylactic vasopressors	Scheduled Nonopioid Analgesia
5-HT3 Antagonists	Not exteriorizing the uterus during surgery	Rescue Antiemetics[b]
Metoclopramide	Acupressure PC6	
Corticosteroid[a]	Rescue Antiemetics[b]	
	Haloperidol/droperidol	
	Antihistamine	
	NK1 receptor antagonists	
	Midazolam	

[a]If dexamethasone is used for prophylaxis, it should be administered after the spinal anesthetic to prevent perineal irritation.
[b]Rescue antiemetics should be an agent from another class of antiemetics not already used for prophylactic or rescue treatment.

Infection Prevention for Cesarean Delivery

SSIs complicate 2% to 7% of CDs[26] which translates to a significant health burden for women and a significant resource and financial burden for payors and hospital systems. Several risk factors are reported in the literature, including: subcutaneous hematomas, chorioamnionitis, ASA physical classification $\geq$3, smoking history, large incision, few prenatal visits, body mass index (BMI) >30 kg/m2, teaching service oversight, and lack of antibiotic prophylaxis and many others.[26] The Centers for Disease Control have guidelines for the prevention of SSI that are discussed later in discussion.[27]

Glycemic control

Parturients with diabetes mellitus (DM) and their neonates have higher rates of morbidity and mortality.[28] Tight maternal glucose control is desirable in the prenatal period to prevent maternal morbidity associated with large for gestational age infants.[28,29] The National Institute for Health and Care Excellence (NICE) emphasizes achieving maternal euglycemia during labor in pregnant women with DM to decrease the risk of neonatal hypoglycemia.[30] However, in the postoperative period, maternal glucose readings must be closely monitored as a rapid decline in insulin requirements puts her at risk for hypoglycemic episodes.

ERAS data on perioperative hyperglycemic outcomes recommend target glucose levels of less than 180 to 200 mg/dL in nonobstetric populations to reduce perioperative morbidity including SSI risk, but no optimal hemoglobinA1C "cut-off" to reduce SSI risk has been established.[27] Future studies should focus on glucose targets and SSI in the peripartum period to guide glycemic management in the CD population.

Glycemic control should begin in prenatal visits by educating patients about the impact of poor glucose control, for both mothers and their babies.[29,30] Furthermore, the future implications of a gestational diabetes diagnosis on their risk of cardiovascular, renal, and ocular health should be discussed. Dietary, weight, and exercise counseling should be offered in the peripartum period.

Skin preparation
Patients should shower the night before and cleanse the surgical area with soap or an antiseptic solution.[27] An alcohol-based solution is recommended for skin preparation and clippers instead of razors for hair removal to reduce the risk of SSI in CD.[31] Vaginal preparation with iodine is recommended to reduce the risk of postoperative endometritis, but does not reduce the risk of SSI.[31,32]

Prophylactic antibiotic administration
Antibiotic administration for SSI is beneficial and SSI should be in all ERAC protocols.[33,34] A first- or second-generation cephalosporin, given 30 to 60 minutes before incision is recommended. Many institutions use weight-based dosing though this is not proven in obstetrics. Azithromycin, given for unscheduled CDs, may further reduce the risk of postpartum infections of all causes.[33] Based on other surgical populations, antibiotics should be redosed at appropriate intervals and cephalosporins after 1500 mL of blood loss.[35,36]

Maintenance of normothermia
The benefits of active warming for the prevention of SSI are well-established in the general surgery population. Active warming during elective CD, with the combination of forced air and intravenous fluid warming is the most effective way to minimize a drop in core temperature; in addition, active warming has been shown to increase maternal comfort,[37] but its effectiveness in reducing SSI remains unproven. Unlike the general surgery population, higher temperature in the PACU has been linked with SSI in CD, likely due to underlying infections acquired during labor.[38] Neonatal hypothermia increases morbidity due to increased rates of respiratory distress syndrome and hypoglycemia, particularly in preterm and low birth weight babies.[39] The World Health Organization (WHO) recommends that operating room (OR) temperature be > 25° Celsius,[40] but the benefits to maternal or neonatal outcomes of implementing this recommendation have not been proven.[41]

Surgical technique for wound closure
A variety of surgical techniques are cited to enhance healing, but the number and quality of studies is limited.[42] The use of subcuticular closure is recommended to prevent wound separation because staple removal ≤4 days can lead to wound separation.[42] Other recommendations for surgical technique include: blunt expansion of a transverse uterine hysterotomy to reduce surgical blood loss, closure of the hysterotomy in 2 layers to reduce the risk of uterine rupture in future pregnancies, not closing the peritoneum to reduce operative times, and reapproximating tissue layers if the woman has more than 2 cm of subcutaneous tissue.[42]

UTEROTONIC ADMINISTRATION

An exhaustive review of risk factors for uterine atony and uterotonic agent use, dosing, and side effects is outside the scope of this review.[43,44] The uterotonics most commonly used include oxytocin or carbetocin, ergometrine, or methylergonovine, and prostaglandins (carboprost or misoprostol).[44] Most international agencies invested in women's health, including WHO, FIGO, and NICE recommend prophylactic use of uterotonics for all CDs to reduce the risk of PPH. The International consensus statement for use of uterotonics during CD was published by the Association of Anaesthetists in 2019 and recommends oxytocin and carbetocin as prophylactic first-line uterotonic agents to prevent PPH.[44] Ergonovine, methylergonovine, and prostaglandin agents can be used for the treatment of PPH and considered early if first-line agents fail.[44]

DELAYED UMBILICAL CORD CLAMPING

Performing delayed umbilical cord clamping for greater than 60 seconds in preterm infants (<37 weeks gestation), reduced incidence of newborn blood transfusions, length of hospital stay, and mortality.[45] Maternal hemorrhage and transfusion were not affected by delayed cord clamping.[45] For infant benefit, delayed cord clamping is recommended during preterm CD.

APPROACH TO MULTIMODAL ANALGESIA

Multimodal analgesia is a key component of every ERAS protocol, including CD.[7,46] CDs are performed primarily under neuraxial anesthesia to facilitate family–infant bonding, early breastfeeding,[47] minimize placenta transfer of systemic anesthetic medication, and avoid instrumenting the potentially difficult airway of pregnancy.[48] Postcesarean analgesia has been refined over time using low-dose neuraxial opioid analgesia and nonopioid multimodal analgesia.

Low dose, long-acting neuraxial opioid, (morphine, hydromorphone, or diamorphine) is considered the "gold standard" for postcesarean analgesia.[49,50] Neuraxial opioid is easily administered during the neuraxial technique, and maximizes analgesia while minimizing the usual side effects of high-dose systemic opioids required after major abdominal surgery. The minimization of pain, sedation, and nausea and vomiting is a critical requirement for new mothers to breastfeed and care for their infants quickly after major abdominal surgery.

If neuraxial anesthesia or neuraxial opioid is contraindicated, postcesarean analgesia can still be effective and systemic opioid-related side effects reduced using regional analgesic blocks paired with multimodal analgesia.[51,52] Effective regional blocks include fascial plane blocks, either transversus abdominis plane (TAP) blocks or quadratus lumborum (QL) blocks, or surgical wound infiltration techniques.[51,52] Although TAP blocks are effective in reducing pain and opioid consumption than placebo, overall analgesia is still inferior to long-acting neuraxial opioid analgesia.[51] TAP blocks and QL blocks are superior to surgical wound infiltration.[51] These techniques have shown no additional analgesic benefit when used in combination with neuraxial opioid analgesia.

Multimodal nonopioid analgesia in combination with neuraxial opioid minimizes the need for breakthrough systemic opioids and their related side effects.[46] Opioid side effects can delay recovery due to sedation, respiratory depression,[50] slowed gastric motility delaying return of bowel function, and nausea and vomiting.[46] An example of a common preoperative, intraoperative, and postoperative multimodal analgesic regimen is shown in Clinical Care Point 2. Scheduled combination therapy with acetaminophen and nonsteroidal antiinflammatory drugs (NSAIDs) is used.[46,53] The quantity of systemic opioid required during admission can be used to create an individualized outpatient opioid prescription and reduce the number of unused opioid tablets.[54] More unused opioid tablets postoperatively correlate with higher rates of opioid dependence for patients and their community,[55] so institutional protocols and patient education on this topic should be included in ERAS protocols.[56]

Clinical Care Point 2: Example of a multimodal analgesic regimen for cesarean delivery

Preoperative Analgesic Regimen	Intraoperative Analgesic Regimen	Postoperative Analgesic Regimen
Acetaminophen	Neuraxial Anesthetic Technique	NSAIDS (ie, ketorolac, diclofenac)
	Spinal Opioid	Acetaminophen
	Epidural Opioid	Rescue TAP block
	OR Regional Anesthetic Technique[a]	Oral opioid for breakthrough pain[b]
	Transversus Abdominis Plane Block	
	Quadratus Lumborum Block	
	Surgical Wound Infiltration	

[a]Regional anesthetic techniques can be used following a general anesthetic or as a rescue in those who fail neuraxial opioid analgesia.
[b]Protocols to reduce the number of opioid tablets prescribed on discharge should be used

PROMOTING EARLY MOBILIZATION

Early mobilization has been associated with lower thromboembolic risks, reduced insulin resistance levels, decreased muscle atrophy, and shorter lengths of stay. Excellent pain control using a multimodal analgesic regimen[57] and limiting factors such as ongoing intravenous infusions and indwelling urinary catheters[58] is critical to early mobilization. The SOAP consensus statement on ERAS for CDs recommends graduated mobilization following the recovery of motor strength after spinal anesthesia.[7] For example, a woman 0 to 8 hours postcesarean may sit on the edge of her bed, or get out of her bed to chair, or ambulate in her room whereas a woman on postcesarean day 2 should aim to walk the halls 3 to 4 times per day. Educating and setting expectations for patients regarding early mobilization starts in the preoperative patient education visit and materials.

EARLY URINARY CATHETER REMOVAL

Early removal of urinary catheters postcesarean allows patients to achieve early mobility goals as mentioned above, but also carries the added benefits of increased patient comfort, shorter lengths of stay and lower rates of urinary tract infections.[58–60] Current ERAS Society recommendations support immediate removal of urinary catheters postcesarean, but a Cochrane review demonstrated that urinary catheter placement itself was associated with increased time to first void, higher incidence of patient discomfort, delayed postoperative ambulation, and prolonged length of stay in uncomplicated CDs.[18,61] Not placing a urinary catheter may not be an option because the majority are placed to decompress the bladder to reduce the risk of bladder injury and postpartum uterine atony, but future ERAS protocols for CD may recommend immediate removal of urinary catheters in women not requiring close urine output monitoring. ERAS protocols should include strategies to manage urinary retention as long-acting neuraxial opioids and local anesthetics can cause detrusor muscle dysfunction.[61] Urinary catheters should be removed 6 to 12 hours post-CD per current SOAP recommendations.[7]

VENOUS THROMBOEMBOLISM PROPHYLAXIS

Maternal mortality from thromboembolism is preventable, and thromboprophylaxis protocols reduce maternal mortality associated with VTE.[62] VTE prophylaxis strategies can include either mechanical or pharmacologic techniques. One large US health system study demonstrated a reduction in mortality post-CD from VTE after implementation of universal mechanical compression.[63] The ERAS Society, ACOG, and the American College of Chest Physicians recommend mechanical prophylaxis in all ERAS patients and those undergoing CD regardless of pharmacologic therapy until the resumption of ambulation; they caution against the routine use of heparin in low-risk patients.[64,65] Institutions should risk-stratify women throughout the peripartum period to determine their ongoing risk of VTE as some risk factors, such as acute renal injury, may be dynamic and change throughout their hospitalization.[64,65] If a patient qualifies as high risk for VTE (1 or 2 risk factors present), chemoprophylaxis with heparin, or low-molecular-weight heparin should be prescribed.[62]

PROMOTING RESTING PERIODS

Women undergoing CD report higher levels of exhaustion and less sleep than women who deliver vaginally.[66,67] Sleep deprivation following CD has been associated with poor cognitive function, postpartum depression, more pain complaints, and breastfeeding problems.[67–69] Therefore, it is imperative for maternal recovery to minimize or consolidate interruptions from visitors and health care providers to facilitate maternal rest.[70] Although absent from the recommendations from the ERAS Society, the promotion of maternal rest is recommended by the SOAP ERAS for CD consensus statement.[7]

FACILITATING BREASTFEEDING

Prenatally, institutions should offer lactation and feeding educational materials and robust in-person support in the immediate hours after birth through discharge. ERAC protocols should provide patients early access to educational materials such as the WHO "Ten Steps for Successful Breastfeeding."[47] Studies demonstrate that adherence to these 10 step recommendations increases the early initiation of breastfeeding, exclusive breastfeeding, total duration of breastfeeding and lowers rates of maternal anxiety, and depression.[71] Research suggests that breastfeeding within the first "golden hour" of life is associated with longer duration of breastfeeding and lower infant death rates.[72]

FACILITATING EARLY DISCHARGE

Patient empowerment is critical to achieving enhanced recovery goals because patients who are empowered and educated about their care beforehand can play an active role in the decision-making processes during their peripartum care. Patient-oriented analgesic and discharge goals can be established preoperatively in birth classes and appointments with their care providers. Standardized preoperative education for patients and their support persons should encompass neonatal care plans, lactation education and support, and contraceptive planning[73] so that discharge can be facilitated as soon as care goals are achieved. Discharge instructions should be written in a standardized, succinct, and clear fashion and should be available in print in the patient's native language. A 2016 systematic review of 30 RCTs evaluating early discharge planning standardization across multiple patient groups in multiple medical specialties found a reduced risk of readmission in some patient groups as well as increased satisfaction in both the medical professionals and their patients.[74] Discharge planning should inform patients about appropriate recovery metrics such as The Perceived Readiness for Discharge After Birth Scale,[75] a validated scale that assesses a mothers' perception of readiness for discharge and identifies mothers at risk for postdischarge problems. Most postpartum visits occur 6 weeks after discharge, so patients should be educated on monitoring for postpartum complications[76] such as infection, preeclampsia, breast engorgement, vaginal hemorrhage, and postpartum depression and when to call their physicians or present for emergency care. Discharge planning should also consider neonatal readiness for discharge.

OUTCOME STUDIES FOR ERAC

The latest review on ERAC included 11 published studies and demonstrated a reduction in hospital stay and costs with no difference in readmission rates and mixed outcomes for breastfeeding success rates and opioid consumption.[6] The GRADE level of evidence for ERAC outcomes in systematic reviews is low or very low given the protocol heterogeneity among institutions and the inability to randomize patient care pathways for study purposes.[6,77]

SUMMARY

CD is a challenging surgical pathway to develop with ERAS strategies. There are essential components for 2 patients: a mother and a neonate (at times more than one). One patient must recover quickly enough to care for a newborn in 72 hours or less. For these reasons, CD is the optimal surgical pathway to be strengthened by ERAS pathways aiming to improve both maternal and neonatal outcomes and safety. Institutions with existing protocols for ERAC should have ongoing interdisciplinary quality improvement projects aimed at auditing outcomes and robust systems in place for continuous improvement within these protocols.

After establishing robust ERAC pathways for uncomplicated CD, innovation should turn toward optimizing ERAC for more challenging patient populations with appropriate pathway modifications. For example, with the rising rates of opioid-dependent mothers[78] this population will require unique modifications to the postcesarean analgesic regimens within ERAC. The complexity of maternal clinical care in labor and delivery units cannot be underestimated with rising complexity of obstetric cases, rising maternal and neonatal comorbidities, and worsening socioeconomic patient burden further challenge clinicians. The implementation of ERAC pathways requires highly functional relationships between all stakeholders involved in maternal clinical care and hospital system buy-in to support each element of the pathway.[1]

Successful implementation of ERAC pathways has been associated with improved patient satisfaction.[1] When women are pleased with their hospital delivery experience, they are more likely to return to that hospital system for care. In a recent survey, 82% of patients ranked customer service as the most influential factor for provider selection and brand loyalty.[79]

CLINICS CARE POINTS

- Many of the ERAS components for the general surgery population apply to ERAC and also improve maternal and hospital-related outcomes.

- ERAC also include components that improve infant outcomes, such as antepartum maternal anemia management, maintenance of infant normothermia, delayed cord clamping and breastfeeding facilitation.
- In ERAC, considerations for the use of non-sedating medications as first-line therapies in the mother for antiemetic prophylaxis and treatment and multimodal analgesic regimens are essential to facilitate maternal recovery and care of the infant.

DISCLOSURE

The authors have nothing to disclose.

REFERENCES

1. Ljungqvist O, Scott M, Fearon KC. Enhanced recovery after surgery: a review. JAMA Surg 2017;152(3):292–8.
2. Bisch SP, Wells T, Gramlich L, et al. Enhanced Recovery After Surgery (ERAS) in gynecologic oncology: system-wide implementation and audit leads to improved value and patient outcomes. Gynecol Oncol 2018;151(1):117–23.
3. Gibbons LBJ, Lauer JA, Betran AP, et al. The global numbers and costs of additionally needed and unnecessary caesaran sections performed per year: overuse as a barrier to universal coverage. In: World health report, background Paper No 30. 2010. Available at: https://www.who.int/healthsystems/topics/financing/healthreport/30C-sectioncosts.pdf.
4. White RS, Matthews KC, Tangel V, et al. Enhanced recovery after surgery (ERAS) programs for cesarean delivery can potentially reduce healthcare and racial disparities. J Natl Med Assoc 2019;111(4):464–5.
5. Hospital admission prices for a C-section delivery in selected countries in 2017 (in U.S. dollars). IFHP. Available at: https://www.statista.com/statistics/312028/cost-of-hospital-and-physician-for-a-c-section-delivery-by-country/. Accessed October 21, 2021.
6. Sultan P, Sharawi N, Blake L, et al. Enhanced recovery after caesarean delivery versus standard care studies: a systematic review of interventions and outcomes. Int J Obstet Anesth 2020;43:72–86.
7. Bollag L, Lim G, Sultan P, et al. Society for obstetric anesthesia and perinatology: consensus statement and recommendations for enhanced recovery after cesarean. Anesth Analg 2020;132(5):1362–77.
8. Breymann C. Iron deficiency anemia in pregnancy. Semin Hematol 2015;52(4): 339–47.
9. Milman N. Postpartum anemia II: prevention and treatment. Ann Hematol 2012; 91(2):143–54.
10. American College of O, Gynecologists. ACOG Practice Bulletin No. 95: anemia in pregnancy. Obstet Gynecol 2008;112(1):201–7.
11. Sultan P, Bampoe S, Shah R, et al. Oral vs intravenous iron therapy for postpartum anemia: a systematic review and meta-analysis. Am J Obstet Gynecol 2019;221(1):19–29.e3.
12. Munoz M, Pena-Rosas JP, Robinson S, et al. Patient blood management in obstetrics: management of anaemia and haematinic deficiencies in pregnancy and in the post-partum period: NATA consensus statement. Transfus Med 2018;28(1):22–39.
13. Carli F. Physiologic considerations of Enhanced Recovery After Surgery (ERAS) programs: implications of the stress response. Can J Anaesth 2015;62(2):110–9.

14. Practice guidelines for preoperative fasting and the use of pharmacologic agents to reduce the risk of pulmonary aspiration: application to healthy patients undergoing elective procedures: an updated report by the American Society of Anesthesiologists Task Force on preoperative fasting and the use of pharmacologic agents to reduce the risk of pulmonary aspiration. Anesthesiology 2017;126(3): 376–93.

15. Chooi C, Cox JJ, Lumb RS, et al. Techniques for preventing hypotension during spinal anaesthesia for caesarean section. Cochrane Database Syst Rev 2020;7: CD002251.

16. Thiele RH, Raghunathan K, Brudney CS, et al. American Society for Enhanced Recovery (ASER) and Perioperative Quality Initiative (POQI) joint consensus statement on perioperative fluid management within an enhanced recovery pathway for colorectal surgery. Perioper Med (Lond) 2016;5:24.

17. Ngan Kee WD. The use of vasopressors during spinal anaesthesia for caesarean section. Curr Opin Anaesthesiol 2017;30(3):319–25.

18. Macones GA, Caughey AB, Wood SL, et al. Guidelines for postoperative care in cesarean delivery: Enhanced Recovery After Surgery (ERAS) Society recommendations (part 3). Am J Obstet Gyneco 2019;221(3):247.e1–9.

19. Hsu YY, Hung HY, Chang SC, et al. Early oral intake and gastrointestinal function after cesarean delivery: a systematic review and meta-analysis. Obstet Gynecol 2013;121(6):1327–34.

20. Huang H, Wang H, He M. Early oral feeding compared with delayed oral feeding after cesarean section: a meta-analysis. J Matern Fetal Neonatal Med 2016;29(3): 423–9.

21. Charoenkwan K, Phillipson G, Vutyavanich T. Early versus delayed (traditional) oral fluids and food for reducing complications after major abdominal gynaecologic surgery. Cochrane Database Syst Rev 2007;(4):CD004508.

22. Gan TJ, Belani KG, Bergese S, et al. Fourth consensus guidelines for the management of postoperative nausea and vomiting. Anesth Analg 2020;131(2): 411–48.

23. Griffiths JD, Gyte GM, Paranjothy S, et al. Interventions for preventing nausea and vomiting in women undergoing regional anaesthesia for caesarean section. Cochrane Database Syst Rev 2012;(9):CD007579.

24. Drugs and Lactation Database (LactMed) [Internet]. Bethesda (MD): National Library of Medicine (US); 2006. Available at: https://www.ncbi.nlm.nih.gov/books/NBK501922/.

25. Zaphiratos V, George RB, Boyd JC, et al. Uterine exteriorization compared with in situ repair for Cesarean delivery: a systematic review and meta-analysis. Can J Anaesth 2015;62(11):1209–20.

26. Kawakita T, Landy HJ. Surgical site infections after cesarean delivery: epidemiology, prevention and treatment. Matern Health Neonatol Perinatol 2017;3:12.

27. Berrios-Torres SI, Umscheid CA, Bratzler DW, et al. Centers for disease control and prevention guideline for the prevention of surgical site infection, 2017. JAMA Surg 2017;152(8):784–91.

28. Negrato CA, Mattar R, Gomes MB. Adverse pregnancy outcomes in women with diabetes. Diabetol Metab Syndr 2012;4(1):41.

29. Dude A, Niznik CM, Szmuilowicz ED, et al. Management of diabetes in the intrapartum and postpartum patient. Am J Perinatol 2018;35(11):1119–26.

30. (UK) LNIfHaCE. Diabetes in pregnancy: management from preconception to the postnatal period. National Institute for Health and Care Excellence: Clinical Guidelines; 2020. Available at: https://www.nice.org.uk/guidance/ng3/

resources/diabetes-in-pregnancy-management-from-preconception-to-the-postnatal-period-pdf-51038446021. Accessed October 21, 2021.

31. American College of Obstetricians and Gynecologists Women's Health Care P, Committee on Gynecologic P. Committee Opinion No. 571: Solutions for surgical preparation of the vagina. Obstet Gynecol 2013;122(3):718–20.

32. Haas DM, Morgan S, Contreras K. Vaginal preparation with antiseptic solution before cesarean section for preventing postoperative infections. Cochrane Database Syst Rev 2014;(9):CD007892.

33. Practice Bulletin No. 199: Use of prophylactic antibiotics in labor and delivery: correction. Obstet Gynecol 2019;134(4):883–4.

34. Smaill FM, Grivell RM. Antibiotic prophylaxis versus no prophylaxis for preventing infection after cesarean section. Cochrane Database Syst Rev 2014;(10):CD007482.

35. Bratzler DW, Dellinger EP, Olsen KM, et al. Clinical practice guidelines for antimicrobial prophylaxis in surgery. Surg Infect (Larchmt) 2013;14(1):73–156.

36. Fay KE, Yee L. Applying surgical antimicrobial standards in cesarean deliveries. Am J Obstet Gynecol 2018;218(4):416 e1–4.

37. Sultan P, Habib AS, Cho Y, et al. The effect of patient warming during Caesarean delivery on maternal and neonatal outcomes: a meta-analysis. Br J Anaesth 2015; 115(4):500–10.

38. Edwards RK, Madani K, Duff P. Is perioperative hypothermia a risk factor for post-Cesarean infection? Infect Dis Obstet Gynecol 2003;11(2):75–80.

39. Allen TK, Habib AS. Inadvertent perioperative hypothermia induced by spinal anesthesia for cesarean delivery might be more significant than we think: are we doing enough to warm our parturients? Anesth Analg 2018;126(1):7–9.

40. WHO. Thermal Protection of the newborn: a practical guide. 1997:68. Available at: http://apps.who.int/iris/bitstream/handle/10665/63986/WHO_RHT_MSM_97.2. pdf;jsessionid=0C38C8BF019BF2CA67738C9954D04B1C?sequence=1. Accessed October 21, 2021.

41. Duryea EL, Nelson DB, Wyckoff MH, et al. The impact of ambient operating room temperature on neonatal and maternal hypothermia and associated morbidities: a randomized controlled trial. Am J Obstet Gynecol 2016;214(4):505.e1–7.

42. Caughey AB, Wood SL, Macones GA, et al. Guidelines for intraoperative care in cesarean delivery: enhanced recovery after surgery society recommendations (Part 2). Am J Obstet Gynecol 2018;219(6):533–44.

43. Ende HB, Lozada MJ, Chestnut DH, et al. Risk factors for atonic postpartum hemorrhage: a systematic review and meta-analysis. Obstet Gynecol 2021;137(2): 305–23.

44. Heesen M, Carvalho B, Carvalho JCA, et al. International consensus statement on the use of uterotonic agents during caesarean section. Anaesthesia 2019;74(10): 1305–19.

45. Fogarty M, Osborn DA, Askie L, et al. Delayed vs early umbilical cord clamping for preterm infants: a systematic review and meta-analysis. Am J Obstet Gynecol 2018;218(1):1–18.

46. Sutton CD, Carvalho B. Optimal pain management after cesarean delivery. Anesthesiol Clin 2017;35(1):107–24.

47. WHO. Ten steps to successful breastfeeding. Available at: www.who.int/activities/promoting-baby-friendly-hospitals/ten-steps-to-successful-breastfeeding. Accessed October 21, 2021.

48. Mushambi MC, Kinsella SM, Popat M, et al. Obstetric Anaesthetists' Association and Difficult Airway Society guidelines for the management of difficult and failed tracheal intubation in obstetrics. Anaesthesia 2015;70(11):1286–306.

49. Practice guidelines for obstetric anesthesia: an updated report by the American Society of Anesthesiologists Task Force on obstetric anesthesia and the society for obstetric anesthesia and perinatology. Anesthesiology 2016;124(2):270–300.

50. Bauchat JR, Weiniger CF, Sultan P, et al. Society for obstetric anesthesia and perinatology consensus statement: monitoring recommendations for prevention and detection of respiratory depression associated with administration of neuraxial morphine for cesarean delivery analgesia. Anesth Analg 2019;129(2):458–74.

51. Sultan P, Sultan E, Carvalho B. Regional anaesthesia for labour, operative vaginal delivery and caesarean delivery: a narrative review. Anaesthesia 2021;76(Suppl 1):136–47.

52. Gabriel RA, Burton BN, Curran BP, et al. Regional anesthesia abdominal blocks and local infiltration after cesarean delivery: review of current evidence. Curr Pain Headache Rep 2021;25(5):28.

53. ACOG Committee Opinion No. 742: postpartum pain management. Obstet Gynecol 2018;132(1):e35–43.

54. Osmundson SS, Raymond BL, Kook BT, et al. Individualized compared with standard postdischarge oxycodone prescribing after cesarean birth: a randomized controlled trial. Obstet Gynecol 2018;132(3):624–30.

55. Jones CM, Paulozzi LJ, Mack KA. Sources of prescription opioid pain relievers by frequency of past-year nonmedical use United States, 2008-2011. JAMA Intern Med 2014;174(5):802–3.

56. Shinnick JK, Ruhotina M, Has P, et al. Enhanced recovery after surgery for cesarean delivery decreases length of hospital stay and opioid consumption: a quality improvement initiative. Am J Perinatol 2020. https://doi.org/10.1055/s-0040-1709456.

57. Kehlet H, Wilmore DW. Multimodal strategies to improve surgical outcome. Am J Surg 2002;183(6):630–41.

58. Ahmed MR, Sayed Ahmed WA, Atwa KA, et al. Timing of urinary catheter removal after uncomplicated total abdominal hysterectomy: a prospective randomized trial. Eur J Obstet Gynecol Reprod Biol 2014;176:60–3.

59. Phipps S, Lim YN, McClinton S, et al. Short term urinary catheter policies following urogenital surgery in adults. Cochrane Database Syst Rev 2006;(2):CD004374.

60. Rousseau A, Sadoun M, Aime I, et al. [Comparative study about enhanced recovery after cesarean section: what benefits, what risks?]. [Etude comparative sur la rehabilitation amelioree postcesarienne : quels benefices, quels risques ?] Gynecol Obstet Fertil Senol 2017;45(7–8):387–92.

61. Abdel-Aleem H, Aboelnasr MF, Jayousi TM, et al. Indwelling bladder catheterisation as part of intraoperative and postoperative care for caesarean section. Cochrane Database Syst Rev 2014;(4):CD010322.

62. D'Alton ME, Friedman AM, Smiley RM, et al. National partnership for maternal safety: consensus bundle on venous thromboembolism. Anesth Analg 2016;123(4):942–9.

63. Clark SL, Christmas JT, Frye DR, et al. Maternal mortality in the United States: predictability and the impact of protocols on fatal postcesarean pulmonary embolism and hypertension-related intracranial hemorrhage. Am J Obstet Gynecol 2014;211(1):32, e1–9.

64. American College of Obstetricians, Gynecologists' Committee on Practice B-O. ACOG Practice Bulletin No. 196: thromboembolism in pregnancy. Obstet Gynecol 2018;132(1):e1–17.

65. Kearon C, Akl EA, Comerota AJ, et al. Antithrombotic therapy for VTE disease: Antithrombotic Therapy and Prevention of Thrombosis, 9th ed: American College of Chest Physicians Evidence-Based Clinical Practice Guidelines. Chest 2012; 141(2 Suppl):e419S–96S.

66. Lee SY, Lee KA. Early postpartum sleep and fatigue for mothers after cesarean delivery compared with vaginal delivery: an exploratory study. J Perinat Neonatal Nurs 2007;21(2):109–13.

67. Thompson JF, Roberts CL, Currie M, et al. Prevalence and persistence of health problems after childbirth: associations with parity and method of birth. Birth 2002; 29(2):83–94.

68. Clout D, Brown R. Sociodemographic, pregnancy, obstetric, and postnatal predictors of postpartum stress, anxiety and depression in new mothers. J Affect Disord 2015;188:60–7.

69. Dias CC, Figueiredo B. Breastfeeding and depression: a systematic review of the literature. J Affect Disord 2015;171:142–54.

70. ACOG Committee Opinion No. 766: approaches to limit intervention during labor and birth. Obstet Gynecol 2019;133(2):e164–73.

71. Perez-Escamilla R, Martinez JL, Segura-Perez S. Impact of the Baby-friendly Hospital Initiative on breastfeeding and child health outcomes: a systematic review. Matern Child Nutr 2016;12(3):402–17.

72. Group NS. Timing of initiation, patterns of breastfeeding, and infant survival: prospective analysis of pooled data from three randomised trials. Lancet Glob Health 2016;4(4):e266–75.

73. Ferguson S, Davis D, Browne J. Does antenatal education affect labour and birth? A structured review of the literature. Women Birth 2013;26(1):e5–8.

74. Goncalves-Bradley DC, Lannin NA, Clemson LM, et al. Discharge planning from hospital. Cochrane Database Syst Rev 2016;(1):CD000313.

75. Weiss ME, Ryan P, Lokken L. Validity and reliability of the Perceived Readiness for Discharge After Birth Scale. J Obstet Gynecol Neonatal Nurs 2006;35(1):34–45.

76. Provision of Care, Treatment, and Services standards for maternal safety. The Joint Commission. Available at: https://www.jointcommission.org/standards/r3-report/r3-report-issue-24-pc-standards-for-maternal-safety/. Accessed October 21, 2021.

77. Corso E, Hind D, Beever D, et al. Enhanced recovery after elective caesarean: a rapid review of clinical protocols, and an umbrella review of systematic reviews. BMC Pregnancy Childbirth 2017;17(1):91.

78. Patrick SW, Schumacher RE, Benneyworth BD, et al. Neonatal abstinence syndrome and associated health care expenditures: United States, 2000-2009. JAMA 2012;307(18):1934–40.

79. Available at: https://www.healthcaredive.com/news/new-hospital-ranking-looks-at-customer-loyalty/530930/. Accessed October 21, 2021.

Caring for Parturients with Substance Use Disorders

David L. Stahl, MD[a,*], Leslie J. Matthews, MD, PharmD[a,b]

KEYWORDS

- Substance use disorder • Medication-assisted treatment • Opioid use disorder
- Overdose • Maternal mortality • Maternal substance use
- Neonatal abstinence syndrome • Neonatal opioid withdrawal syndrome

KEY POINTS

- Substance use disorder, in particular opioid use disorder, is an increasingly common co-morbidity among obstetric patients.
- It is important to screen patients for substance use disorders throughout the prenatal period and connect patients with resources for treatment and support.
- Obstetric anesthesiologists must be familiar with the effects of acute intoxication and chronic use of various substances.
- Pain management can be challenging in this population, and nonconventional strategies, such as postpartum neuraxial analgesia, regional anesthesia, and multimodal pain control, may be beneficial.

NATURE OF THE PROBLEM

Imagine a group of dedicated professionals committed to reducing maternal mortality who meet two to three times per year to review all the cases of women who died while pregnant or within a year of being pregnant. Now consider the group realizing they would need to hold an entirely separate meeting just to review cases of unintentional overdose deaths: harrowing stories of toddlers finding pulseless mothers, case after case.

This was Ohio shortly before the COVID-19 pandemic, when the death rate from unintentional overdose among women of reproductive age jumped from 16.3 per 100,000 to 37.8 per 100,000 in 4 years (2012–2016), and pregnancy-associated deaths rose during the same time period, from 8 to 46.[1] This mirrors a Centers for Disease Control and Prevention (CDC) report, documenting a national 4-fold increase in opioid use disorder in pregnancy from 1999 to 2014.[2] One of the major public health concerns that have developed in the United States is the rise in substance use

[a] Department of Anesthesiology, The Ohio State University, 410 West 10th Avenue, Columbus, OH 43210, USA; [b] Department of Anesthesiology and Pain Medicine, Nationwide Children's Hospital, 700 Children's Drive, Columbus, OH 43205, USA
* Corresponding author.
E-mail address: david.stahl@osumc.edu
Twitter: @DoctorStahl (D.L.S.)

Anesthesiology Clin 39 (2021) 761–777
https://doi.org/10.1016/j.anclin.2021.08.006
1932-2275/21/© 2021 Elsevier Inc. All rights reserved.

anesthesiology.theclinics.com

disorders (SUDs). Particularly concerning is the rise in substance abuse in vulnerable patient populations, including adolescents and pregnant patients.[3]

Before clinical strategies to better care for parturients with SUD are discussed, it is important note the opportunities for awareness and advocacy around this issue. There is a 50-fold variability regarding state-specific prevalence of opioid use disorder documented at delivery hospitalization, with further in-state variability.[1,2] It is critical for providers to understand their local community, type of substance use, and prevalence of substance use to best care for these parturients. Given the persistent racial and ethnic disparities seen in treating pregnant patients with SUD, however, community understanding must include understanding these disparities and should not limit universal screening.[4] SUD in pregnancy also offers an outstanding opportunity for public health advocacy. Many states and communities have designed programs to target the multi-faceted nature of the disease (**Fig. 1**), but the need for ongoing advocacy persists.[5]

INTRODUCTION: DEFINITIONS AND HISTORY
Definitions

The *Diagnostic and Statistical Manual of Mental Disorders* (Fifth Edition) (*DSM-5*) uses 11 diagnostic criteria to define SUD.[6] Older literature describes substance use and

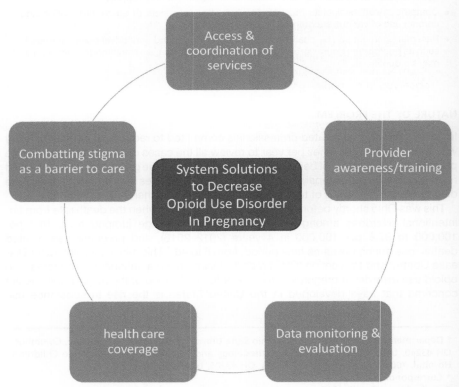

Fig. 1. Public health strategies to decrease rates of opioid use disorder in pregnancy have targeted access to care and funding, stigma, and the associated ethical/legal concerns, including requirements to involve child protective services, provider awareness and training, and access to and coordination of high-quality services. Increasingly, monitoring of data allows for assessment of programmatic successes.

dependence separately, and the *DSM-5* combines these into a single diagnosis with mild, moderate, or severe gradations based on the number of symptoms (**Fig. 2**).[6] For parturients, it may be particularly important to note the classifications of early remission and late remission because these may represent outcome-based treatment milestones.[7] Early remission is defined as no longer meeting criteria for SUD for 3 months to 12 months, and sustained remission as 12 months or longer.

For fetuses and neonates, a few definitions are worth reviewing. Fetal alcohol spectrum disorder is a broad description of the range of physical, developmental, behavioral, and cognitive effects that can occur in those exposed to prenatal alcohol. Neonatal abstinence syndrome (NAS) is an umbrella term that describes neonates at risk of withdrawal from multiple substances. Neonatal opioid withdrawal syndrome (NOWS) refers specifically to infants at risk for opioid withdrawal. Like rates of opioid-related deaths in

A **problematic pattern** of use of an intoxicating substance leading to ***clinically significant impairment or distress***, as manifested by ***at least two of the following***, occurring within a 12-month period. SUD is described by the substance and the severity (defined by the number of symptoms):
• The substance is often taken in larger amounts or over a longer period than was intended
• There is a persistent desire or unsuccessful efforts to cut down or control use of the substance.
• A great deal of time is spent in activities necessary to obtain the substance, use the substance, or recover from its effects.
• Craving, or a strong desire or urge to use the substance.
• Recurrent use of the substance resulting in a failure to fulfill major role obligations at work, school, or home.
• Continued use of the substance despite having persistent or recurrent social or interpersonal problems caused or exacerbated by the effects of its use.
• Important social, occupational, or recreational activities are given up or reduced because of use of the substance.
• Recurrent use of the substance in situations in which it is physically hazardous.
• Use of the substance is continued despite knowledge of having a persistent or recurrent physical or psychological problem that is likely to have been caused or exacerbated by the substance.
• Tolerance (either of the following):   i) A need for markedly increased amounts of the substance to achieve intoxication or desired effect.   ii) A markedly diminished effect with continued use of the same amount of the substance.
• Withdrawal (either of the following):   i) The characteristic withdrawal syndrome for other (or unknown) substance.   ii) The substance (or a closely related substance) is taken to relieve or avoid withdrawal symptoms.

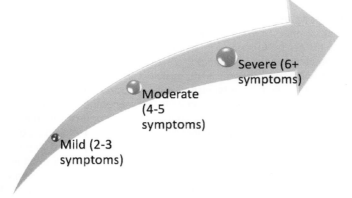

Severe (6+ symptoms)

Moderate (4-5 symptoms)

Mild (2-3 symptoms)

Fig. 2. Diagnostic criteria for SUD as described in the *DSM-5*. (*Reprinted with permission from* the Diagnostic and Statistical Manual of Mental Disorders, Fifth Edition, 2013:xliv, 947 p. (Copyright ©2013). American Psychiatric Association. All Rights Reserved.)

pregnancy, rates of NAS have increased significantly in the past decade with similar geographic heterogeneity, ranging from 1.3 per 1000 birth hospitalizations in Nebraska to 53.5 per 1000 birth hospitalizations in West Virginia.[8]

History

A cursory understanding of the history of both the public health and criminal justice systems can better inform providers in caring for parturients with SUD. Beginning with tobacco in the 1950s, there has been an increased understanding of the public health risks of substance use in pregnancy.[9] Unfortunately, this understanding has been enmeshed in enforcing the criminality of substance use, to both deter and punish people from using substances while pregnant.[10] These efforts are entwined in the debate about fetal personhood as well as pursuit of charges of child abuse against pregnant people who use drugs. Unfortunately, rather than deter substance use, these criminal justice efforts serve primarily as barriers to accessing care.[10] Mandatory reporting laws vary widely and providers should educate themselves on how these requirements have an impact on their patients.[11] Obstetric anesthesiologists should be aware of the legal concerns, societal stigma, and barriers to care faced by patients and how these may influence patients' disclosures of substances use. Fear of detection may lead, in the worst case, to isolation, pregnancy denial, avoidance of prenatal care, and withholding of information from providers.[10] These fears do not affect all patients uniformly. A descriptive study evaluated the criminal cases from 1973 to 2005, where pregnant people were criminally prosecuted for substance use, demonstrating a disproportionate enforcement against those who were poor or of color.[12] This history of racism can inform the social determinants of health as well as disparities in health care to better understand the risk factors of modern SUD. For example, many studies identify variables, such as race, or late initiation of prenatal care and missed appointments as risk factors for SUD. These factors themselves may be the results of decades of discriminatory criminal justice patterns that have left profound effects on the diagnosis, access to care, and treatment of pregnant people. Therefore, although the public health and criminal justice systems intersect at the uterus of parturients with SUD, it is critical for providers to be informed, be open, and maintain a universal screening program for substance use.

CURRENT EVIDENCE
Screening

As with any anesthetic encounter, a thorough preoperative or intrapartum evaluation of a patient is critical for effective management but also for anticipation and prevention of complications in the peripartum period. The Society for Maternal-Fetal Medicine, American College of Obstetricians and Gynecologists (ACOG), and American Society of Addiction Medicine (ASAM) report recommends routine screening for substance use for all pregnant patients at the first prenatal visit, but it is important to do a thorough history upon presentation for delivery, because patients with substance use history often have limited access to prenatal care and may not have been appropriately identified and optimized prior to delivery.[13,14] ACOG specifically notes that screening based on factors, such as poor adherence to prenatal care, may lead to stereotyping and stigma.[15] Several evidence-based screening tools exist, including the 4 Ps, National Institute on Drug Abuse Quick Screen, and CRAFFT.[15] These tools may take the form of a verbal conversation between patient and physician or nonphysician caregiver or can be part of the electronic medical record. These tools are superior to universal urine drug screens, which both are insensitive and can have false-positive results. Obstetric anesthesiologists should be aware of these tools and of motivational interviewing techniques that may be leveraged to utilize the perioperative period as teachable moments.[16,17] It also is important to be aware of treatment resources (or how to connect patients to knowledgeable team members); the adage, "ask, advise, connect" has been proposed to screen patients for substance use, advise quitting, and connect them to resources.[17]

Tobacco

Tobacco is the substance used most commonly during pregnancy, with reported smoking rates varying from 3% to 10% but possibly as high as 16%.[18,19] Smoking during pregnancy is associated with a plethora of negative outcomes, including spontaneous abortion (miscarriage), intrauterine growth restriction, premature rupture of membranes, and preterm labor.[20,21]

Anesthetic considerations are related primarily to the risk of respiratory complications, including reactive airway disease/bronchospasm.[20] Less common effects include altered hepatic enzyme function, metabolism of induction drugs, and induction of the cytochrome P450 system, which may speed the metabolism of drugs, such as haloperidol.[20,22] Fortunately, the conduct of obstetric anesthesiology focuses primarily on regional/neuraxial anesthesia so may avoid airway manipulation and offer relatively low risks of airway complications. Where general anesthesia is required, careful consideration of airway management and postoperative monitoring are critical.

Where possible, the obstetric anesthesiologist also should emphasize the benefits of quitting smoking. ACOG recommends the use of nicotine replacement and/or additional pharmacotherapeutic options, including bupropion, so anesthesiologists should be aware that parturients may present in labor using these treatment options.[23] Finally, the use of e-cigarettes and vaping is on the rise, with a recent CDC report demonstrating 7% of women have used e-cigarettes at any time during their pregnancy, including as a perceived tool to quit smoking.[24] The anesthetic and perioperative implications of e-cigarettes are relatively unknown, with potential risks including lung injury and altered cardiovascular effects of anesthetics.[25] At the current time, there are no data to support the use of e-cigarettes to quit smoking, and counseling should mirror the focus on quitting for traditional cigarettes.

Marijuana

When discussing e-cigarettes or vaping, it is critical to identify which substances the patient is using. Marijuana vaping is more common among those who use e-cigarettes than those who smoke cigarettes and could be missed during history taking[26]; 2% to 5% of pregnant women self-report using marijuana during pregnancy, and 18% of those women meet criteria for SUD.[27,28] Similar to cigarette smoke, marijuana contains a multitude of components with various levels of the active psychotropic delta-9-tetrahydrocannabinol. Acute intoxication can have additive sedative effects and may result in variable hemodynamic effects, depending on whether sympathetic or parasympathetic effects predominate.[29] With increasing state-level legalization of medical marijuana for indications, such as neuropathic pain, it is important to consider there may be increased anesthetic requirements in patients with chronic use similar to patients with chronic alcohol or benzodiazepine use.[30–32] In addition for those who smoke marijuana, it is important to consider neuraxial anesthesia to avoid airway manipulation and careful postoperative planning for patients who require general anesthesia to minimize and identify perioperative respiratory complications.

Alcohol

Alcohol use in pregnancy is common, with 11.5% of pregnant women reporting current drinking and 3.9% report binge drinking in the past 30 days.[33] Acute intoxication may result in behavioral problems due to both the sedative and stimulant properties of alcohol.[14] The sedative effects of alcohol can be additive with many anesthetics and in pregnant women, and alterations of consciousness should prompt concerns for airway protection and aspiration risk. Alcohol may compete for cytochrome P450 in the short term and increase levels in the long term, resulting in decreased drug concentrations (or increased toxic metabolites, in the case of cocaine).[29]

Chronic alcohol use should prompt concern for organ dysfunction, including but not limited to cognitive deficits (Wernicke-Korsakoff syndrome), cerebellar atrophy, cardiomyopathy, hepatopulmonary syndrome, esophagitis/gastritis, varices, portal hypertension/cirrhosis, malnutrition, hypoglycemia, hepatorenal syndrome, and pancytopenia.[14] Aside from the most extreme cases, a majority of these are candidates for standard neuraxial anesthesia. In cases of general anesthesia, however, special care should be given for increased minimum alveolar concentration (MAC) requirements and possible increased risk of awareness.[34] Plans for additional benzodiazepines and/or hypnotic use as well as discussion before and screening after for awareness should be considered. For parturients at risk of, or actively experiencing, alcohol withdrawal, ASAM recommends inpatient treatment of women with at least moderate alcohol withdrawal in consultation with an obstetrician using either benzodiazepines or barbiturates.[35] Albeit limited, some data suggest chlordiazepoxide or clonazepam both appear safe, and dexmedetomidine also may have utility in the management of alcohol withdrawal delirium.[36,37]

Stimulants: Cocaine and Amphetamines

Survey data from 2019 suggested the use of cocaine in the past month of pregnancy was 2 per 1000 pregnant women.[38] Acute intoxication presents as behavioral disturbances—euphoria and increased energy—and as cardiovascular stimulation, including hypertension and tachycardia.[29] Cocaine also may increase the risk of thrombotic complications and may explain the association with preterm birth and placental abruption.[39] Management of acute intoxication should be focused on hemodynamic stability, with hydralazine and labetalol the first-line agents in the management of hypertension.[20] Hypotension should be treated with fluids and phenylephrine, as is common on labor and delivery units. The need for invasive arterial blood pressure monitoring depends on the concomitant obstetric and surgical issues, because more recent data suggest the inherent instability commonly associated with cocaine may be unfounded.[40] Several drugs should be avoided, including ketamine, because of the indirect cardiovascular effects, and etomidate, because of the high rate of myoclonus in this population.[20]

Methamphetamine use during pregnancy is less than one-third as common as cocaine although it may be a marker for polysubstance use.[38] This class includes methamphetamine (speed or crystal meth), 3,4-methylenedioxymethamphetamine [MDMA]) (ecstasy), and 3,4,-methylenedioxypyrovalerone (bath salts) as well as other indirect-acting sympathomimetic drugs. The clinical presentation is clinically indistinguishable from cocaine, including the obstetric complications of preterm birth and abruption.[20] Neuraxial anesthesia is preferred but may be accompanied by hypotension, which can be treated with fluids and phenylephrine. If general anesthesia is required, acute intoxication increases MAC whereas chronic use may decrease MAC.[20] Another special consideration is the risk of poor dentition among chronic methamphetamine users ,which may impact airway management.[41] Ketamine and etomidate should be used similarly, with caution in this population.

Uncommon Drugs: Hallucinogens and Solvents

There are almost no data on the prevalence of hallucinogen (lysergic acid diethylamide, phencyclidine, psilocybin, and mescaline) use during pregnancy. Similarly, solvents (eg, toluene) are poorly documented in this population. Hallucinogens may lead to exaggerated response to sympathomimetics and prolonged effects of opioids.[20] Neuraxial analgesia with phenylephrine for treating hypotension is reasonable if a patient is cooperative. There is no evidence that neuraxial opioids should be avoided. Long-term use of solvents may lead to autonomic and equilibrium disorders but is unlikely to have a direct impact on anesthetic planning except in rare circumstances.[20]

Opioids

As discussed previously, the most significant rise in substance use among parturients in the past decade has been opioids. Heroin (diacetylmorphine), oxycodone, and hydrocodone are common drugs of misuse, but fentanyl, the highly potent synthetic opioid, and carfentanil (which is 100 times more potent than fentanyl) increasingly have been implicated in overdose deaths.[42]

Acute intoxication results in euphoric central nervous system changes and increased parasympathetic activity as well as profound respiratory depression. Patients presenting while actively intoxicated should be monitored closely with naloxone immediately available to administer if signs of respiratory depression emerge. In addition, neonates must be evaluated and monitored for NOWS. For patients with chronic opioid use, a thorough history should assess risk of intravenous administration (endocarditis, skin and soft tissue infections, human immunodeficiency virus, hepatitis, and so forth) as well as risk of organ dysfunction, including but not limited to malnutrition and aspiration. Parturients with SUD should be offered treatment in lieu of supervised withdrawal because of lower relapse rates.[15] Neonatal data in the past 10 years suggest that the partial agonist buprenorphine may have superior neonatal outcomes and fewer medical complications or overdoses compared with methadone. As such, the buprenorphine monoproduct (Subutex) or Suboxone (when combined with naloxone—designed to reduce diversion/injection) may be the first-line agent, although patients stable on methadone should not transition to buprenorphine because of pregnancy due to concerns for withdrawal.[15] Limitations of buprenorphine include the requirement to self-administer, the risk of diversion/misuse, and potential fetal exposure to naloxone if injected (Suboxone).[15] Conversely methadone requires a structured daily visit, dose adjustments during pregnancy, and many pharmacokinetic interactions.[15]

Pain control is the most challenging aspect and primary goal of the care for the parturient with opioid use history. Opioid maintenance therapy should be continued in almost all cases. Early involvement with social work and case management resources to plan a postdelivery course is critical because the highest-risk period for overdose is postpartum.[43] Postpartum prescription or access to naloxone should be considered for all pregnant people with opioid prescriptions or at risk for relapse.[43] For vaginal deliveries, evidence suggests that analgesic requirements are similar for parturients maintained on methadone compared with those nonopioid-using parturients, adding support to the use of a standard labor epidural and adjuncts when opioid maintenance therapy is continued in this population.[44] For women with a cesarean delivery, analgesic requirements are likely to be increased for patients maintained on buprenorphine or on methadone.[45] Increased intrathecal doses of morphine or intraoperative intravenous methadone have been described as methods to improve pain control in this population, but overall more work needs to be done before recommendations deviate from standard protocols.[46–48]

DISCUSSION
Anesthetic Considerations

Prenatal care
Historically, obstetric anesthesiologists primarily managed intrapartum pain control for laboring patients and intraoperative management during cesarean deliveries, but this role has evolved in many institutions to be a collaboration with the obstetricians in care planning and management of all obstetric patients, regardless of delivery type beginning in the prenatal period. When a patient with SUD presents to care, it is an opportunity to plan to a successful delivery that minimizes risk to the mother and fetus. It is important also to elicit the chronicity of the patient's substance use, because management of obstetric patients with acute intoxication varies from anesthetic management of chronic substance users and those in treatment. Patients with SUD not only are at increased risk of obstetric complications and emergencies, such as fetal growth restriction, intrauterine fetal demise, preterm labor, and placental abruption, but also may be at higher risk of cardiovascular or pulmonary complications in the peripartum period. Obstetric anesthesiologists must be able to recognize and manage these complications. **Box 1** summarizes anesthetic implications of all substances, discussed previously, and **Table 1** lists common challenges to parturients with SUDs.

Vaginal deliveries
Patients who screen positive for SUDs ideally should be identified by an obstetric team to facilitate care planning. Unless acutely intoxicated, tobacco and marijuana are unlikely to change the acute anesthetic management for an anticipated vaginal delivery, and interactions instead should focus on the readiness and opportunity for quitting and assessing which resources are available. The primary concern for alcohol use in this scenario is the risk of withdrawal, and appropriate planning to treat withdrawal delirium is essential. Cocaine, amphetamines, and other stimulants may require interventions for management of hypertension and tachycardia; if desired, labor epidural

Box 1		
Anesthetic implications of acute and chronic substance use in pregnancy[15,20,29]		
Substance	**Acute Intoxication**	**Chronic Use**
Tobacco	N/A	Perioperative respiratory complications, carboxyhemoglobin
Marijuana	Additive sedation	Perioperative respiratory complications, increased MAC requirements
Alcohol	Behavioral change, aspiration, decreased MAC requirements	Organ system complications, Withdrawal, increased MAC requirements
Cocaine, amphetamines, stimulants	Hypertension, tachycardia, and hypotension after neuraxial anesthesia, increased MAC requirements	Neurologic sequalae, cardiomyopathy, poor dentition (risk for airway management), decreased MAC requirements
Hallucinogens, solvents	Exaggerated response to sympathomimetics (avoid ephedrine), prolonged opioid effects	Autonomic and equilibrium disorders
Opioids	Respiratory depression, additive sedation	Increased analgesic requirements, risk of postpartum relapse

Table 1
Key challenges in the anesthetic management of parturients with substance use disorder

Issue	Clinical Example
Understanding the increase in risk of obstetric emergencies caused by substance use	Cocaine use causing placental abruption
Appraising the anesthetic implications of acute intoxication	Hypertension in methamphetamine intoxication
Identifying organ dysfunction resulting from chronic substance use	Alcohol-related cirrhosis
Predicting the effects of substance use treatment	Higher postcesarean analgesic requirements in a patient on MAT (Suboxone)
Determining which medications should be avoided due to SUD	Ketamine contraindicated with active stimulant use
Assembling an appropriate pain control plan that takes into account substance use and treatment plans	Multimodal approach necessary for postcesarean analgesia in a patient with polysubstance use (MDMA, cocaine, opioids)
Educating and advocating for resources when caring for parturients with SUD	Reporting requirements differing between states; finding ways to advocate for decriminalization of medical care
Recognizing the disparities and social determinants of health that have an impact on SUD	Unique geographic and racial distribution SUD
Encouraging universal screening for SUDs	Creating partnerships with obstetric colleagues to complete appropriate screening for all parturients
Advocating for patients to quit, connect them to resources	Utilizing health care contacts as teachable moments in quitting smoking

analgesia may provide an appropriate sympathectomy, although a plan should be in place to treat resultant hypotension with fluids and phenylephrine. In addition, close hemodynamic monitoring should be practiced after placement or bolus of an epidural catheter due to the up-regulation of sympathetic activity and risk of ischemia in this patient population. Because the presentation of cocaine intoxication (ie, hypertension, tachycardia, placental abruption, intracranial hemorrhage, or proteinuria from hypertensive nephropathy) overlaps with symptoms of preeclampsia and eclampsia, a multidisciplinary discussion should occur to facilitate the appropriate diagnosis and management.[49] Both alcohol and cocaine and result in thrombocytopenia; thus, platelet screening prior to neuraxial anesthesia should be completed. Patients with a history of opioid use who are being treated with medication assistance therapy, specifically buprenorphine or methadone, should be continued on maintenance doses throughout delivery and the postpartum period to avoid withdrawal symptoms and fetal distress.[47] Care also should be taken to avoid partial agonists commonly used to treat neuraxial opioid-induced itching (eg, nalbuphine and butorphanol) to avoid precipitating withdrawal as well.[50] Neuraxial analgesia is recommended for patients with a history of opioid use disorder because the development of opioid tolerance over time can make pain control challenging with standard parenteral doses of medications during labor. Little is known about postpartum pain requirements post–vaginal delivery in patients with chronic opioid use.

Cesarean delivery

For elective or urgent cesarean deliveries, spinal and/or epidural anesthesia generally is the standard of care to allow for surgical anesthesia with the patient awake to experience delivery and bonding, with general anesthesia an alternative in emergency settings or if neuraxial anesthesia is contraindicated or unsuccessful. A patient's history of substance use should be considered when developing an anesthetic plan for cesarean delivery under general or neuraxial anesthesia.

Because general anesthesia generally is avoided in this population already, when required for patients who smoke cigarettes or marijuana, special attention should be paid to the postoperative period and risk of respiratory complications. Patients who have a cesarean delivery and have alcohol use disorder may stay long enough in the hospital to be at risk of withdrawal, so an early plan should be put into place. During a cesarean delivery, a patient with risk of or known varices still may have gastric tubes placed because the risk of bleeding is low, albeit data specific to pregnancy are limited.[51] Cocaine and amphetamines create an up-regulation in maternal sympathetic activity due to the inhibition of neurotransmitter reuptake.[29] Intrathecal administration of local anesthetic may induce a sympathectomy that can result in significant hypotension in these patients. In patients with chronically elevated sympathetic tone secondary to cocaine or amphetamine use, catecholamine stores become depleted, and ephedrine is minimally effective. Phenylephrine is a more appropriate choice for treatment of hypotension after neuraxial anesthesia in these patients.[52] Hypertension in patients with a history of cocaine or amphetamine use also should warrant urgent treatment due to vasoconstriction of coronary arteries and risk of myocardial ischemia. Selective blockade of β-receptors in hypertension may result in unopposed α-adrenergic vasoconstriction and worsening of ischemia. Labetalol blocks both α-adrenergic receptors and β-adrenergic receptors and thus mediates this unopposed alpha agonism. Vasodilators, such as hydralazine and nitroglycerin, are appropriate alternatives in the treatment of hypertension in these patients.[29] With a history of cocaine use, it also is important to consider the effect of cocaine on the pharmacodynamics of the anesthetic. Cocaine use over time alters mu-opioid and kappa-opioid receptor density, making adequate pain control challenging in a similar manner to that in patients with opioid use disorder. Cocaine also induces a shorter duration of intrathecal opioid effect, which should be considered when administering spinal anesthesia for cesarean delivery.[53]

In patients undergoing cesarean delivery under general anesthesia, it also is important to tailor the anesthetic management according to a patient's substance use history. In patients with a history of cocaine or amphetamine use, agents that potentiate sympathetic activity, such as ketamine, should be avoided. Propofol may be administered safely to these patients with cocaine use and is the agent of choice for induction of anesthesia in a nonhypotensive patient.[53]

Postoperative pain control may be challenging in patients with a history of SUD. In patients with chronic opioid use, standard doses of opioids may be ineffective, resulting in a challenging and distressing postoperative period. The Society for Obstetric Anesthesia and Perinatology has released a consensus statement with recommendations for enhanced recovery after cesarean delivery section. This consensus statement highlights that the key goals after cesarean delivery section are maternal and infant bonding, encouragement of mobility to prevent venous thromboembolic events, and preservation of maternal ability to care for the infant with adequate pain control and minimal side effects.[54] These goals also apply to parturients who have a history of SUDs. Patients on chronic buprenorphine or methadone should be continued on their baseline dose through the postoperative recovery period.[54] Higher doses of opioids may be required in patients with history of chronic opioid use and even intermittent intravenous doses or patient-controlled administration may be subtherapeutic in these patients. Whereas spinal anesthesia or removal of an epidural catheter at the conclusion of a cesarean delivery is common practice in opioid-naïve patients, it may be beneficial to continue epidural analgesia postoperatively in opioid-tolerant patients, provided the epidural is appropriately sited and dosed for incisional and intra-abdominal coverage (rather than lower extremities). A low-density local anesthetic combined with an opioid can provide excellent postoperative analgesia, but the presence of local anesthetic may preclude postoperative ambulation if a lumbar epidural is used postoperatively and may inhibit mobility goals from being reached. An alternative approach would be continuation of the epidural catheter with an opioid-only infusion, allowing for greater efficacy from reduced doses of opioid and minimizing adverse effects.[55] Individual patients should be evaluated for the appropriateness of continuing an indwelling catheter based on concern for high-risk behaviors if left unsupervised. Contaminated epidural catheters can lead to life-threatening complications, so the risks and benefits for each patient must be considered. Multimodal analgesia, such as a combination of acetaminophen and nonsteroidal anti-inflammatory drugs, is helpful; gabapentin no longer is recommended in most postcesarean protocols.[48,56]

Regional anesthesia is an excellent strategy in patients with a history of SUD who undergo cesarean delivery section, especially after general anesthesia if neuraxial anesthesia was not utilized. Transversus abdominus plane block has been shown to improve postoperative pain significantly in patients who underwent cesarean delivery without neuraxial opioid administration.[57] Quadratus lumborum and erector spinae plane blocks also are techniques that have been shown to provide effective analgesia after cesarean delivery.[58,59] Although neuraxial opioids may have greater efficacy than regional anesthesia alone, the side-effect profile of regional techniques is favorable and should be considered in combination with neuraxial opioids or as an adjunct to perioperative oral and parenteral analgesics.[60] The implementation of regional anesthesia techniques is a promising alternative or adjunct in patients with SUD, because truncal and fascial blocks have been shown to have benefit with a very low incidence of adverse effects. Further investigation as to the benefits of regional techniques specifically in this patient population would be beneficial.

CASE STUDY
Case Presentation

A 30-year-old G_6P_{3023} presented for repeat cesarean delivery at 37 weeks' gestational age. She had a history of intravenous opioid and amphetamine abuse and has been on medication-assisted therapy with buprenorphine/naloxone for the past 12 months. She reports no other substance use during this pregnancy apart from tobacco. Preoperative blood cell counts were unremarkable, with a platelet count of 221 (10^9/L) as well as a normal coagulation profile. The decision was made to use a combined spinal-epidural technique, with the epidural catheter to be left in place postoperatively for continued analgesia, given her history of chronic opioid use and current buprenorphine/naloxone therapy. An intrathecal injection of 12 mg of 0.75% hyperbaric bupivacaine, 10 μg of fentanyl, and 0.1 mg of morphine was administered, and an epidural catheter was secured. No additional local anesthetic was administered via the epidural catheter. In the recovery room, the patient was started on a continuous epidural infusion of hydromorphone 100 μg/h with a patient-controlled epidural bolus of 20 μg every 30 minutes as needed. She also had orders for intravenous hydromorphone every 3 hours as needed, and oral oxycodone 10 mg to 15 mg every 4 hours as needed. Ketorolac and acetaminophen were given on a scheduled basis.

On postoperative day 1, the patient had excellent analgesia with epidural hydromorphone, acetaminophen, and ketorolac and was continued on her home dose of buprenorphine/naloxone. She required zero doses of opioids for breakthrough pain. She was tolerating a regular diet, ambulating, and voiding without difficulty. She was encouraged to take oral oxycodone throughout the day, and the epidural hydromorphone was discontinued on postoperative day 2. She continued to have good pain control thereafter, using oral oxycodone, acetaminophen, and ibuprofen. She was discharged home on postoperative day 4 and reported being very satisfied with her hospital course and pain control.

Clinical Questions

- What is the best practice for management of medication-assisted treatment (MAT) (eg, buprenorphine/naloxone, buprenorphine, or methadone) in the peridelivery period?
  - In almost all cases, buprenorphine/naloxone, buprenorphine, and methadone should be continued at the patient's usual dose throughout pregnancy and delivery. The consensus is that the potential risks of relapse and withdrawal are more significant than the risks of continuing the medication. Patients may choose to discontinue MAT during pregnancy but should be counseled on the risk of relapse and should be followed closely.
- What are the risks and benefits of continuing a lumbar epidural for postoperative pain control in the parturient with opioid SUD?
  - Epidural catheters should not be continued in patients who display high-risk behaviors that could contaminate the catheter and increase the risk of infection. For example, if a patient wants to leave the building to smoke frequently, or if they have shown diversion behaviors, leaving an indwelling catheter in place may be too high an infectious risk.
- Are there regional anesthesia techniques that could be used in lieu of a postoperative epidural for this population?
  - Yes—transversus abdominus plane, quadratus lumborum, and erector spinae plane blocks all have shown benefit in postcesarean pain.
- When using neuraxial opioids, how do you assess the risk of additional systemic opioids in a parturient with opioid SUD?
  - Patients with SUD have a higher requirement for pain control following cesarean delivery section but are at increased risk of adverse respiratory events as well. Discretion should be used when dosing opioids in this population, and all opioids may be titrated upward to effect. When neuraxial opioids are given, patients should be monitored for respiratory depression and somnolence when additional systemic opioids are given. Naloxone should be ordered and readily available as a precaution.
- What is an appropriate analgesic postdelivery discharge plan for a woman with opioid SUD?
  - When prescribing discharge medications, it is important to assess a patient's opioid usage in the hospital prior to discharge. It is reasonable to determine how many doses were used in the 24 hours prior to discharge and then extrapolate to a postdischarge supply to avoid overprescribing. Patients also should

be encouraged to continue nonopioid analgesics, such as acetaminophen and/or ibuprofen, for discomfort after discharge. Naloxone should be prescribed at discharge due to the high risk of relapse postdelivery.

SUMMARY

Care of the parturient with SUDs is becoming increasingly common and poses significant challenges, particularly with opioid use disorder. Management of MAT during the peripartum period is essential along with a multimodal plan for intrapartum and postpartum analgesia. Because of the wide geographic variation in both prevalence and type of substance use occurring, anesthesiologists must partner with obstetricians and delve into their local public health data to best understand what types of SUD they should expect. Multidisciplinary preparation can better manage the wide range of substances and conditions, including acute intoxication, chronic use, withdrawal, and treatment. There also remain significant disparities in the care for these women as well as opportunities for advocacy to improve identification, resources, and care.

CLINICS CARE POINTS

- It is critical for providers to understand their local community, prevalence, and type of substances used to best care for affected parturients.
- The United States has seen a 4-fold increase in opioid use disorder in pregnancy, with significant geographic variability.
- Historical and racial biases in the public health and criminal justice systems affect the way pregnant women with SUD interact with the health care system.
- Screening for substance use should be a universal tool as part of comprehensive obstetric care. Targeted screening based on risk factors, such as adherence to prenatal care, may worsen stereotyping and stigma.
- *DSM-5* combines substance use and dependence into SUD, which can be classified as mild, moderate, or severe, based on symptoms.
- E-cigarette and vaping use is rising, with 7% of pregnant women endorsing use; because the potential risks are incompletely understood, vaping should not be recommended as a tool to quit smoking.
- Particular care should be giving to parturients who require general anesthesia for delivery and who smoke tobacco or marijuana because of an increased risk of postoperative pulmonary complications.
- Cocaine or stimulants may lead to hemodynamic lability. Hypertension should be treated with hydralazine or labetalol. Hypotension after neuraxial analgesia is common and should be treated with phenylephrine and fluid resuscitation.
- MAT with buprenorphine, buprenorphine/naloxone, or methadone should be continued throughout pregnancy and delivery.
- Parturients with opioid use disorder on MAT do not have different analgesic requirements from non–opioid-using parturients while laboring for anticipated vaginal deliveries.
- Parturients with opioid use disorder on MAT have significantly increased analgesic requirements following cesarean delivery; however, current data are limited on varying from standard practice neuraxial anesthesia.
- The postpartum period is the highest risk of relapse and opioid overdose; therefore. naloxone should be prescribed on discharge from the hospital after delivery.

DISCLOSURE

The authors have nothing to disclose.

REFERENCES

1. Ohio Department of Health. Special Topics Report on Pregnancy-Associated Deaths Due to Unintentional Overdose in Ohio, 2008-2016. 2020. Available at: https://odh.ohio.gov/wps/portal/gov/odh/know-our-programs/pregnancy-associated-mortality-review/media/pamr-brief-overdose.
2. Haight SC, Ko JY, Tong VT, et al. Opioid Use Disorder Documented at Delivery Hospitalization - United States, 1999-2014. MMWR Morb Mortal Wkly Rep 2018;67(31). https://doi.org/10.15585/mmwr.mm6731a1.
3. National Institute on Drug Abuse. Monitoring the Future Study: Trends in Prevalence of Various Drugs for 8th Graders, 10th Graders, and 12th Graders; 2017-2020. Available at: https://www.drugabuse.gov/drug-topics/trends-statistics/monitoring-future/monitoring-future-study-trends-in-prevalence-various-drugs.
4. Schiff DM. Division of General Academic Pediatrics MHfC, Boston, Massachusetts, Nielsen T, et al. Assessment of Racial and Ethnic Disparities in the Use of Medication to Treat Opioid Use Disorder Among Pregnant Women in Massachusetts. JAMA Netw Open 2021;3(5). https://doi.org/10.1001/jamanetworkopen.2020.5734.
5. Kroelinger CD, Rice ME, Cox S, et al. State strategies to address opioid use disorder among pregnant and postpartum women and infants prenatally exposed to substances, including infants with neonatal abstinence syndrome. MMWR Morb Mortal Wkly Rep 2019;68(36). https://doi.org/10.15585/mmwr.mm6836a1.
6. American Psychiatric Association. Diagnostic and Statistical Manual of Mental Disorders. Fifth Edition. Arlington, VA: American Psychiatric Association; 2013. p. 947.
7. Hasin DS, O'Brien CP, Auriacombe M, et al. DSM-5 criteria for substance use disorders: recommendations and rationale. Am J Psychiatry 2013;170(8):834–51.
8. Hirai AH, Ko JY, Owens PL, et al. Neonatal abstinence syndrome and maternal opioid-related diagnoses in the US, 2010-2017. JAMA 2021;325(2):146–55.
9. Simpson WJ. A preliminary report on cigarette smoking and the incidence of prematurity. Am J Obstet Gynecol 1957;73(4):807–15.
10. Stone R. Pregnant women and substance use: fear, stigma, and barriers to care. Health Justice 2015;3(1). https://doi.org/10.1186/s40352-015-0015-5.
11. Institute G. Substance Use During Pregnancy. 2021. Available at: https://www.guttmacher.org/state-policy/explore/substance-use-during-pregnancy. Accessed July 20, 2021.
12. Paltrow LM, Flavin J. Arrests of and forced interventions on pregnant women in the United States, 1973-2005: implications for women's legal status and public health. J Health Polit Policy Law 2013;38(2):299–343.
13. Ecker J, Abuhamad A, Hill W, et al. Substance use disorders in pregnancy: clinical, ethical, and research imperatives of the opioid epidemic: a report of a joint workshop of the Society for Maternal-Fetal Medicine, American College of Obstetricians and Gynecologists, and American Society of Addiction Medicine. Am J Obstet Gynecol 2019;221(1):B5–28.
14. Pulley DD. Preoperative Evaluation of the Patient with Substance Use Disorder and Perioperative Considerations. Anesthesiol Clin 2016;34(1):201–11.
15. Committee Opinion No. 711: Opioid Use and Opioid Use Disorder in Pregnancy. Obstet Gynecol 2017;130(2):e81–94.

16. Shi Y, Yu C, Luo A, et al. Perioperative tobacco interventions by Chinese anesthesiologists: practices and attitudes. Anesthesiology 2010;112(2):338–46.

17. Yousefzadeh A, Chung F, Wong DT, et al. Smoking Cessation: The Role of the Anesthesiologist. Anesth Analg 2016;122(5):1311–20.

18. Avsar TS, McLeod H, Jackson L. Health outcomes of smoking during pregnancy and the postpartum period: an umbrella review. BMC Pregnancy Childbirth 2021; 21(1):254.

19. Forray A. Substance use during pregnancy. F1000Res 2016;5. https://doi.org/10. 12688/f1000research.7645.1.

20. Kuczkowski KM. Anesthetic implications of drug abuse in pregnancy. J Clin Anesth 2003;15(5):382–94.

21. Warner DO. Perioperative abstinence from cigarettes: physiologic and clinical consequences. Anesthesiology 2006;104(2):356–67.

22. Carrick MA, Robson JM, Thomas C. Smoking and anaesthesia. BJA Educ 2019; 19(1):1–6.

23. Tobacco and nicotine cessation during pregnancy: ACOG Committee Opinion, Number 807. Obstet Gynecol 2020;135(5):e221–9.

24. Kuehn B. Vaping and Pregnancy. JAMA 2019;321(14):1344.

25. Feinstein MM, Katz D. Sparking the Discussion about Vaping and Anesthesia. Anesthesiology 2020;132(3):599.

26. Baldassarri SR, Camenga DR, Fiellin DA, et al. Marijuana Vaping in U.S. Adults: Evidence From the Behavioral Risk Factor Surveillance System. Am J Prev Med 2020;59(3):449–54.

27. Ryan SA, Ammerman SD, O'Connor ME. Committee on substance USE, prevention, section on B. marijuana use during pregnancy and breastfeeding: implications for neonatal and childhood outcomes. Pediatrics 2018;142(3). https://doi. org/10.1542/peds.2018-1889.

28. Ko JY, Farr SL, Tong VT, et al. Prevalence and patterns of marijuana use among pregnant and nonpregnant women of reproductive age. Am J Obstet Gynecol 2015;213(2):201.e1–10.

29. Chestnut DH. Chestnut's Obstetric Anesthesia: Principles and Practice. 6th edition. Philadelphia (PA): Elsevier; 2020.

30. Sarrafpour S, Urits I, Powell J, et al. Considerations and implications of cannabidiol use during pregnancy. Curr Pain Headache Rep 2020;24(7):38.

31. Urits I, Gress K, Charipova K, et al. Use of cannabidiol (CBD) for the treatment of chronic pain. Best Pract Res Clin Anaesthesiol 2020;34(3):463–77.

32. Imasogie N, Rose RV, Wilson A. High quantities: Evaluating the association between cannabis use and propofol anesthesia during endoscopy. PLoS One 2021;16(3):e0248062.

33. Denny CH, Acero CS, Naimi TS, et al. Consumption of Alcohol Beverages and Binge Drinking Among Pregnant Women Aged 18-44 Years - United States, 2015-2017. MMWR Morb Mortal Wkly Rep 2019;68(16):365–8.

34. Ghoneim MM, Block RI, Haffarnan M, et al. Awareness during anesthesia: risk factors, causes and sequelae: a review of reported cases in the literature. Anesth Analg 2009;108(2):527–35.

35. The ASAM clinical practice guideline on alcohol withdrawal management. J Addict Med 2020;14(3S Suppl 1):1–72.

36. Iqbal MM, Sobhan T, Ryals T. Effects of commonly used benzodiazepines on the fetus, the neonate, and the nursing infant. Psychiatr Serv 2002;53(1):39–49.

37. Mueller SW, Preslaski CR, Kiser TH, et al. A randomized, double-blind, placebo-controlled dose range study of dexmedetomidine as adjunctive therapy for alcohol withdrawal. Crit Care Med 2014;42(5):1131–9.

38. Center for Behavioral Health Statistics and Quality. Results from the 2019 National Survey on Drug Use and Health: Detailed tables. Rockville, MD: Substance Abuse and Mental Health Services Administration. 2020. Retrieved from https://www.samhsa.gov/data/.

39. Sharma T, Kumar M, Rizkallah A, et al. Cocaine-induced Thrombosis: Review of Predisposing Factors, Potential Mechanisms, and Clinical Consequences with a Striking Case Report. Cureus 2019;11(5):e4700.

40. Moon TS, Pak TJ, Kim A, et al. A Positive Cocaine Urine Toxicology Test and the Effect on Intraoperative Hemodynamics Under General Anesthesia. Anesth Analg 2021;132(2):308–16.

41. Shetty V, Mooney LJ, Zigler CM, et al. The relationship between methamphetamine use and increased dental disease. J Am Dent Assoc 2010;141(3):307–18.

42. Scholl L, Seth P, Kariisa M, et al. Drug and Opioid-Involved Overdose Deaths - United States, 2013-2017. MMWR Morb Mortal Wkly Rep 2018;67(5152):1419–27.

43. Schiff DM, Nielsen T, Terplan M, et al. Fatal and Nonfatal Overdose Among Pregnant and Postpartum Women in Massachusetts. Obstet Gynecol 2018;132(2):466–74.

44. Meyer M, Wagner K, Benvenuto A, et al. Intrapartum and postpartum analgesia for women maintained on methadone during pregnancy. Obstet Gynecol 2007;110(2 Pt 1):261–6.

45. Reno JL, Kushelev M, Coffman JH, et al. Post-cesarean delivery analgesic outcomes in patients maintained on methadone and buprenorphine: a retrospective investigation. J Pain Res 2020;13:3513–24.

46. Russell T, Mitchell C, Paech MJ, et al. Efficacy and safety of intraoperative intravenous methadone during general anaesthesia for caesarean delivery: a retrospective case-control study. Int J Obstet Anesth 2013;22(1):47–51.

47. Booth JL, Harris LC, Eisenach JC, et al. A randomized controlled trial comparing two multimodal analgesic techniques in patients predicted to have severe pain after cesarean delivery. Anesth Analg 2016;122(4):1114–9.

48. Roofthooft E, Joshi GP, Rawal N, et al. PROSPECT guideline for elective caesarean section: updated systematic review and procedure-specific postoperative pain management recommendations. Anaesthesia 2021;76(5):665–80.

49. Kain ZN, Rimar S, Barash PG. Cocaine abuse in the parturient and effects on the fetus and neonate. Anesth Analg 1993;77(4):835–45.

50. Harrison TK, Kornfeld H, Aggarwal AK, et al. Perioperative considerations for the patient with opioid use disorder on buprenorphine, methadone, or naltrexone maintenance therapy. Anesthesiol Clin 2018;36(3):345–59.

51. Al-Obaid LN, Bazarbashi AN, Cohen ME, et al. Enteric tube placement in patients with esophageal varices: Risks and predictors of postinsertion gastrointestinal bleeding. JGH Open 2020;4(2):256–9.

52. Kuczkowski KM. Cocaine abuse in pregnancy–anesthetic implications. Int J Obstet Anesth 2002;11(3):204–10.

53. Ludlow J, Christmas T, Paech MJ, et al. Drug abuse and dependency during pregnancy: anaesthetic issues. Anaesth Intensive Care 2007;35(6):881–93.

54. Bollag L, Lim G, Sultan P, et al. Society for Obstetric Anesthesia and Perinatology: Consensus Statement and Recommendations for Enhanced Recovery After Cesarean. Anesth Analg 2021;132(5):1362–77.

55. Stanislaus MA, Reno JL, Small RH, et al. Continuous epidural hydromorphone infusion for post-cesarean delivery analgesia in a patient on methadone maintenance therapy: a case report. J Pain Res 2020;13:837–42.
56. Raymond BL, Kook BT, Richardson MG. The opioid epidemic and pregnancy: implications for anesthetic care. Curr Opin Anaesthesiol 2018;31(3):243–50.
57. Mishriky BM, George RB, Habib AS. Transversus abdominis plane block for analgesia after Cesarean delivery: a systematic review and meta-analysis. Can J Anaesth 2012;59(8):766–78.
58. Blanco R, Ansari T, Girgis E. Quadratus lumborum block for postoperative pain after caesarean section: A randomised controlled trial. Eur J Anaesthesiol 2015;32(11):812–8.
59. Hamed MA, Yassin HM, Botros JM, et al. Analgesic efficacy of erector spinae plane block compared with intrathecal morphine after elective cesarean section: a prospective randomized controlled study. J Pain Res 2020;13:597–604.
60. Champaneria R, Shah L, Wilson MJ, et al. Clinical effectiveness of transversus abdominis plane (TAP) blocks for pain relief after caesarean section: a meta-analysis. Int J Obstet Anesth 2016;28:45–60.

Trauma-Informed Care on Labor and Delivery

Tracey M. Vogel, MD[a],*, Erica Coffin, MD[b]

KEYWORDS

- Trauma informed • Obstetrics • Anesthesia • Peripartum • Mental health • PTSD

KEY POINTS

- General trauma-informed care principles are based on 4 Rs: realize the widespread nature of interpersonal trauma, recognize chronic and acute traumatic stress in our patients and ourselves, respond with policy and protocol changes, and resist retraumatization.
- Eight percent of all maternal deaths are due to trauma-related and mental health conditions.
- Establishment of a trauma-informed service is essential, but lack of leadership support, lack of consistent training, and production pressure are significant barriers to implementation.
- The obstetric anesthesia provider is crucial in recognizing and responding to acute stress responses and safeguarding emotional well-being in the labor and delivery unit and in the operating room.

INTRODUCTION

Trauma in obstetrics is not a new phenomenon. In 1957, journalists from the *Ladies' Home Journal* published an article revealing the inhumane treatment of women in labor and delivery rooms and included commentary from women, nurses, and other professionals from around the country.[1] Interestingly, the sources of suffering that many women described 6 decades ago are strikingly similar to what women report today, including the loss of control and forced restraint, feelings of powerlessness, loss of autonomy and lack of true informed consent, actual physical harm, and negative interactions with caregivers.[2–4] It was not until the 1990s, however, that perinatal mental health experts recognized that negative events surrounding childbirth could be a

[a] Department of Anesthesiology, West Penn Hospital/Allegheny Health Network, 4800 Friendship Avenue, Pittsburgh, PA 15224, USA; [b] Obstetric Anesthesia, Department of Anesthesiology, West Penn Hospital/Allegheny Health Network, 4800 Friendship Avenue, Pittsburgh, PA 15224, USA
* Corresponding author.
E-mail address: tracey.vogel@ahn.org
Twitter: @TraceyVogelMD (T.M.V.); @coffin_erica (E.C.)

Anesthesiology Clin 39 (2021) 779–791
https://doi.org/10.1016/j.anclin.2021.08.007
1932-2275/21/© 2021 Elsevier Inc. All rights reserved.

cause of significant emotional distress, and that this extreme stress could directly contribute to the development of post-traumatic stress disorder (PTSD). Our understanding of how women view their delivery experiences and what they feel are factors associated with traumatic births has increased greatly with qualitative studies,[2–4] however, how we as providers address these issues is still not clearly defined. For more than 60 years, women have been voicing their concerns about treatment in maternity wards, yet universal cultural changes in medical practices have been slow to evolve. We are also more informed now about how chronic traumatic stress from previous (or current) life experiences negatively impacts a woman's physical and psychological responses surrounding childbirth. The concept of trauma and trauma-focused interventions, "trauma-informed care" (TIC) is finally receiving attention in various health care settings as a way forward to address these issues.

The Substance Abuse and Mental Health Services Administration (SAMHSA) defines TIC using 4 R general principles of care: realize the pervasive and widespread nature of trauma in our society, recognize what unresolved trauma looks like in adult survivors, respond by incorporating knowledge into practices, protocols and principles, and resist retraumatization.[5] These important, yet nonspecific guidelines are fundamental to the incorporation of trauma-informed services in our communities, schools, law enforcement, and health care arenas, but they do not fully define what such an approach to care would look like specifically in the setting of current obstetric practices. Although organizations such as the National Health Service in the UK and the American College of Obstetricians and Gynecologists (ACOG) in the United States have put forth statements supporting the inclusion of trauma-informed principles into obstetrics and have offered recommendations on how to care for survivors of trauma, no single accepted construct has yet been developed outlining exactly how screening for a history of trauma should be done, who should do it, how we should train providers in this care, how we would assess for the incorporation of such principles over time, and how we would assess for outcomes once organizations adopt this new culture of care.[6,7] Protocols to minimize psychological morbidity after known traumatic obstetric events are also lacking. Various government organizations have also shown interest in mandating the incorporation of TIC principles into various aspects of society. The US Digital Health Services has developed task forces and collaborated with mental health experts and other medical providers to brainstorm barriers and possible solutions to the issue of integrating this new type of approach in health care settings. In Pennsylvania, the governor has convened a similar task force with the goal of making it a trauma-informed state.[8] Unfortunately, these institutions also do not define how trauma-informed principles should be executed in the health care setting.

Equally important to how we should implement TIC practices, is why we should do it. The increasing rate of maternal mortality in the United States coupled with the fact that we rank at the bottom when compared with other high-income nations[9] has prompted intense scrutiny into possible preventable etiologies. Although significant effort has been applied to decrease the mortality due to physical complications such as hemorrhage, hypertensive crises, or cardiovascular events, the same approach to mental health and trauma-related conditions is lacking. The Centers for Disease Control and Prevention recently published a study looking at data from 14 state Maternal Mortality and Review Committees over a 9-year period examining the deaths of women who had given birth within the previous year (study dates 2008–2017.)[10] Because they extended their review to include a full postpartum year and not merely 6 weeks, they revealed that deaths owing to suicide, overdose, and homicide related to intimate partner violence (IPV), substance use disorder, and mental health conditions account for 8% to 9% of all maternal deaths. And, importantly, 67% of those deaths due to trauma and/or mental health-related issues occur after the 6-week postpartum window. The link between trauma-related conditions and maternal mortality is undeniable; not only do we see it in the increasing rates of suicide, overdose, and homicide, but we now also recognize the role implicit bias plays in the treatment of women of color who are 2.5 times more likely to die in childbirth than White women.[11] Trauma-informed principles not only serve to mitigate or eliminate preventable causes of intrapartum and postpartum emotional trauma, but address antepartum psychological trauma, such as that associated with substance use disorders, structural and cultural racism, domestic violence, a history of childhood abuse, and/or sexual trauma that may be part of a woman's cultural context.

The proper implementation of the 4R bundles of readiness, recognition, response, and reporting for postpartum hemorrhage and hypertensive disorders of pregnancy has been shown to improve outcomes in the peripartum period. An adaptation of a similar TIC bundle for obstetrics could function in a similar way to decrease morbidity and mortality associated with maternal mental health issues and trauma-related conditions.[12] The successful implementation of these evidence-based care bundles, although effective, is challenging. It requires administrative and leadership support, specific resources, ongoing training to improve communication between all staff members, appropriate staff education, simulation training with opportunities for staff to discuss decision-making, effective interfacing with electronic medical records, and methods for evaluating effectiveness of training. With the significant contribution of mental health and trauma-related conditions to the overall maternal mortality rate it is imperative that at the minimum, we push for trauma-awareness in all areas of obstetric care. A care bundle for depression and anxiety in the peripartum period has been developed; however, it has not yet been accepted widely and does not include trauma-specific concerns.[13] It is a stepping stone, nonetheless, to a more comprehensive approach to the recognition and understanding of how trauma impacts obstetric patients throughout the peripartum period, as well as how we can respond to it to allow for the best outcomes.

DISCUSSION
Trauma Aware or Trauma Denied?

Adapting the 4 Rs from SAMHSA's general principles to any health care discipline requires substantial understanding of how trauma impacts the lives of specific patient populations. In the past decade, numerous articles have documented the impact of innovative TIC clinics and services for many unique groups of trauma survivors in health care settings. Primary care trauma-informed integrated care for children and youth,[14] services for women living with HIV,[15] and for violently injured patients in emergency departments[16] are some of the health care environments that have implemented and tailored the 4 Rs to their patients' needs. Although these different clinics are uniquely suited for their populations and use slightly different adaptations of these principles, they all share a fundamental goal of understanding the impact that interpersonal violence and victimization have on a person's life and development. According to some authors this is what it means to be a trauma-informed service. In fact, they suggest that a service that is not trauma informed is trauma denied. In other words, the "absence of this understanding of the impact of trauma on a woman's life is the equivalent of denying the existence and significance of trauma in women's lives."[17]

The following 4 *R*s are an adaptation of the general principles within an obstetric context.

R1: Realize

One of the first crucial steps in becoming a trauma-informed provider is to become trauma-aware. That requires a realization that trauma not only exists and is pervasive in our society, but also the frequency at which different types of interpersonal trauma affect women. The following statistics are sobering, and would imply that a significant portion of women presenting for obstetric care have a history of trauma.

- Approximately 20% to 33% of women will be the victims of childhood sexual trauma.[2,18–20]
- Approximately 33% of female veterans will self-report a history of military sexual trauma.[21]
- Approximately 25% of women will experience severe physical violence from IPV in their lifetimes.[22]
- Up to 44% of women report their birth experiences as traumatic.[23]
- Adolescent parturients have a mean Adverse Childhood Experience score of 5.1.[24]

Many women who are survivors of trauma have never disclosed their experiences or sought treatment and thus do not present with a diagnosis. The peripartum period provides an opportunity for obstetric providers to inquire about traumatic histories and to offer support. This practice can often be challenging because most providers currently are untrained in how to elicit a history of certain types of interpersonal trauma such as sexual assault or rape, or IPV, and are, as important, lacking a framework for responding to a woman's disclosure. Screening for specific types of trauma is either required or recommended by multiple agencies and organizations, including the ACOG,[7] the Joint Commission, the Women's Preventive Services Initiative, the National Academy of Medicine (formerly the Institute of Medicine), the American Medical Association, and the US Preventive Services Task Force, yet it is not performed routinely.

Eliciting these histories is not the responsibility exclusively of obstetricians. Obstetric anesthesiologists may find themselves in a position to either elicit a trauma history or respond to a patient disclosure. Even if a provider has not yet achieved a level of competency in this area, basic approaches to all women offering validation for and belief of her previous negative experience, establishment of safety, and mutual development of care plans can be offered by anyone. A recent meta-analysis examining health care providers' responses to disclosures of intimate partner abuse recommends using the LIVES mnemonic as a best practice model: listen without judging, inquire about and respond to concerns and needs, validate experiences, and enhance safety, support, and follow-up.[25] The National Health Service England and the Center for Early Child Development, in their efforts to implement TIC, put forth useful guidelines to aid providers in this process. Some of the authors' recommendations that may be particularly useful for anesthesia providers include (1) asking women how their traumatic past continues to affect them generally and what they might need from you, (2) avoid triggering PTSD reactions by learning potential triggers, (3) assume, in the absence of disclosure, but in the presence of PTSD reactions, that the woman could be a survivor, and (4) acknowledge the long-term effects of trauma, and that they are not alone and that you and/or others can help. An alternative approach would be for providers to assume that all women have a history of trauma, thereby eliminating the need for screening, and as a result never failing to identify survivors.

R2: Recognize

The recognition of trauma in the peripartum period is vital if we are to provide trauma-informed interventions to minimize or mitigate potential harm. The absence of consistent, universal screening for survivors of trauma, as mentioned previously, makes it difficult for providers to accurately identify individuals with preexisting trauma. Consequently, providers are left to rely on other methods for identification, including recognizing the physical, mental health, and behavioral symptoms and signs that are associated with unresolved trauma in adult survivors. Women who have a history of interpersonal trauma (ie, sexual assault or abuse, IPV, rape) are at an increased risk of having a negative birth experience and developing postpartum mental health conditions, such as PTSD.[26] Other antenatal risk factors, including a lack of social support, maternal mental health conditions (anxiety and/or depression), or fear of childbirth, may also increase a woman's vulnerability to negative birth experiences and the development of PTSD.[27] If providers can recognize those individuals at highest risk early in the antepartum period, alternative tailored care plans can be implemented to improve the likelihood of a positive birth outcome (**Box 1**).[2,3,20,26,28–33]

Trauma is not limited to a woman's life experience before pregnancy. It can coexist during the pregnancy, occur de novo during labor or delivery, or surface in the postpartum period, or it can occur at multiple time points with one trauma superimposed on another. Thus, it is imperative that providers know how to recognize not only chronic traumatic stress in adult survivors, but also the symptoms of acute stress in the peripartum period.

In addition to preexisting risk factors and conditions associated with chronic traumatic stress, several intrapartum events have been identified as traumatic events and have been associated with an increased risk for the development of postpartum PTSD. These include operative birth (assisted vaginal delivery with forceps or vacuum or cesarean delivery), obstetric emergencies including the response of emergency teams to these emergencies, maternal medical complications, infant complications, fetal death, and early pregnancy loss.[26] Anesthesia-related events identified as traumatic include severe nausea and vomiting, failed neuraxial anesthesia leading to

---

Box 1
Physical, psychological and behavioral manifestations of chronic unresolved trauma

- Physical
  - Hypertension, cardiovascular disease
  - Gastrointestinal problems
  - Chronic pain states including chronic migraines, fibromyalgia syndrome, interstitial cystitis/bladder pain syndrome
  - Poor immune function
  - Fatigue

- Psychological
  - Depression/suicidal ideation
  - PTSD
  - Anxiety
  - Extreme fear of childbirth

- Behavioral
  - Substance use disorders
  - Eating disorders
  - Sleeping difficulties
  - Request for no male providers

intraoperative pain requiring rescue medications, unintentional dural puncture followed by severe postpartum postdural puncture headache, traumatic needle insertion with pain, residual cutaneous hematoma, or both, and neurologic injuries.[34] The occurrence of any of these peripartum events should prompt hypervigilance by the providers to monitor patients for signs of acute stress responses (**Box 2**).[35,36] It is only when we are adept at recognizing when a traumatic event has occurred and how a woman might manifest her response to it that we will be able to provide the vital psychological safety that these patients require.

R3: Respond

SAMHSA states that we should all strive to respond to trauma in our workplaces and environments by incorporating knowledge into practices, protocols, and principles. The realizations and recognition of trauma's impact in the lives of our patients (and ourselves) is essential, and a good first step. These skills must be developed in parallel with sustainable policy changes if we are to reframe the way all providers approach care for these individuals and their families.

Box 2
Signs and symptoms of acute stress disorder

- Intrusion symptoms
  - Recurrent images, thoughts, illusions, dreams/nightmares or flashbacks related to the event leading to:
    - Sleep disruption
    - Exacerbation of underlying anxiety/depression
    - Poor concentration
    - Exaggerated startle, agitation
- Hyperarousal/distress with exposure to stimuli
  - Intense reaction to exposure to stimuli related to the event
    - Physical: hypertension, tachycardia, perspiration
    - Psychological: fear, irritability, inability to comply with care recommendations
    - Can include hospital sounds, certain providers, smells, procedures, the infant
    - Sleep disturbance
    - Poor concentration
    - Exaggerated startle, agitation
      - Jumping, flinching, shaking in response to unexpected movements by others, noises, alarms, physical touch
- Negative mood
  - The woman may show no positive emotion or joy when she is with her baby or family
    - She may seem withdrawn, numb, or detached from the event
    - She may exhibit a flat affect
    - She may exhibit a wide range of negative emotions, including fear, sadness, guilt, shame, embarrassment, and disappointment
- Dissociative symptoms
  - The woman may exhibit an altered sense of reality or disturbance in memory
    - She may seem like she is "out of it," dazed, or confused
    - Some women speak of an "out-of-body" experience
- Avoidance symptoms
  - The woman may avoid any distressing memories, thoughts, or feelings or external reminders of the event
    - This could include procedures, parts of the hospital, providers, even the baby
    - Minimal postpartum follow-up care

There are no universally accepted protocols currently for the implementation of TIC in obstetric practices. There is ample research, however, detailing what is important to survivors of trauma. This insight can serve as a foundation for the types of protocols necessary for best outcomes. In one qualitative study, the authors outlined the specific needs of sexual assault survivors.[2] Some of the themes elucidated in this study include the need for a trusting environment, clear explanations of all providers' roles, control over the timing of examinations, respect for her privacy, and communication of her history in a consistent way, especially in the medical record. In another article that highlighted the needs of survivors of childhood trauma, similar themes were identified, but these authors also included concepts of valuing diversity to enrich communication and understanding and a team approach to mental health care and support.[37] An example of how a protocol could address these needs would be one where designated signage (ie, a picture of a flower) could be placed on the door of all trauma survivors to remind providers to knock before entering and to have their name badge visible with the expectation that they will need to introduce themselves every time. Another straightforward protocol would address how patients' histories are communicated during any change of shift or provider. Many obstetric units use a common display board for use during scheduled safety rounds. An added column to this board to allow for comments about mental health and trauma could also be incorporated into daily practices.

Other qualitative narratives discussed factors that influence a patient's overall subjective birth experience, including wanting control over exposure of their bodies, fear of restraints and oxygen masks in the operating room, nausea and vomiting, and separation of loved ones for procedures.[2,3] Policies that address nausea and vomiting have already been established in many institutions as part of Early Recovery After Cesarean protocols, but policies that allow flexibility in having a significant other in their operating room for the placement of neuraxial blocks are not as widely accepted, despite evidence that doing so would decrease anxiety levels for survivors. Some policies, such as those concerning the use of restraints, may need to be reviewed and adapted to the unique needs of obstetric patients. The use of restraints must balance the potential physical harm that a patient could do to themselves or others, and the potential for psychological harm to the patient as a result of retraumatization.

Additional research looking at trauma-informed services for the emergency department setting outlines other recommended policy changes. These could also be adapted to the care of obstetric patients.[38] They suggest that trauma-informed systems should include mandatory training for providers focusing on trauma prevention and intervention strategies, and an understanding of the social determinants of health, implicit bias, and racism. Additionally, they recommend routine screening protocols for PTSD or histories of trauma and the establishment of extended follow-up policies. For obstetric patients, these extended follow-up periods should continue up to one year postpartum and would aid in the diagnosis of mental health complications. Finally, they encourage institutional-level acceptance and support through policy development, support protocols for providers who are at risk for secondary trauma, and funding for education.

R4: Resist Retraumatization

To resist retraumatization means adapting our practices to prevent further psychological trauma for survivors. Trauma is unique to each person and thus individualized, tailored approaches may be required. Additionally, each medical discipline may have their own unique responsibilities in the care of these patients. Because chronic traumatic stress and PTSD may leave many patients feeling extremely vulnerable, having difficulty trusting providers, and struggling for control—usually a surrogate for safety—changes in practices need to focus on these underlying principles.[29] The following recommendations are rooted in these basic needs and focus on shared approaches to care, which include allowing patients to participate in care decisions as much as possible, respecting a woman's autonomy and rights during the peripartum period, working on giving the patient a sense of control over her situation, offering choices when possible, providing as much consistency in care as possible for the establishment of trust, and allowing for professional adaptability for creative solutions. Some of these recommendations are straightforward and can be used in any system, but others, such as the establishment of trusting relationships, especially between disciplines, takes time and may not be implemented as easily.

The following practice recommendations are based on general TIC principles and these authors' extensive work with trauma survivors in the peripartum period (**Box 3**).[36,39]

Barriers

TIC specific to anesthesia providers is an unexplored area of research, and barriers to TIC are not investigated specifically in the anesthesia literature. The emergency medicine literature lists challenges such as time, the need to handle more immediate priorities, and compassion fatigue often due to secondary traumatic stress.[38] Across the trauma literature, training is also cited as inconsistent or lacking, both for residents and for active practitioners. Results of a September 2019 survey published in ACOG of all US and Canadian obstetrics and gynecology residencies indicated that only just more than 20% of programs have formal TIC training, and 15.5% of programs reported no TIC training, citing "lack of facilitators" and "lack of time" as the top reasons.[40] A 2018 survey of Family Medicine residency programs reported similar results.[41] Their programs met patients' TIC needs only about 5% of the time, also citing "lack of a champion" and "lack of time" as the top reasons.

Organizations and systems are notoriously resistant to change. Without effective administrative support, changes will not last and individual health providers wishing to implement TIC may find themselves trying to create system work-arounds on an individual patient level.[42] A child welfare system wishing to implement TIC at an operational level observed a number of systems challenges, including a dearth of trained TIC mental health providers, lack of affordable treatment options, a lack of funding, and a lack of time spent on implementation.[43] This same system mentioned "limited staff time," which could translate to what we consider production pressure in a labor and delivery unit or operating room.

Inherent patient characteristics may make recognition of a trauma difficult or may result in additional challenges to TIC implementation. Patients may not feel a trauma history is relevant to disclose, even when directly asked or have concerns about retriggering when it is discussed.[44] Serious mental health pathology may interfere with eliciting a trauma history.[45] African American patients may be less likely to self-report personal trauma, may have increased rates of institutional mistrust, a desire to underplay a trauma history, as well as feel an inability to connect with health care providers.[46–48] Age may also play a role. More than 80% of pregnant teenagers may have a history of trauma, but research suggests that these patients may not be willing to discuss this history with providers with whom they do not have an ongoing relationship. Multiple appointments may be needed to elicit a history and engage in care.[24] Cultural differences may present unique challenges to the recognition of a trauma history and there are additional challenges in the implementation of culturally sensitive TIC.[49] Socioeconomic factors may affect the ability of patients to afford or show up to appointments.[43]

Box 3
TIC principles to prevent retraumatization in obstetric patients

- Antepartum period
  - Plan for early consultation during pregnancy
    - Elucidate fears or concerns of the upcoming delivery
    - Identify known triggers, history of panic, and any successful nonpharmacologic and pharmacologic coping mechanisms for stressful situations
    - Explain the risks and benefits of low-dose anxiolytics
    - Discuss pain expectations and pain management options, opiate maintenance and withdrawal prevention strategies, and nicotine management (especially for any women with substance use disorders)
    - Discuss the role of the significant other and level of social support, and any need for private preoperative and/or recovery space
    - Offer an opportunity for patients to familiarize themselves with the hospital environment, including the operating room (live or virtual tours) so patients can process information and ask questions in advance of delivery
    - Plan for early selection and introduction of team members to foster trusting positive therapeutic relationships
    - Establish best practice for communicating her history and plan to her care team when she presents to the obstetric unit

- Intrapartum and intraoperative periods
  - Minimize the number of providers assigned to the patient
  - Eliminate positions that promote the authoritative hierarchy between patient and provider (ie, sit at eye level with the patient) to foster a more collaborative relationship; sitting also implies that you are taking time to listen to a patient
  - Focus on culturally sensitive, compassionate, and respectful language at all times
  - Frequent "check-ins" to inquire about the patient's emotional state and planned use of nonpharmacologic (ie, breathing techniques, music) or pharmacologic anxiolytics
  - Minimize harsh and loud stimuli and allow for compassionate measures (ie, warm blankets, mouth swabs, and clear surgical drapes) if desired
  - Communicate with a calm voice with focus on her, avoid nonrelevant sidebar discussions with other staff members
  - Avoid separation of the patient and her significant other when possible if the patient desires, the use of arm straps (unless she meets criteria for restraints), unnecessary oxygen masks, severe nausea and vomiting, and severe shaking; these events can all trigger acute stress responses
  - Respect a patient's modesty and privacy by keeping her body covered as much as possible and asking before entering her room
  - Designate the most advanced anesthesia provider to perform any neuraxial procedures
  - Insist on vigilance and consistency with neuraxial block evaluation for surgery and rapid conversion to other forms of anesthesia when deemed inadequate
  - Support an environment that allows for early skin-to-skin contact with the neonate

- Postpartum period
  - Observe for any changes in affect or mood and refer early to perinatal mental health specialists
  - Recognize that any complications, including difficult block placement or conversion to general anesthesia could be perceived as a traumatic experience, and acknowledge any such reports with understanding, validation and support, and offer referrals for mental health experts

---

SUMMARY

The need for a more trauma-aware, holistic approach to obstetric care is needed. This approach must incorporate not only the woman's current medical status physically and psychologically, but also realize how her cultural context and past experiences influence her current experience. We now understand the role of trauma in the maternal mortality rate in this country, but its impact on maternal, fetal, and neonatal morbidity cannot be overstated. Whether it is chronic traumatic stress contributing to a premature delivery and extended neonatal intensive care unit stay or an unexpected anesthesia-related event resulting in PTSD, a traumatic birth experience comes at a high cost to the woman, her child, her family, and to society. Decreased maternal–infant bonding, decreased breastfeeding success, relationship difficulties, and maternal mental health conditions as a result of a traumatic birth have all been well described in the literature.[50] Some trauma survivors experience dissociation during a traumatic event and grieve the loss of memory of the birth experience itself. Authors have also noted the potential for generational transmission of oxytocin deficiency—an implication of maternal trauma— that can contribute to the higher rates of behavioral and psychiatric disorders among the offspring.[51] Patient narratives have also highlighted the distrust and anger toward providers and health care institutions after traumatic events during childbirth, with some patients refusing to return for any postpartum care or antepartum care in future pregnancies.[52] In a recent review, authors have identified the potential for altered pain perception for women who have a history of trauma and other mental health conditions. Patients who are not treated adequately may suffer increased pain after surgical delivery and be at risk for chronic pain states.[39]

We must explore ways to build trust with our patients and provide safe spaces for them to disclose and share any traumatic past events. We may need to reallocate time so that extra time is spent developing relationships with patients early in pregnancy and creating plans that optimize a positive birth experience. The extra time (and cost) spent early in pregnancy is recouped when a traumatic birth with its inherent consequences is avoided. When time is not available, our responses during an acute event need to reflect our realization and recognition of the potential difficulties a woman is experiencing during her delivery experience. For anesthesia providers, our expertise in managing acute physical crises must be expanded to incorporate the acute management of psychological crises as well, but this process requires training and practice. Consistency in education for all the staff is essential so that women, especially those who are survivors of trauma, feel validated and safe throughout the peripartum period. With the understanding that trauma-related mental health conditions are contributing significantly to the maternal mortality rate in this country, we now have even more reason to adopt TIC into our obstetric practices. Innovative patient-centered approaches that prevent traumatic peripartum experiences or retraumatization can not only decrease maternal, fetal, and neonatal morbidity and mortality, but also mitigate the extensive and expensive burdens placed onto society, health care systems, and health care providers as a result of this trauma.

CLINICS CARE POINTS

- It is essential that providers realize that trauma exists and understand the impact that violence and victimization can have on a person's life.

- Failure to recognize and respond appropriately to an individual who has survived past trauma, or who has suffered an acutely traumatizing birth experience, can have long term physical, psychological and behavioral impacts on mothers and their children.

- The development of individualized trauma services that prevent re-traumatization can improve patient outcomes and decrease expensive burdens placed onto society, healthcare systems and healthcare providers.

- Consistent training of all maternal care providers in trauma-informed care practices requires institutional level acceptance and support and prioritized funding.

DISCLOSURE

The authors have nothing to disclose.

REFERENCES

1. Schultz GD. Cruelty in maternity wards. Ladies Home J 1958;44–5, 152–155.
2. Sobel L, O'Rourke-Suchoff D, Holland E, et al. Pregnancy and childbirth after sexual trauma. Patient perspectives and care preferences. Obstet Gynecol 2018; 132:1461–8.
3. Simpkin P, Klaus P. When survivors give birth. Seattle, WA: Classic Day Publishing; 2004.
4. Futura M, Sandall J, Bick D. Women's perceptions and experiences of severe maternal morbidity-a synthesis of qualitative studies using a meta-ethnographic approach. Midwifery 2014;30:158–69.
5. SAMHSA's concept of trauma and guidance for a trauma-informed approach prepared by SAMHSA's trauma and justice strategic initiative July 2014. Available at: https://ncsacw.samhsa.gov/userfiles/files/SAMHSA_Trauma.pdf. Accessed May 30, 2021.
6. Law C, Wolfenden L. A good practice guide to support implementation of trauma-informed care in the perinatal period. The Centre for Early Child Development (Blackpool, UK). Commissioned by NHS England and NHS Improvement in 2019.
7. Caring for patients who have experienced trauma: ACOG committee opinion summary, number 825. Obstet Gynecol 2021;137(4):757–8.
8. Heal PA. Available at: https://www.pacesconnection.com/resource/heal-pa-leadership-and-action-teams-pdf. Accessed May 30, 2021.
9. Hoyert LD. Maternal mortality rates in the United States, 2019. National Center for Health Statistics; 2021. https://doi.org/10.15620/cdc:103855.
10. Pregnancy-related deaths: data from 14 U.S. maternal mortality review committees, 2008-2017. https://www.cdc.gov/reproductivehealth/maternal-mortality/erase-mm/MMR-Data-Brief_2019-h.pdf. Accessed May 30, 2021.
11. Singh GK. Trends and social inequalities in maternal mortality in the United States, 1969-2018. Int J MCH AIDS 2021;10(1):29–42.
12. Eppes CS, Han SB, Haddock AJ, et al. Enhancing obstetric safety through best practices. J Womens Health 2021;30(2):265–9.
13. Kendig S, Keats JP, Hoffman MC, et al. Consensus bundle on maternal mental health: perinatal depression and anxiety. Obstet Gynecol 2017;129(3):422–30.
14. Brown JD, King MA, Wissow LS. The central role of relationships with trauma-informed integrated care for children and youth. Acad Pediatr 2017;17(7): S94–101.
15. Cuca YP, Shumway M, Machtinger EL, et al. The association of trauma with the physical, behavioral, and social health of women living with HIV: pathways to guide trauma-informed health care interventions. Womens Health Issues 2019; 29(5):376–84.
16. Fischer KR, Bakes KM, Corbin TJ, et al. Trauma-informed care for violently injured patients in the emergency department. Ann Emerg Med 2019;73(2):193–202.
17. Elliott DE, Bjelajac P, Fallot RD, et al. Trauma-informed or trauma-denied: principles and implementation of trauma-informed services for women. J Community Psychol 2005;33(4):461–77.
18. Singh M, Parsekar S, Nair S. An epidemiological overview of child sexual abuse. J Fam Med Prim Care 2014;3(4):430.

19. Seng JS, Sperlich M, Low LK, et al. Childhood abuse history, posttraumatic stress disorder, postpartum mental health, and bonding: a prospective cohort study. J Midwifery Womens Health 2013;58(1):57–68.

20. Felitti VJ, Anda RF, Nordenberg D, et al. Relationship of childhood abuse and household dysfunction to many of the leading causes of death in adults. Am J Prev Med 1998;14(4):245–58.

21. Sadler AG, Mengeling MA, Syrop CH, et al. Lifetime sexual assault and cervical cytologic abnormalities among military women. J Womens Health 2011;20(11): 1693–701.

22. Preventing intimate partner violence |violence prevention|injury center|cdc. 2021. Available at: https://www.cdc.gov/violenceprevention/intimatepartnerviolence/ fastfact.html. Accessed June 1, 2021.

23. de Graaff LF, Honig A, van Pampus MG, et al. Preventing post-traumatic stress disorder following childbirth and traumatic birth experiences: a systematic review. Acta Obstet Gynecol Scand 2018;97:648–56.

24. Millar HC, Lorber S, Vandermorris A, et al. "No, you need to explain what you are doing": obstetric care experiences and preferences of adolescent mothers with a history of childhood trauma. J Pediatr Adolesc Gynecol 2021;34(4):538–45.

25. Tarzia L, Bohren MA, Cameron J, et al. Women's experiences and expectations after disclosure of intimate partner abuse to a healthcare provider: a qualitative meta-synthesis. BMJ Open 2020;10:e041339.

26. Vogel TM, Homitsky S. Antepartum and intrapartum risk factors and the impact of PTSD on mother and child. BJA Educ 2020;20(3):89–95.

27. Dekel S, Stuebe C, Dishy G. Childbirth induced posttraumatic stress syndrome: a systematic review of prevalence and risk factors. Front Psychol 2017;8:560.

28. Herman JL. Trauma and recovery. 2015 edition. New York: BasicBooks; 2015.

29. Van der Kolk BA, McFarlane AC, Weisæth L, editors. Traumatic stress: the effects of overwhelming experience on mind, body, and society. New York: Guilford Press; 2007.

30. Hellou R, Häuser W, Brenner I, et al. Self-reported childhood maltreatment and traumatic events among Israeli patients suffering from fibromyalgia and rheumatoid arthritis. Pain Res Manag 2017;2017:3865249.

31. Gerber MR, Bogdan KM, Haskell SG, et al. Experience of childhood abuse and military sexual trauma among women veterans with fibromyalgia. J Gen Intern Med 2018;33(12):230–1.

32. Tietjen GE, Peterlin BL. Childhood abuse and migraine: epidemiology, sex differences, and potential mechanisms. Headache 2011;51(6):869–79.

33. McKernan LC, Johnson BN, Reynolds WS, et al. Posttraumatic stress disorder in interstitial cystitis/bladder pain syndrome: relationship to patient phenotype and clinical practice implications. Neurourol Urodyn 2019;38(1):353–62.

34. Lopez U, Meyer M, Loures V, et al. Post-traumatic stress disorder in parturients delivering by caesarean section and the implication of anaesthesia: a prospective cohort study. Health Qual Life Outcome 2017;15(1-13):118.

35. American Psychiatric Association, American Psychiatric Association. In: Diagnostic and statistical manual of mental disorders. Fifth edition. Arlington (VA): American Psychiatric Association; 2013.

36. OB HemorrhageToolkit v 2. 0 | California Maternal Quality Care Collaborative. Available at: https://www.cmqcc.org/resources-tool-kits/toolkits/ob-hemorrhage-toolkit. Accessed June 1, 2021.

37. Muzik M, Ads M, Bonham C, et al. Perspectives on trauma-informed care from mothers with a history of childhood maltreatment: a qualitative study. Child Abuse Neglect 2013;37(12):1215–24.
38. Fischer KR, Bakes KM, Corbin TJ, et al. Trauma-informed care for violently injured patients in the emergency department. Ann Emerg Med 2019;73(2):193–202.
39. Vogel TM. Unique pain management needs for pregnant women with pre-existing PTSD and other mental health disorders. Curr Anesthesiol Rep 2021;11(1):1–11.
40. DeAndrade S, Pelletier A, Bartz D, et al. Trauma informed care training in ob/gyn residency programs [26g]. Obstet Gynecol 2020;135:77S.
41. Dichter ME, Teitelman A, Klusaritz H, et al. Trauma-informed care training in family medicine residency programs results from a cera survey. Fam Med 2018;50(8): 617–22.
42. Weinger MB, Gaba DM. Human factors engineering in patient safety. Anesthesiology 2014;120(4):801–6.
43. Donisch K, Bray C, Gewirtz A. Child welfare, juvenile justice, mental health, and education providers' conceptualizations of trauma-informed practice. Child Maltreat 2016;21(2):125–34.
44. Gokhale P, Young MR, Williams MN, et al. Refining trauma-informed perinatal care for urban prenatal care patients with multiple lifetime traumatic exposures: a qualitative study. J Midwifery Womens Health 2020;65(2):224–30.
45. Mihelicova M, Brown M, Shuman V. Trauma-informed care for individuals with serious mental illness: an avenue for community psychology's involvement in community mental health. Am J Community Psychol 2018;61(1–2):141–52.
46. Armstrong K, Putt M, Halbert CH, et al. Prior experiences of racial discrimination and racial differences in health care system distrust. Med Care 2013;51(2): 144–50.
47. Armstrong K, McMurphy S, Dean LT, et al. Differences in the patterns of health care system distrust between blacks and whites. J Gen Intern Med 2008;23(6): 827–33.
48. Liebschutz J, Schwartz S, Hoyte J, et al. A chasm between injury and care: experiences of black male victims of violence. J Trauma Inj Infect Crit Care 2010; 69(6):1372–8.
49. Ranjbar N, Erb M, Mohammad O, et al. Trauma-informed care and cultural humility in the mental health care of people from minoritized communities. Focus (Am Psychiatr Publ) 2020;18(1):8–15.
50. Fenech G, Thomson G. Tormented by ghosts from their past: a meta-synthesis to explore the psychosocial implications of a traumatic birth on maternal well-being. Midwifery 2014;30:185–93.
51. Toepfer P, Heim C, Entringer S, et al. Oxytocin pathways in the intergenerational transmission of maternal early life stress. Neurosci Biobehav Rev 2016;73: 293–308.
52. Stanford SER, Bogod DG. Failure of communication: a patient's story. Int J Obstet Anesth 2016;28:70–5.

Decision Making in Obstetric Anesthesia

Rebecca D. Minehart, MD, MSHPEd[a],*, Daniel Katz, MD[b]

KEYWORDS

- Cognitive biases • Metacognition • Shared mental models
- Crisis resource management • Clinical decision support • Teamwork • Simulation

KEY POINTS

- Decision making is a complex and dynamic process vulnerable to external forces that need examining.
- Obstetric anesthesiologists can lead their teams in establishing robust preventative and recovery behaviors aimed at improving decision making by both individuals and teams.
- Team training using simulation improves team performance through sharing information and collaborating, crucial for decision making in obstetric care

INTRODUCTION

Caring for obstetric patients can be straightforward or profoundly complex, even when a pregnant patient's clinical course appears to be unfolding as the team expects. As any obstetric anesthesiologist knows, emergencies can manifest at any time, necessitating clear and coordinated team responses representing complex decision making in the moment. Forecasting how one may react and make decisions during an emergency is difficult. On the labor floor, interprofessional obstetric care teams have varied training backgrounds and practice patterns, adding a layer of complexity to decision making. This often leads people to thinking and acting in ways that may be misunderstood, especially when examined in hindsight. Critically examining all these decision-making processes,[1] and the influences that can lead individuals and teams astray on a wrong treatment course or create problematic teamwork more generally, is therefore fundamental to the practice of obstetric anesthesia.

Famed economists Daniel Kahneman and Amos Tversky created the field of behavioral economics in the late 1980s by investigating why humans' decisions did not

[a] Obstetric Anesthesia Division, Department of Anesthesia, Critical Care, and Pain Medicine, Massachusetts General Hospital, Harvard Medical School, 55 Fruit Street, GRJ 440, Boston, MA 02114, USA; [b] Department of Anesthesiology, Perioperative & Pain Medicine, The Mount Sinai Hospital, 1 Gustave L. Levy Place, New York City, NY 10029, USA
* Corresponding author.
E-mail address: rminehart@mgh.harvard.edu
Twitter: @RDMinehart (R.D.M.)

Anesthesiology Clin 39 (2021) 793–809
https://doi.org/10.1016/j.anclin.2021.08.013
1932-2275/21/© 2021 Elsevier Inc. All rights reserved.

always appear to be rational,[2–5] culminating in Kahneman winning the Nobel Prize for Economics in 2002.[6] Together, their in-depth examination of what drove human decision making incorporated empiric evidence and revealed a vast and integrated web of risk calculation, framing effects, and cognitive short-cuts (or heuristics) to explain what seemed to be an otherwise enigmatic or arbitrary process. These processes are necessary to function in the clinical environment where circumstances can change from second to second; however, reflexive use of such processes may leave one falling prey to erroneous decision making, especially when stress is high. As such, arming oneself with deliberate strategies to preserve thinking and rational decision making may reduce cognitive errors and enhance patient safety.

This article aims to introduce modern concepts of cognitive decision making fundamental to behavioral economics and applies them in the context of rapidly evolving team-based approaches that characterize obstetric care. It will consider the ways in which humans are hard-wired to make assumptions and perform short-cuts to save time and effort, although these may not serve people in every circumstance. Finally, the authors will share strategies to promote better, team-based thinking through enhanced shared mental models that keep practitioners fresh and patients safe from harm.

INDIVIDUAL COGNITIVE DECISION-MAKING PROCESSES

In a general sense, the decision-making process in the obstetric anesthesia setting is no different than what is encountered in other areas. As such, this article will first discuss cognitive processes involved in decision making and what influences these processes (for a review including historic models of decision making that have been since disproven, please refer to Stiegler and Tung's paper[1]).

Dual Process Reasoning: System 1 and System 2 Thinking

Many researchers have reaffirmed and expounded on Kahneman and Tversky's original work, which has culminated in identifying 2 distinct pathways by which people come to decisions.[7] A dual-process theory has been described, which comprises 2 types of decision making (**Table 1**).[8,9] System 1 is a pathway that relies on cognitive shortcuts, or heuristics, to arrive at a decision more quickly (and is more cognitively efficient). Commonly referred to as gut thinking, system 1 is valuable for its efficiency and is thought to produce highly reliable decisions; in fact, most decisions use this system. However, system 1 also relies on repeated, timely, high-quality feedback for fine tuning, and therefore is vulnerable when feedback is delayed, erroneously interpreted, or outright absent.

In contrast, system 2 is a slow, deliberate process that carefully analyzes ideas in a logical procession, culminating in a decision that is thought to be more air tight in reasoning. System 2 is thought to be inherently valuable for producing quality decisions yet is cognitively more cumbersome and time consuming than system 1. It is also worth noting that cognitive errors may also occur within system 2 thinking. Researchers postulate that both types of processing are necessary for decision making, and fluidly moving between system 1 and system 2 allows one to adapt decision making to each situation.

There is no 1 right way to process information under the dual process model. In certain circumstances, a rapidly deteriorating patient will not allow for deliberation over each data point (meaning that pattern-based, system 1 thinking is more appropriate). However, when time allows and a decision is high stakes, system 2 thinking may be more reliable for avoiding disastrous mistakes. In either case, developing

Table 1
Characteristics of system 1 and system 2

System 1	System 2
Automatic	Analytical
Unintentional	Deliberate
Effortless	Effortful
Free-associating	Orderly
Low awareness	High awareness
Reflexive	Rule-based
More vulnerable to bias	Less vulnerable to bias
More influenced by emotions	Less influenced by emotions
Low predictive power	High predictive power
Low scientific rigor	High scientific rigor
Context is critically important	Context is less important
Multiple parallel cognitive channels for processing	Single linear cognitive channel for processing
Quick	Slow

Adapted from Croskerry.[7]

awareness of each system's merits helps one be more intentional applying selected decision-making approaches.

The Ladder of Inference

On a practical note, organizational psychologist Chris Argyris created a schematic representation approximating system 1 thinking with his "Ladder of Inference," specifically noting how one's assumptions, if left unchecked, can leave one vulnerable to misinterpreting data (**Fig. 1**).[10,11] In this schematic, which incorporates acquiring information in addition to processing it, the data (at the bottom rungs of the ladder) are unconsciously selected through filters based on an individual's prior experiences, preferences, training, and other influences. Meaning is then applied automatically

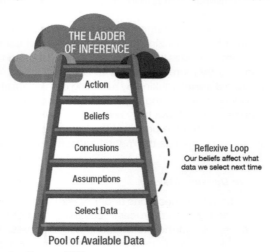

Fig. 1. The ladder of influence.[10,11]

(assumptions), and if these data are left unchecked and undergo further unconscious processing, meaning continues to be assumed until actions are taken.[10,11]

This type of reasoning is important when applied to aspects of the physical world (eg, assuming a steaming cup of dark liquid is hot coffee, and one should not drink it quickly to protect against burns) and is reliant on the development of stable and accurate patterns. However, when applied to behaviors or situations in which not all data fit together, cumulative misinterpretations up the ladder can lead to flawed decisions and erroneous actions. In addition, past assumptions often drive one's predilection for certain kinds of data, leading to prematurely discarding important data points during future decision making for the sake of efficiency. Only by critically examining one's assumptions, Argyris argues, can one be protected against making incorrect inferences.[10,11] The key question to ask is, "What am I missing here?" More strategies for pausing and deliberately evaluating one's thinking (known as cognitive forcing strategies) will be described later in this article.

INFLUENCES ON INDIVIDUAL DECISION MAKING

Individual decision making is not invulnerable to external influences; in fact, as described previously, there are multiple potential ways that the same individuals witnessing a situation may process information differently and arrive at disparate conclusions. Here the authors will review some of these factors influencing decision making.

Cognitive Biases in Obstetric Anesthesia

As noted previously, data acquisition is subject to biases, or unconscious processes that filter and shift how one interprets information, especially when one applies cognitive heuristics (or short-cuts) to arrive at a decision.[1,12–15] Awareness of these biases is the first step in guiding one's thinking. Although multiple researchers have studied cognitive debiasing strategies,[16,17] it is unclear whether any thinking can be truly unbiased. Certain conditions may predispose one to biased thinking, such as when one is fatigued, feeling strong emotions, or in unfamiliar circumstances.[1,13–15] In addition, there are many team-based factors that can predispose to erroneous decision making, including leadership behaviors (most notably authoritative or authoritarian leadership within a team)[18] and diversity that is inadequately managed.[19] The team's role will be discussed later in this article.

Although all decision making in obstetric anesthesia may be subject to bias, one can detect these biases earlier by familiarizing oneself with the most common biases present (**Table 2** lists common biases encountered during obstetric anesthesia). By recognizing when one may be more vulnerable to biased thinking, one can double-check assumptions during decision making by retracing data acquisition and processing to reveal gaps or inaccuracies. Being explicit in one's decision making by saying out loud what one is considering allows thinking to be reviewed, likely catching errors in the act. This also demonstrates the power of the independent observer during any obstetric emergency, as he or she has the mental capacity to examine these circumstances above the fray.

How Emotions Influence Decision Making

It is clear to anyone who has made decisions under pressure that emotions play a role in decision making, and although dual-process reasoning did not originally explicitly include emotions as influences, further adaptations based on research have shown they play a clear role,[20,21] especially in risky situations.[22] Emotions come in 2 distinct categories in the context of decision making: integral and incidental. Integral emotions

Table 2
Common cognitive biases in obstetric anesthesia

Cognitive Bias	Definition	Illustration
Anchoring	Focusing on 1 issue at the expense of understanding the whole situation	While troubleshooting an alarm on an infusion pump, one is unaware of sudden surgical bleeding and hypotension
Availability bias	Choosing a diagnosis because it is in the forefront of one's mind due to an emotionally charged memory of a bad experience	Misdiagnosing hypotension as anaphylaxis because of a prior case of anaphylaxis that had a poor outcome
Premature closure	Accepting a diagnosis prematurely, failure to consider reasonable differential of possibilities	Assuming that hypotension during a Cesarean delivery is from bleeding and missing septic shock
Feedback bias	Misinterpretation of no feedback as positive feedback	Believing that one has never had a case of unintentional awareness during emergency Cesarean delivery under general anesthesia, because one has never received a complaint about it
Confirmation bias	Seeking or acknowledging only information that confirms the desired or suspected diagnosis	Repeatedly cycling a noninvasive blood pressure cuff, changing cuff sizes, and locations, because one "does not believe" the low reading
Framing effect	Subsequent thinking is swayed by leading aspects of initial presentation	After being told by a colleague, "this patient was extremely anxious preoperatively," one attributes postoperative agitation to her personality rather than low blood glucose
Commission bias	Tendency toward action rather than inaction; performing unindicated maneuvers, deviating from protocol; may be due to overconfidence, desperation, or pressure from others	"Better safe than sorry" insertion of additional unnecessary invasive monitors or access; potentially resulting in a complication
Overconfidence bias	Inappropriate boldness, not recognizing the need for help, tendency to believe one is infallible	Delay in calling for help when one has trouble intubating, believing in eventual success
Omission bias	Hesitation to start emergency maneuvers for fear of being wrong or causing harm, tendency toward inaction	Delay in performing front-of-neck airway access during a cannot-intubate, cannot-ventilate situation, because it seems too invasive despite profound hypoxemia
Sunk costs	Unwillingness to let go of a failing diagnosis or decision, especially if much time/resources have	Having decided that a patient needs an awake fiberoptic intubation, refusing to consider

(continued on next page)

Table 2 (continued)		
Cognitive Bias	**Definition**	**Illustration**
	already been allocated; ego may play a role	alternative plans despite multiple unsuccessful attempts
Visceral bias	Countertransference; one's negative or positive feelings about a patient influencing decisions	Not troubleshooting on epidural for a laboring patient, because she is "high maintenance," a "complainer," or has "unrealistic expectations" about her pain relief
Zebra retreat	Rare diagnosis figures prominently among possibilities, but physician is hesitant to pursue it	Trying to "explain away" hypercarbia during nonobstetric surgery under general anesthesia when MH should be considered
Unpacking principle	Failure to elicit all relevant information, especially during transfer of care	Omission of key test results, medical history, or surgical event

Adapted from Patino Montoya and Minehart.[12]

are directly attributable to the decision making, such as anxiety or fear experienced during high-stakes decision making. Incidental emotions are unrelated to the decisions at hand but may still influence decision making, such as the frustration felt by being stuck in a traffic jam on the way to work; this then influences decisions made that day.[23] The authors will first consider integral emotions and how they may influence decision making.

Research in marketing has revealed that appealing to consumers' integral emotions rather than logic may lead to influencing consumers to cognitively appraise products or messages differently. This leads to changes in behavior.[24] The common strategy of framing messages in gains (rather than losses) can lead consumers to accept advertising messages more readily. For example, in antidrinking public service campaigns, guilt induced by showing the public what they can gain by reducing binge drinking led to more effective binge drinking avoidance when contrasted with the shame induced by messages focused on losses from binge drinking.[25] Although both guilt and shame are negative emotions, researchers propose that guilt focuses the individual on behaviors that can be changed, while shame is more focused on the self, which is experienced by some as more immutable.[26] In clinical situations, guilt may enhance (and shame may reduce) empathy between patients and clinicians, leading to altered decision making—in this case, with guilt broadening decision making capability and shame blunting it.[27]

Although certain integral emotions described previously have been found to generally enhance decision making,[27] even incidental (unrelated) emotions can play a role during decision making, as they can spill over from prior interactions and influence more broadly.[23] A recent study revealed that subjects in whom fear was invoked by having them recall a prior fear-inducing situation had a weaker preference for risky situations than the other groups who recalled happiness or anger.[23] Katz and colleagues[28] demonstrated that medical decision making was highly vulnerable to incidental emotions during a randomized, controlled trial involving anesthesia residents who were exposed to incivility during a simulated operative case, as judged by expert raters. Although the exact emotions experienced by the residents were not directly assessed,[28] the incivility between the simulated surgeon and the rest of the team was designed to evoke intimidation and possibly fear in the participants. Conversely, Crane and colleagues[29] found that anesthesiologists who reported generally positive emotions (or affect) 3 days preceding their involvement in a medical simulation demonstrated lower rates of cognitive fixation than those who reported more negative affect, indicating the incidental positive affect was protective. Although incidental emotions may seem to bluntly impact decision making, they can also have subtle yet significant effects. In 1 study, scores for medical school interviewees were lower when interviewed on rainy versus sunny days. On regression analysis, this had an equivalent impact of about a 10% lower score on the Medical College Admission Test.[30] These provocative findings indicate that one should focus on clinicians' emotional intelligence and emotional management strategies, as they seem paramount to ensuring accurate situational awareness and appraisal. However, to date there are no formal curricular expectations for emotional management strategies within either graduate medical training or maintenance of certification in anesthesiology.

Individual Situation Awareness

Individual situation awareness (SA), a model first proposed by Mica Endsley in 1995, is a "state of knowledge, from the processes used to achieve that state."[31,32] Endsley created a model for conceptualizing how people form and update SA (**Fig. 2**). Conceptually, SA may be analogous to a mental visual field, with low levels of SA akin to tunnel vision and high levels of SA as gaining the 1000 foot view.

Although some argue that SA is not dynamic, Endsley submits that SA can be updated nearly continuously as part of incorporating feedback and newer assessments.[32] A recent American Society of Anesthesiologists (ASA) closed claims review indicated that loss of SA, defined as failures in perceiving relevant information (level 1 SA), comprehending its meaning (level 2 SA), or projecting possible outcomes (level 3

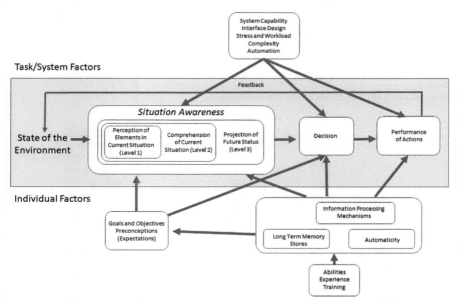

Fig. 2. Endsley's 1995 model of situation awareness, *Adapted from* Endsley.[32,33]

SA), frequently contributed to serious morbidity or mortality in claims from 2002 to 2013.[33] Obstetric anesthesia cases were not included; however, 74% of claims made during that time involved errors in one of the levels of SA during anesthetic care and were not more common in emergency compared with routine cases.[33] One may still learn from these cases, as there are many analogous situations in obstetric care that can be diagrammed according to Endsley's model.[32] **Table 3** provides examples of SA levels for a few potential obstetric situations. Although individual SA is key for accurate decision making, the entire SA process is more robust with multiple team members.

TEAM INFLUENCES ON DECISION MAKING

While examining individual decision-making processes remains critically important, equally valuable is to review team processes. Team decision-making processes involve much more than a single pathway, such as one of those models represented earlier. Instead, influences such as leadership behaviors,[1,18,34] team diversity of all kinds (including skill levels and training backgrounds),[19] and stress levels[23,35,36] all shape the team's willingness to engage in decision making via robust team shared mental models. In this way, the team influence on decision making is inherently more complex than the sum of the decision-making processes of the individuals on the team. Team dynamics can independently enhance or stifle the quality of decisions depending on the environment and functioning of the team.

The Role of Psychological Safety

Psychological safety of the team and environment play crucial roles in making it safer to discuss how one makes sense of a clinical situation. For most, the act of publicly sharing one's thinking can feel risky; allowing others to examine one's own reasoning feels like an exposure if one is wrong. Teams with a strong sense of psychological safety perform better in part because of the beliefs that members are safe to take interpersonal risks by sharing ideas and concerns, and that they will be valued and respected despite potentially being wrong at times.[34,37] Psychological safety is promoted by inclusive leadership behaviors:

Table 3
Examples of Endsley's levels of situation awareness.[33]

Perception (Level 1)	Comprehension (Level 2)	Projection (Level 3)
Sudden low blood pressure, urticaria	Anaphylactic shock	Continued airway and cardiovascular compromise if epinephrine is not administered
Small mouth opening, Mallampati 4 examination, short thyromental distance, obstructive sleep apnea	Possible obstetric difficult airway	Potential for hypoxia or anoxia during emergent induction of general anesthesia
Fever, tachycardia in labor	Evolving maternal sepsis	Multiorgan system dysfunction from untreated septic shock
Acute hypoxia, hypotension, and anxiety during a Cesarean delivery	Acute phase of amniotic fluid embolism	Potential for disseminated intravascular coagulopathy and maternal cardiac arrest

1. Specifically inviting others to speak up and share ideas
2. Responding constructively when others share their thoughts (often by thanking them for doing so, despite potentially disagreeing with the idea shared)
3. Incorporating (where possible) others' ideas into the action plans
4. Motivating the team through encouragement rather than threats or rewards[18,34,37]

When teams feel they can share their concerns and evaluate the decision making together, more shared data can inform better SA, and opportunities for discovering flawed thinking arise.[18] Leadership within teams that promotes psychological safety and inclusive decision making lowers a team's burnout and increases team members' organizational commitment,[38] both essential to team members' engaging in patient care. Although inclusive leadership does not appear to be a well-established model in the operating room environment,[18] obstetric units may be suited to adopting an inclusive culture given the high level of teamwork needed to provide care.

Psychological safety is a powerful concept with a robust research base and should not be confused with niceness.[39] Imposing a culture of being nice to each other encourages conformity and eventually groupthink, an extremely flawed decision-making state where team members do not actively seek additional information and instead seek excessive and uncritical concurrency for all decisions.[35] A team is vulnerable to groupthink under extremely stressful conditions, authoritarian or authoritative leadership models (where team members are encouraged to defer to the leader), and in situations where allegiance to the team and promoting team harmony are encouraged above all else.[18,35] In contrast to what may be expected, psychological safety is likely low under those conditions and can have drastic consequences. One of the most memorable examples is Korean Air flight 801. In this circumstance a failure of the copilot and flight crew to question the clearly erroneous decisions made by the pilot led a crash that killed 229 people.[39]

Team Situation Awareness

As noted previously, cognitive decision making relies upon acquiring robust data. This involves not only individuals capturing information and directing their attention (which is imperfect, as shown by studies of inattentional blindness,[40] where individuals miss even important information if they are not expecting to see it), but also team sharing information to build better team SA.[34,36,41] Endsley and Jones proposed specific processes that promote team SA:

- Self-checking, and checking against others at each step of SA formation
- Coordinating together to share information with each other
- Prioritizing with the team to set up contingencies and rejoin
- Questioning as a group to ensure SA fidelity[32]

Many other factors contribute to team SA, such as verbal and nonverbal communication, shared audio and visual displays (and alerts), and a shared environment with multiple potential cues.[32] Regular invitations or structured updates can lower the barriers some have for speaking up to provide additional information.

Effects of Team Diversity on Speaking up

Team diversity is a strength for decision making[42,43] and a vulnerability to speaking up.[19] Diverse teams are especially prone to conflict, which can be categorized per subject: either task, process, or relational conflict.[18,44] Relational (or interpersonal) conflict is magnified by supporting the hierarchical model of health care and mitigated by familiarity, prodiversity environments, minimizing the hierarchy, and inclusivity.[19,45]

Teams should strive to cultivate membership diversity, selecting members additionally for age, experience, and educational background, as these promote different perspectives of a same situation, which lead to enhanced creativity and decision making.[19] Another helpful construct is the idea of collective competence, which promotes interdependence among team members with the idea that the whole team is worth more than the sum of its parts.[46] Teams that demonstrate high levels of collective competence can overcome an individual member who may be incompetent, and teams comprised of many highly competent members can be wildly dysfunctional.[46] Leaders who promote collective competence can invite unique and valuable contributions that each member must share, which may compel diverse teams to demonstrate more openness.

STRATEGIES TO PRESERVE AND ENHANCE DECISION MAKING IN OBSTETRIC ANESTHESIA

Despite vulnerabilities inherent in human decision making, applying strategies may help avoid some common pitfalls associated with biased thinking, incomplete information, flawed SA processing, and emotional influences. It is important to note that these strategies often involve the utilization of system 2 processes. However, the authors are not suggesting that the best decision making strategy is to always utilize system 2 pathway. Instead, one should use these tools to decide when it is appropriate to shift from a system 1 decision pathway to a system 2 decision pathway. In other words, the authors encourage learning the circumstances under which a person should double check his or her gut.

High-Risk Situations for Biased Thinking

As discussed previously, certain situations can engender biased thinking more than others, which should prompt a person to double-check his or her decision making. Graber and colleagues created a checklist for emergency room physicians to use and mitigate diagnostic errors, which included rare and "don't miss" diagnoses.[47] What was most unique about such a checklist is that it included a list of high-risk situations for diagnostic error to alert clinicians to possibly biased decision making.[47] Alerting obstetric anesthesiology team members to potential pitfalls in decision making, paired with recovery strategies, can boost the team's cognitive flexibility to prevent errors (**Fig. 3**).

Metacognition and Cognitive Debiasing Strategies

Metacognition, or thinking about thinking, encompasses a host of skills such as reflecting on cognitive processes, self-awareness of one's areas of strengths and of growth, and mindfulness about influences on one's emotional state to help plan and monitor decision making.[48] Gaining awareness of these processes deserves invested time and energy, like learning a new technical skill within anesthesiology. Specifically practicing reflection and mindfulness can promote metacognition. Essential steps for reflection include:

1. Noticing (through self-monitoring thoughts and emotions)
2. Processing (by reviewing whether all information and skills are possessed)
3. Altering future action (by planning for changed responses based on reflections)[49]

In addition to these steps, metacognition includes slowing down one's thinking (potentially allowing for system 2 reasoning) and acknowledging – and accepting – uncertainty, which is uncomfortable for most obstetric anesthesiologists.[1,18] Deliberately

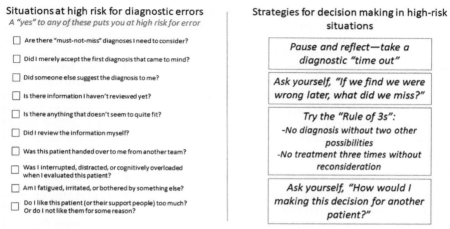

Fig. 3. Selected high-risk conditions under which biased thinking may occur in obstetric anesthesia and suggested cognitive forcing strategies. (*Adapted from* Graber, et al., and Stiegler and Tung[1,47])

practicing these allows better recovery in high-risk decision-making settings.[1] Furthermore, this practice should occur outside of the emergent circumstance. It should not be expected that these strategies would perform well on their first few utilizations. Likewise, their performance should not be judged on the first few implementations.

Other cognitive debiasing strategies have been proposed and have found to be effective. In a recent systematic review, Ludolph and Schulz found that over 70% of all included studies revealed partial or complete success for debiasing decision making.[50] Such debiasing strategies, also known as cognitive forcing strategies, require a definitive trigger for initiation. **Fig. 3** also provides some cognitive forcing strategies the authors have used in their obstetric anesthesiology practices. One such trigger could be recognizing a high-risk situation that prompts a cognitive forcing strategy (such as asking, "Am I fatigued? If so, I should choose a strategy to help my thinking."). Another trigger might be encountered with the third dose of phenylephrine for the obstetric post-operative patient who is hypotensive, which should prompt re-evaluating the assumed etiology for the hypotension, per the rule of threes.[1] This strategy can also be deployed diagnostically, disallowing the closing of a diagnostic loop until at least 3 diagnoses are considered, which may enhance SA.

Methodical approaches to individual data collection are critical for not missing important information and avoiding confirmation bias and anchoring. Applying systematic methods can enhance data collection, such as deliberately evaluating patients during an anesthetic by double-checking all elements within one's visual field sweeping from left to right, or evaluating problems using mnemonics, such as applying the primary and secondary surveys conducted during trauma assessments.[51] Additionally, using emergency manuals or cognitive aids ensures that other diagnoses are considered, and reduces the number of missed steps when diagnosing and treating an acutely unstable patient.[52–54] Goldhaber-Fiebert and colleagues have shown that perceived safety culture improved after adopting cognitive aids in an anesthesiology department.[55] Importantly, a set of obstetric anesthesiology-specific cognitive aids produced by Abir and colleagues may be freely downloaded.[54,56]

Teams interested in adopting cognitive aids to improve team decision making should consider following best implementation science strategies, where shortcutting extensive training prior to emergent events may lead to poor adoption.[54,57] Cognitive aids should be dual purposed for teaching during calmer times, which will serve to familiarize team members with these tools in addition to refreshing knowledge.[57] Although cognitive aids are not a salvo for every situation, teams that use them regularly report lower levels of stress and better teamwork.[54] Finally, cognitive aids are best used as part of a team approach and require an independent utilizer to function effectively. For example, one should not utilize a cognitive aid for a difficult airway while simultaneously managing a difficult airway. This again underpins the importance of calling for help early.

A Focus on Teaming as a Strategy for Better Decision Making

Team decision making has outperformed individual decision making in studies, specifically regarding problems related to cognition, coordination, and cooperation.[58,59] To that end, building and maintaining a team are active strategies—hence the word "teaming." Edmondson's work in complex health care teams[34,37] has revealed 4 distinct behaviors present in high-performing teams:

1. Speaking up
2. Collaboration
3. Experimentation and
4. Reflection[40]

Obstetric anesthesiology leaders should familiarize themselves with these concepts to promote each of these behaviors, boosting team connectedness, creativity, and flexibility for dynamic situations.[40] Often, obstetric anesthesiologists may work in small anesthesiology teams, but teaming should be the goal for all interprofessional obstetric caregivers. Teaming takes deliberate effort and pays off through improved relational coordination, the idea that familiarity and connectedness (achieved through training [eg, using simulation]) can improve the team's communication and shared knowledge.[19,60] Other formats to improve teaming such as escape rooms may also be utilized and be an effective tool to enhance teamwork and reduce burnout.

Explicitly Teaching Situation Awareness Processes and Name/Claim/Aim Through Full-Team Simulation

In addition to improving relational coordination, teams can improve their SA through deliberate training.[61,62] Morgan and colleagues reported using the Situation Awareness Global Assessment Technique (SAGAT) within interprofessional teams undergoing simulation training.[61] The SAGAT employs distinct pauses during an interprofessional simulation session, during which facilitators ask questions aimed at evaluating the team's SA. They found this technique to be feasible with some iteration; interestingly, the pauses enacted during this technique were associated with anesthesiologists feeling less stressed.[61] In another randomized controlled simulation-based trial, Jonsson and colleagues assessed intensive care unit (ICU) team SA training through 3 distinct teamwork and SA assessment tools; of these, 1 tool, the TEAM tool, highlighted improved leadership and task management.[62] Overall, simulation training has been shown to improve obstetric medical malpractice claims, as evidenced by a recent study by Schaffer and colleagues.[63]

The mnemonic Name/Claim/Aim is used by the authors as a tool to facilitate rapid team organization and developing shared team SA.[12] Teams are taught to explicitly Name out loud what signs and symptoms they perceive, and what a potential diagnosis might be, followed by designating roles aloud (Claim) and then sharing which steps the team should enact in a coordinated manner (Aim) (**Fig. 4**).[12] Although this strategy may seem initially simplistic, organizing one's thinking this way is difficult in moments of high stress; it involves encapsulating only need-to-know information and sharing it succinctly, which takes deliberate practice.

Name/Claim/Aim incorporates multiple crisis resource management principles under the spirit of inclusivity to promote teams' improved decision making and treatment skills.[12,18] Anecdotally (in the authors' institution), teams seem to readily adopt this mnemonic, and it appears to help the team's stress levels; more research here is needed.

Emotion Management Strategies to Reduce Incidental Emotional Biases

As mentioned, stress levels felt in the team can disrupt cognition in multiple ways, mostly through altering executive functioning.[64] Mindfully taking a few deep breaths in the moment can restore functional neural connections, as can noticing one's emotional responses in the moment ("I'm feeling stressed" rather than "I am stressed"), also known as affect labeling. This is akin to the adage, "before treating the patient, take your own pulse."[20,65] These techniques have a robust functional neuroscientific base[20] and are easy to adopt over time when practiced deliberately. Although much of obstetric and anesthesiology training may not regularly incorporate these techniques, a growing interest in them signals potential wider adoption.

FUTURE DIRECTIONS

Thus far, research in improving team-based obstetric care is robust, yet there is much more to be done regarding effects of the previously mentioned training strategies on improved decision making both for individuals and for teams. Referencing Prochaska and DiClemente's Transtheoretical Model of Change, Croskerry and colleagues submit that clinicians need to move through

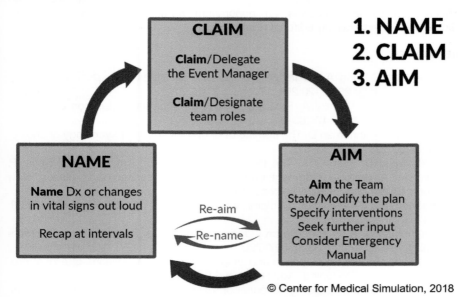

© Center for Medical Simulation, 2018

Fig. 4. Name/Claim/Aim mnemonic for rapidly organizing obstetric teams.[12]

1. Precontemplating changing their decision-making strategies, to
2. Contemplating adopting these strategies, to
3. Preparing ways to change their decision-making practices, to
4. Acting using these strategies, and finally to
5. Maintaining those changes over time[15]

Although all change can be challenging, a critical re-examination of how obstetric anesthesiologists and their teams make decisions highlights what strengths exist, and what areas for growth might be. All skills presented in this article are inherently adoptable; dedication and deliberate practice are all that are required to elevate critical decision making. As obstetric anesthesiologists encourage inclusivity and sharing within their teams, they serve as role models for future clinicians who care for obstetric patients when they are at their most vulnerable.

CLINICS CARE POINTS

- Consider examining individual and team decision making, which can highlight areas of vulnerability and growth.
- Review high-risk situations with interprofessional obstetric team members to increase team members' awareness of conditions under which their thinking may likely be flawed.
- Evaluate the obstetric team's capacity for team training in metacognitive strategies and using cognitive aids and team organization frameworks (such as Name/Claim/Aim).

DISCLOSURE

The authors both receive honoraria from their work with the American Society of Anesthesiologists (ASA) Interactive Computer-Based Education Editorial Board, and Minehart additionally receives an honorarium from her work with the ASA Simulation-Based Training Editorial Board.

REFERENCES

1. Stiegler MP, Tung A. Cognitive processes in anesthesiology decision making. Anesthesiology 2014;120:204–17.
2. Kahneman D, Tversky A. Prospect theory: an analysis of decision under risk. Econometrica 1979;47:263–91.
3. Tversky A, Kahneman D. The framing of decisions and the psychology of choice. Science 1981;211:453–8.
4. Kahneman D, Tversky A. The simulation heuristic. In: Kahneman D, Slovic P, Tversky A, editors. Judgment under uncertainty: heuristics and biases. New York: Cambridge University Press; 1982. p. 201–8.
5. Kahneman D, Tversky A. Choices, values, and frames. Am Psychol 1984;39: 341–50.
6. Kahneman D. A perspective on judgment and choice: mapping bounded rationality. Am Psychol 2003;58:697–720.
7. Croskerry P. Clinical cognition and diagnostic error: applications of a dual process model of reasoning. Adv Health Sci Educ 2009;14:27–35.
8. Evans JS. Dual-processing accounts of reasoning, judgment, and social cognition. Annu Rev Psychol 2008;59:255–78.

9. Osman M. An evaluation of dual-process theories of reasoning. Psychon Bull Rev 2004;11(6):988–1010.

10. Argyris C. Overcoming organizational defenses: facilitating organizational learning. 1st edition. Upper Saddle River, (NJ): Pearson Education, Inc; 1990.

11. Senge PM. The fifth discipline: the art and practice of the learning organization. New York: Currency/Doubleday; 2006.

12. Patino Montoya MA, Minehart RD. Safety in anesthesia. In: Pino RM, editor. Clinical anesthesia procedures of the Massachusetts General Hospital. Philadelphia: Wolters Kluwer; 2022. p. 148–57.

13. Blumenthal-Barby JS, Krieger H. Cognitive biases and heuristics in medical decision making: a critical review using a systematic search strategy. Med Decis Making 2015;35(4):539–57.

14. Croskerry P, Singhal G, Mamede S. Cognitive debiasing 1: origins of bias and theory of debiasing. BMJ Qual Saf 2013;22:ii58–64.

15. Croskerry P, Singhal G, Mamede S. Cognitive debiasing 2: impediments to and strategies for change. BMJ Qual Saf 2013;22:ii65–72.

16. Norman GR, Monteiro SD, Sherbino J, et al. The causes of errors in clinical reasoning: cognitive biases, knowledge deficits, and dual process thinking. Acad Med 2017;92(1):23–30.

17. Eichbaum Q. Medical error, cognitive bias, and debiasing: the jury is still out. Acad Med 2019;94(8):1065–6.

18. Minehart RD, Foldy EG, Long JA, et al. Challenging gender stereotypes and advancing inclusive leadership in the operating theatre. Br J Anaesth 2020; 124(3):e148–54.

19. Minehart RD, Foldy EG. Effects of gender and race/ethnicity on perioperative team performance. Anesthesiol Clin 2020;38(2):433–47.

20. Lerner JS, Li Y, Valdesolo P, et al. Emotion and decision making. Annu Rev Psychol 2015;66:799–823.

21. Naqvi N, Shiv B, Bechara A. The role of emotion in decision making: a cognitive neuroscience perspective. Curr Dir Psychol Sci 2006;15(5):260–4.

22. De Martino B, Kumaran D, Seymour B, et al. Frames, biases, and rational decision-making in the human brain. Science 2006;313(5787):684–7.

23. Yang Q, Zhou S, Gu R, et al. How do different kinds of incidental emotions influence risk decision making? Biol Psychol 2020;154:107920.

24. Achar C, So J, Agrawal N, et al. What we feel and why we buy: the influence of emotions on consumer decision-making. Curr Opin Psychol 2016;10:166–70.

25. Duhachek A, Agrawal N, Han D. Guilt versus shame: coping, fluency, and framing in the effectiveness of responsible drinking messages. J Mark Res 2018;49(6):928–41.

26. Wilson TD, Schooler JW. Thinking too much: introspection can reduce the quality of preferences and decisions. J Pers Soc Psychol 1991;60(2):181–92.

27. Ferrer R, Klein W, Lerner J, et al. Emotions and health decision making: extending the appraisal tendency framework to improve health and healthcare. In: Roberto CA, Kawachi I, editors. Behavioral economics and public health. New York: Oxford University Press; 2016. p. 101–32.

28. Katz D, Blasius K, Isaak R, et al. Exposure to incivility hinders clinical performance in a simulated operative crisis. BMJ Qual Saf 2019;28(9):750–7.

29. Crane MF, Brouwers S, Forrest K, et al. Positive affect is associated with reduced fixation in a realistic medical simulation. Hum Factors 2017;59(5):821–32.

30. Redelmeier DA, Baxter SD. Rainy weather and medical school admission interviews. Can Med Assoc J 2009;181(12):933.

31. Endsley MR. Toward a theory of situation awareness in dynamic systems. Hum Factors 1995;37(1):32–64.
32. Endsley MR. Situation awareness misconceptions and misunderstandings. J Cogn Eng Decis Making 2015;9(1):4–32.
33. Schulz CM, Burden A, Posner KL, et al. Frequency and type of situational awareness errors contributing to death and brain damage: a closed claims analysis. Anesthesiology 2017;127(2):326–37.
34. Edmondson A. Psychological safety and learning behavior in work teams. Admin Sci Q 1999;44(2):350–83.
35. Janis I. Groupthink. In: Griffin E,, editor. A first Look at communication theory. New York: McGrawHill; 1991. p. 235–46.
36. Turner ME, Virick M. Threat and group creativity. Soc Influ 2008;3(4):286–303.
37. Edmondson AC. Speaking up in the operating room: how team leaders promote learning in interdisciplinary action teams. J Manag Stud 2003;40(6):1419–52.
38. Manser T. Teamwork and patient safety in dynamic domains of healthcare: a review of the literature. Acta Anaesthesiol Scand 2009;53(2):143–51.
39. National Transportation Safety Board. 2000. Controlled Flight Into Terrain, Korean Air Flight 801, Boeing 747-300, HL7468, Nimitz Hill, Guam, August 6, 1997. Aircraft Accident Report NTSB/AAR-00/01. Washington, DC. Available at: https://www.ntsb.gov/investigations/AccidentReports/Reports/AAR0001.pdf. Accessed August 27, 2021.
40. Edmondson AC. Teaming: how organizations learn, innovate, and compete in the knowledge economy. San Francisco (CA): Jossey-Bass; 2012.
41. Greig PR, Higham H, Nobre AC. Failure to perceive clinical events: an under-recognised source of error. Resuscitation 2014;85(7):952–6.
42. Mannix E, Neale MA. What differences make a difference? Psychol Sci Public Interest 2005;6(2):31–55.
43. Pitcher P, Smith AD. Top management team heterogeneity: personality, power, and proxies. Organ Sci 2001;12(1):1–18.
44. O'Neill TA, Allen NJ, Hastings SE. Examining the "pros" and "cons" of team conflict: a team-level meta-analysis of task, relationship, and process conflict. Hum Perform 2013;26(3):236–60.
45. Greer LL, de Jong BA, Schouten ME, et al. Why and when hierarchy impacts team effectiveness: a meta-analytic integration. J Appl Psychol 2018;103(6):591–613.
46. Lingard L. Paradoxical truths and persistent myths: reframing the team competence conversation. J Contin Educ Health Prof 2016;36(Suppl 1):S19–21.
47. Graber ML, Sorensen AV, Biswas J, et al. Developing checklists to prevent diagnostic error in Emergency Room settings. Diagnosis (Berl) 2014;1(3):223–31.
48. Croskerry P. Adaptive expertise in medical decision making. Med Teach 2018;40(8):803–8.
49. Sandars J. The use of reflection in medical education: AMEE Guide No. 44. Med Teach 2009;31(8):685–95.
50. Ludolph R, Schulz PJ. Debiasing health-related judgments and decision making: a systematic review. Med Decis Making 2017;38(1), 3–13.
51. Runciman WB, Kluger MT, Morris RW, et al. Crisis management during anaesthesia: the development of an anaesthetic crisis management manual. Qual Saf Health Care 2005;14:e1.
52. Burden AR, Carr ZJ, Staman GW, et al. Does every code need a "reader?" improvement of rare event management with a cognitive aid "reader" during a simulated emergency: a pilot study. Simul Healthc 2012;7(1):1–9.

53. Abir G, Austin N, Seligman KM, et al. Cognitive aids in obstetric units: design, implementation, and use. Anesth Analg 2020;130(5):1341–50.
54. Goldhaber-Fiebert SN, Bereknyei Merrell S, Agarwala AV, et al. Clinical uses and impacts of emergency manuals during perioperative crises. Anesth Analg 2020; 131(6):1815–26.
55. Goldhaber-Fiebert SN, Pollock J, Howard SK, et al. Emergency manual uses during actual critical events and changes in safety culture from the perspective of anesthesia residents: a pilot study. Anesth Analg 2016;123(3):641–9.
56. Emergency Manuals Implementation Collaborative (EMIC). Available at: https://www.emergencymanuals.org/tools-resources/free-tools/. Accessed August 27, 2021.
57. Agarwala AV, McRichards LK, Rao V, et al. Bringing perioperative emergency manuals to your institution: a "how to" from concept to implementation in 10 steps. Jt Comm J Qual Patient Saf 2019;45(3):170–9.
58. Surowiecki J. The wisdom of crowds. New York, NY: Anchor Books; 2005.
59. Bornstein G, Yaniv I. Individual and group behavior in the ultimatum game: are groups more "rational" players? Exp Econ 1998;1:101–8.
60. Brazil V, Purdy E, Alexander C, et al. Improving the relational aspects of trauma care through translational simulation. Adv Simulation 2019;4:10.
61. Morgan P, Tregunno D, Ryan B, et al. Using a situational awareness global assessment technique for interprofessional obstetrical team training with high fidelity simulation. J Interprof Care 2015;29(1):13–9.
62. Jonsson K, Brulin C, Härgestam M, et al. Do team and task performance improve after training situation awareness? A randomized controlled study of interprofessional intensive care teams. Scand J Trauma Resusc Emerg Med 2021;29(1):73.
63. Schaffer AC, Babayan A, Einbinder JS, et al. Association of simulation training with rates of medical malpractice claims among obstetrician–gynecologists. Obstet Gynecol 2021;138(2):246–52.
64. Arnsten AF. Stress signalling pathways that impair prefrontal cortex structure and function. Nat Rev Neurosci 2009;10(6):410–22.
65. Doll A, Hölzel BK, Mulej Bratec S, et al. Mindful attention to breath regulates emotions via increased amygdala-prefrontal cortex connectivity. Neuroimage 2016; 134:305–13.

Point of Care Ultrasound on Labor and Delivery

Kaitlyn E. Neumann, MD, MEd*, Jennifer M. Banayan, MD

KEYWORDS

- POCUS - FoCUS - Point of care ultrasound - Focused cardiovascular ultrasound
- Transthoracic echocardiogram - Bedside echocardiogram - Lung ultrasound
- Neuraxial ultrasound

KEY POINTS

- Point of care ultrasound (POCUS) has a role in rapid bedside diagnosis, clinical decision-making, and procedural assistance on labor and delivery.
- Using POCUS in the obstetric population can aid in the airway management and assessment of aspiration risk, the placement of neuraxial analgesia and/or anesthesia, the diagnosis and management of cardiorespiratory dysfunction, and intravascular fluid status evaluation and/or resuscitation.
- Ultrasound findings should be taken into clinical context with the perspective that point-of-care evaluation can help answer clinical questions, but is not fully comprehensive; thus, a low threshold should exist for formal imaging and second opinion.

INTRODUCTION

Prompt diagnosis of pathologic condition is of the utmost importance in the obstetric population as maternal physiology rapidly changes throughout the peripartum period, severe peripartum complications can develop abruptly, and there can be severe consequences for delays in care in terms of maternal and fetal morbidity and mortality. Point of care ultrasound (POCUS) can be performed at the bedside, is noninvasive, safe, and can provide expedited answers to a variety of clinical questions.[1] POCUS is associated with significantly reduced time to correct diagnosis and treatment[2] and improved outcome and potentially survival in the hospital setting.[3] Ideally, POCUS should be used as an extension of the physical examination, akin to the stethoscope, to extend the diagnostic potential of the bedside evaluation, instead of viewed and performed solely as a limited diagnostic test.[4]

In the obstetric population, POCUS can be used for the diagnosis and management of cardiopulmonary dysfunction, evaluation of intravascular fluid status, assessment

Department of Anesthesiology–Northwestern University, Northwestern McGaw Medical Center, Northwestern University–Feinberg School of Medicine, 251 East Huron Street, Suite 5-704, Chicago, IL 60611, USA
* Corresponding author.
E-mail address: kaitlyn.neumann@northwestern.edu

Anesthesiology Clin 39 (2021) 811–837
https://doi.org/10.1016/j.anclin.2021.08.014
1932-2275/21/Published by Elsevier Inc.
anesthesiology.theclinics.com

of aspiration risk, placement of neuraxial analgesia and/or anesthesia, and airway management.

A BRIEF OVERVIEW OF ULTRASOUND DEFINITIONS AND PHYSICS

Ultrasound uses sound waves, typically 2 to 15 MHz, to generate an image. *Acoustic impedance* refers to the measure of the resistance of particles in a medium to mechanical vibrations generated by these ultrasound waves. When ultrasound waves travel between mediums with different acoustic impedances, some waves cross the medium boundary, and some are reflected. The greater the difference in acoustic impedance, the greater the amount of wave reflection.[5]

In clinical application, when imaging tissue that has a similar acoustic impedance to soft tissue, such as fluid, there is minimal wave reflection, and the tissue will appear *hypoechoic* or black. When imaging tissue has different acoustic impedances than soft tissue, such as bone or denser soft tissue, there is increased wave reflection and the tissue will appear *hyperechoic* or white. Air is impenetrable to ultrasound with approximately 99% reflection.[5]

Proficiency in ultrasound requires using the appropriate transducer (**Table 1**) for penetration and resolution optimization,[5,6] as well as fine-tuning image acquisition with probe positioning, angling, and tilting (**Box 1**).[4]

CARDIAC ULTRASOUND
Overview of Cardiac Physiology in Pregnancy and Peripartum Cardiac Disease

A variety of cardiovascular changes take place throughout pregnancy including increased cardiac output secondary to an increase in plasma volume and heart rate, reduction in systemic vascular resistance (SVR), and left ventricular (LV) structural changes.[7] In addition, small (<0.5 cm) pericardial effusions, as well as mild mitral and tricuspid regurgitation are normal findings in pregnant women.[8] Understanding these expected cardiovascular physiologic and structural changes during the peripartum period is vital for the identification of pathologic condition.

Peripartum cardiac disease is a significant contributor to maternal morbidity and mortality (**Table 2**).[6,9–11] Clinicians can use POCUS as a tool to assist in the assessment and management of these potentially preventable contributors (**Box 2**).[6,7,10,12]

Performing Focused Cardiovascular Ultrasound

Focused cardiovascular ultrasound (FOCUS) consists of 5 views: *parasternal long axis*, *parasternal short axis*, *apical 4-chamber*, *subcostal 4-chamber*, and *subcostal inferior vena cava (IVC) long axis*. The goal of FoCUS is not to perform a formal comprehensive echocardiogram, but instead to evaluate for gross abnormalities to inform diagnosis and management. If abnormalities are observed, upon stabilization, the patient should be referred for formal imaging and evaluation by a cardiologist.

Positioning (**Fig. 1**) as well as breathing techniques for spontaneously ventilating patients can aid in adjusting the heart within the thorax to minimize artifact from lung and optimize image windows and resolution. Images are best at end-exhalation at low lung volumes, so patients should be instructed to take small tidal volume breaths.[4]

Parasternal long-axis view
The parasternal long-axis view is obtained by placing the phased array probe to the left of sternum in the third to fifth intercostal space with the indicator pointed toward the patient's right shoulder (**Fig. 2A**).[4]

Table 1
Ultrasound transducer probes overview[a]

Linear (Vascular Access) Probe	Curvilinear (Abdominal) Probe	Phased Array (Cardiac) Probe
High frequency (8–12 MHz)	Low frequency (3–5 MHz)	3–4.5 MHz
High resolution	High Penetration & Large Sector Width	Small probe footprint
Poor penetration	Low resolution	
	Large probe footprint	

[a] Demonstrates the transducer-related image quality trade-off between resolution and penetration. In general, high-frequency probes provide excellent resolution of superficial structures, but lack penetration depth. Conversely, low-frequency probes provide high penetration and large sector width, thus are great at visualizing deep structures, but with poor resolution.

Box 1
Probe manipulation nomenclature[a]

Sliding = translational motion of the probe to a different location on the body
- *"Window shopping"* for the *"window"* or location of the ultrasound probe that will provide the optimal image
- *Example:* moving from one rib interspace to another to best visualize the heart

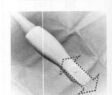

Tilting = rocking motion of the probe (movement is toward or away from probe indicator)
- Obtain images of different structures within the same *plane* (or cross-section of the heart that is made by the ultrasound beam)

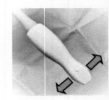

Angulation = angling motion of the probe (movements are perpendicular to the tilting motion)
- Obtain imaging planes parallel to the original plane
- *Example:* angling from parasternal short axis plan image plane to image mitral valve and/or left ventricle apex

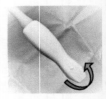

Rotation = while the probe is held still at one location, it is turned around its central axis (similar to turning a key in a lock)
- *Example:* Rotating probe from the parasternal long axis (indicator pointing to R shoulder) to parasternal short-axis view (indicator pointing to L shoulder).

[a]Other textbooks and articles have used different nomenclatures (eg, rocking and fanning) which is equally acceptable. The terminology suggested in **Box 2** is for the consistency of terms within this article.

Although the entirety of both ventricles is not visualized in this view (**Fig. 2**B), gross qualitative dysfunction and/or enlargement of the LV and right ventricle (RV) can be assessed. Additionally, the structure and opening of the aortic (AV) and mitral valve (MV) can be observed. However, the best assessment of global cardiac anatomic structure and function can be determined in this view by comparing the right ventricular outflow tract (RVOT), aortic root, and left atrium (LA) sizes. In normal imaging, the

Table 2
Incidence of peripartum cardiac disease

Peripartum Cardiac Disease	Incidence
Hypertensive Disorders of Pregnancy	10% of pregnancies (14% of maternal deaths)
Peripartum Cardiomyopathy	1/3000 pregnancies (13% severe cardiomyopathy/death)
Peripartum Cardiac Arrest	1/12,000 admissions

Box 2
POCUS in peripartum cardiac disease

Preeclampsia
Obstetric patients with preeclampsia with severe features have demonstratable changes on cardiopulmonary ultrasonography when compared with healthy pregnant women:
- Higher right ventricular systolic pressures (RVSP)
- Abnormal LV diastolic function
- Increased left-sided chamber remodeling (including left atrial (LA) enlargement and LV hypertrophy)
- Higher rates of peripartum pulmonary edema

Peripartum cardiomyopathy
- Severe LV systolic dysfunction (ejection fraction <45%) of unknown cause in the third trimester or within the first month postpartum. Although the pathogenesis is largely unknown, it is thought that an autoimmune inflammatory process triggered by fetal or placental antigens may play a role.
- Presentation similar to other forms of nonischemic cardiomyopathy: dyspnea, hypotension, edema.
- Prognosis is ultimately dependent on LV recovery. Higher left ventricular end-diastolic volumes (LVEDV) and lower ejection fractions on echocardiogram imaging tend to indicate poor LV recovery.

Cardiac arrest
The principal advantages of POCUS during cardiac arrest include the ability to identify potentially reversible mechanical causes of cardiac arrest (eg, profound hypovolemia, pulmonary embolism, tension pneumothorax, or pericardial tamponade), as well as confirm cardiac standstill.

RVOT diameter should roughly be the same size as the aortic root and LA (**Fig. 2**C). Roughly equivalent sizes suggest that right heart strain resulting in RV enlargement, aortic dissection resulting in an enlarged aortic root, and LA dilatation secondary to diastolic dysfunction, MV disease, and/or atrial fibrillation would be unlikely.[4]

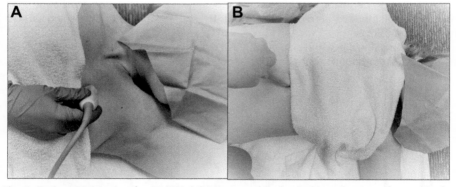

Fig. 1. Patient Positioning for FOCUS. (*A*) Parasternal and apical imaging is performed in the left-lateral decubitus position with the left arm of the patient extended above the head. Clinical situations may present whereby the patient cannot be easily turned from supine positioning. In these scenarios, wedges or manipulation of the bed itself (if electronic) can be used to achieve the same positioning goals. (*B*) Subcostal imaging is obtained in the supine position with a pillow under the knees for a slight bend to relax the abdominal muscles.

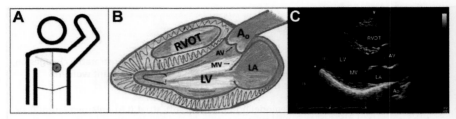

Fig. 2. Parasternal long axis. (*A*) Probe positioning. (*B*) Anatomy of the parasternal long axis—right ventricular outflow tract (RVOT), aortic valve (AV), proximal ascending aorta (Ao), left atrium (LA), mitral valve (MV), and left ventricle (LV). (*C*) Ultrasound image of parasternal long axis without pathologic condition—the size of the RVOT grossly similar in size to the aortic root and LA. (*Adapted from* Sturgess D. Transthoracic echocardiography: An Overview. In: Lumb P. Critical Care Ultrasound Expert Consult. London: Elsevier Health Sciences, 2015. p. 138 to 145; with permission (Figure. 26–2 in original).)

Qualitative function of the walls of the LV can be illustrated by brisk thickening of the myocardium in systole, brisk anterior–posterior motion of the aortic root secondary to the filling-emptying of the LV and LA, brisk opening of the anterior mitral leaflet in diastole, and descent of the base of the LV toward the apex.[4]

Parasternal short-axis view

The parasternal short-axis view is obtained by placing the probe in the same location as a parasternal long-axis view, but rotating the probe 90° clockwise the indicator points toward the patient's left shoulder (**Fig. 3**A).[4] This view transects the LV and RV at the level of the papillary muscles (**Fig. 3**B). Information regarding global and regional LV function, intravascular volume status, and RV strain can be obtained from this view. It is of the utmost importance to have the papillary muscles in view for the proper evaluation of LV volume and function.

Normal global LV function is demonstrated by the symmetric thickening of the entire myocardium; however, this view also provides the visualization of all midsegments of the LV (see **Fig. 3**B), allowing the assessment of regional function. Any disruption of coronary artery perfusion would result in regional wall motion abnormalities in their respective distributive territory, illustrated by the asymmetric thickening of the myocardium.[4]

Evaluation of the filling and size of the LV in diastole, as well as the size in the systole can provide information regarding intravascular volume status. In hypovolemic states,

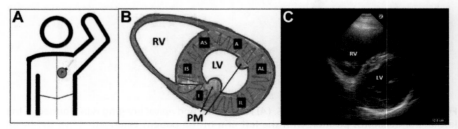

Fig. 3. Parasternal short axis. (*A*) Probe positioning. (*B*) Anatomy of the parasternal short axis—transection of the right ventricle (RV) and left ventricle (LV) at the level of the papillary muscles (PM) with identified midsegments of the LV—anteroseptal (AS), inferoseptal (IS), inferior (I), inferolateral (IL), anterolateral (AL), anterior (*A*). (*D*) Ultrasound image of the parasternal short axis without pathologic condition.

the LV is small in diastole and systole with hyperdynamic systolic function. However, low-afterload states are often misdiagnosed as hypovolemia. In low-afterload states, the LV is full in diastole and empty in systole reflecting increased cardiac output.[4] This discernment in a patient with hypotension could influence management by determining the administration of colloid or blood (eg, postpartum hemorrhage) versus vasopressor (eg, veno/vasodilation in the setting of neuraxial anesthesia).

The RV size and position of the interventricular septum can provide information regarding volume status and the presence and/or of RV strain. In general, if the RV size is significantly larger than the LV, further investigation needs to ensure as there is likely a significant pathologic condition (eg, pulmonary embolus, pulmonary edema, pulmonary arterial hypertension, anaphylactoid syndrome of pregnancy). It is the position of the interventricular septum that can provide insight into the balance of LV and RV pressures. In normal physiology, the LV should be circular throughout the cardiac cycle (**Fig. 3**C), indicating that the LV pressures are greater than the RV pressures. A normal septum should be concave with respect to the LV. An interventricular septum that is flat in diastole and concave in systole indicates an RV volume overload state. An interventricular septum that is flat in both diastole and systole indicates an RV pressure overload state. Persistent septal flattening is concerning for severe pulmonary hypertension.[4]

Apical 4-chamber view

The apical 4-chamber view is obtained by finding the apex of heart with ultrasound, usually at the inferolateral quadrant of the left breast, and then pointing the probe indicator toward 5 o'clock (**Fig. 4**A). Left lateral decubitus positioning can facilitate obtaining this image; however, it also makes it more challenging to place the probe at the true apex. In the apical 4-chamber view, all 4 chambers of the heart can be assessed (**Fig. 4**B). In an ideal apical 4-chamber view, the interventricular septum is centered and oriented vertically such that the interventricular septum runs straight down the middle of the screen (**Fig. 4**C).

The assessment of the global function of the LV and RV, the atria, and the tricuspid valve (TV) and MV can be achieved in this view. In a normal heart, the RV should be smaller than the LV and the apex of the heart should be made entirely by the LV. The apicalization of the RV, or enlargement of the RV such that RV size is greater

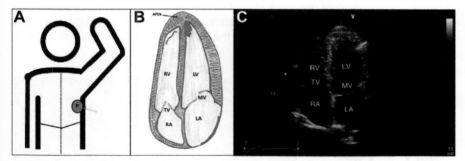

Fig. 4. Apical 4-chamber. (*A*) Probe positioning. (*B*) Anatomy of the apical 4-chamber—left atrium (LA), mitral valve (MV), left ventricle (LV), right atrium (RA), tricuspid valve (TV), and right ventricle (RV). (*C*) Ultrasound image of apical 4-chamber without pathologic condition. (*Adapted from* Sturgess D. Transthoracic echocardiography: An Overview. In: Lumb P. Critical Care Ultrasound Expert Consult. London: Elsevier Health Sciences, 2015. p. 138 to 145; with permission (Figure 26–4 in original).)

than LV size, suggests RV enlargement. A common occurrence is the inability to place the probe at the true apex, resulting in an erroneous overestimation of RV size. The normal function of the RV will be demonstrated by the thickening of the free wall and brisk descent of the base of the TV toward the apex in systole.[4]

Subcostal views. Both subcostal views are performed in the supine position with the probe placed 1–2 cm below the xiphoid process and slightly right of midline. This view can be challenging in the parturient and is often reserved for the postpartum patient once the gravid uterus is no longer obstructing probe placement. Conversely, these views are essential in emergency situations whereby chest compressions are being performed and parasternal views are unobtainable. In this scenario, subcostal views may be the only option to evaluate the heart.

Subcostal 4-chamber view

The subcostal 4-chamber view is performed by placing the probe with the indicator pointing to the patient's left or 3 o'clock (**Fig. 5**A).

As with the apical 4-chamber view, all 4 chambers of the heart can be visualized, although the interventricular septum is now at an angle as opposed to running vertically (**Fig. 5**B), allowing improved visualization of the free wall of the RV (**Fig. 5**C).[4]

Subcostal inferior vena cava long axis

To obtain the subcostal IVC long-axis view, the probe is placed with the indicator pointing to the patient's head or 12 o'clock (**Fig. 6**A). Alternatively, the view can be achieved by a 90-degree rotation counterclockwise from the subcostal 4-chamber view. The subcostal window should be optimized to reveal the IVC entering the RA (**Fig. 6**B, C).

The primary benefit of the subcostal IVC long-axis view is assessing volume status and fluid responsiveness. A large IVC with a minimal change in diameter with ventilation corresponds with greater right atrial pressures and decreased fluid responsiveness.[4] Conversely, progressive narrowing of the IVC diameter and collapsibility (greater than 50%) during inspiration with spontaneous ventilation is associated with hypovolemia, and thus volume responsiveness.[1]

The big picture

Diagnosis or management decisions should not be made based on abnormal findings in *one* FoCUS view. Instead, evidence of pathologic condition should be elucidated and confirmed in multiple views. Similarly, the cardiovascular system does not exist

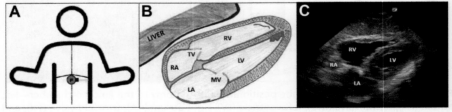

Fig. 5. Subcostal 4-Chamber. (*A*) Probe positioning. (*B*) Anatomy of the subcostal 4-chamber—left atrium (LA), mitral valve (MV), left ventricle (LV), right atrium (RA), tricuspid valve (TV), and right ventricle (RV). (*C*) Ultrasound image of subcostal 4-chamber without pathologic condition.

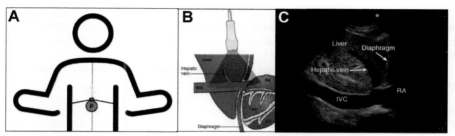

Fig. 6. Subcostal IVC long axis. (*A*) Probe positioning. (*B*) Anatomy of the subcostal IVC long axis - right atrium (RA), inferior vena cava (IVC). (*C*) Ultrasound image of subcostal IVC long axis. (*Images B-C adapted from* Tyler MD, Arntfield R, Roy A, Mallemat H. Inferior Vena Cava. In: Soni NJ, Arntfield R, Kory P. Point-of-Care Ultrasound. Second edition. Philadelphia, PA: Elsevier, 2020. p. 145 to 155; with permission (Figure 17.1 A-B in original).)

in a vacuum, and FoCUS can be combined with lung ultrasound for a more comprehensive evaluation.

LUNG ULTRASOUND
Overview of Pulmonary Physiology and Acute Respiratory Failure in Pregnancy

During pregnancy, there is relaxin-induced anterior–posterior widening of the rib cage. Lung volumes adapt to accommodate a gravid uterus and alterations in the diaphragmatic excursion, including increased tidal volumes and decreased expiratory reserve volume, residual reserve volume, and functional residual capacity. Despite these mechanical and hormonal changes in pulmonary physiology during pregnancy, lung ultrasound images have been shown to remain similar to nonpregnant patients.[13]

The etiologies for acute respiratory failure in pregnancy are numerous (**Box 3**). Lung ultrasound has higher diagnostic accuracy (90.5%) than physical examination and chest radiography combined (75%).[5] Specifically, the sensitivity and specificity of lung ultrasound in detecting pulmonary edema is 100%, whereas up to 500 mL of fluid is easily missed with chest radiography.[5]

Performing Lung Ultrasound

When taken into clinical context, lung ultrasound can provide diagnostic answers to why an obstetric patient is hypoxemic and/or dyspneic and can help guide fluid resuscitation or diuresis. Recognizable patterns of artifacts on lung ultrasound can

Box 3
Etiologies for acute respiratory failure in pregnancy
Cardiogenic and noncardiogenic pulmonary edema
Aspiration pneumonitis
Pneumonia
Pulmonary embolism
Pneumothorax
Exacerbation of obstructive lung diseases
Anaphylactoid syndrome of pregnancy
Acute respiratory distress syndrome (ARDS)
Transfusion-related acute lung injury (TRALI)

distinguish normal lung from pathologic lung (eg, pneumothorax, pleural edema/effusion, interstitial syndrome, and alveolar consolidation). The Blue protocol (**Box 4**)[14] is a brief lung ultrasound examination algorithm for rapid evaluation and diagnosis in patients with acute respiratory failure.[5,15]

Lung ultrasound can be performed in the supine or sitting position with a variety of probes (**Box 5**).

Normal lung

First, it is important to establish ultrasound characteristics that indicate normally aerated lung. Beginning with the evaluation of the anterior lung field (**Fig. 7**A), normal aerated lung will be identified by the *"bat sign,"* rib shadows on either side of a hyperechoic horizontal pleural line (**Fig. 7**B).[5] Center the view on the pleural line to optimize the image. Air below the pleural line reflects the ultrasound waves back to the transducer and an artifact representing aerated lung tissue is produced from the reverberating of ultrasound waves. These artifacts, *A lines*, are horizontal lines below the pleura with the same spacing as the distance between the probe and the pleural line (**Fig. 7**C).[5]

Visceral and parietal pleura are typically closely approximated with a minute amount of fluid between them, allowing them to slide over one another with respiration. *"Lung*

Box 4
The Blue protocol

1. Evaluate the *anterior* portion of each lung.
   Air is nondependent and will collect in the highest point on the anterior chest in a supine patient. If lung sliding is present, pneumothorax as the etiology of acute respiratory failure can quickly be ruled out. If lung sliding is absent and there is an absence of B lines, scan lateral lung fields to find lung point. If a lung point is identified and there is a lack of a lung pulse, the diagnosis of pneumothorax is confirmed.

2. Evaluate the *inferolateral* portion of each lung.
   If A lines are present and there are no (or minimal) B lines, pulmonary effusion and or edema is unlikely. If abundant B lines are identified, scanning the entirety of the lung fields can help identify the extent of pulmonary edema, or if lobular consolidation is more likely.

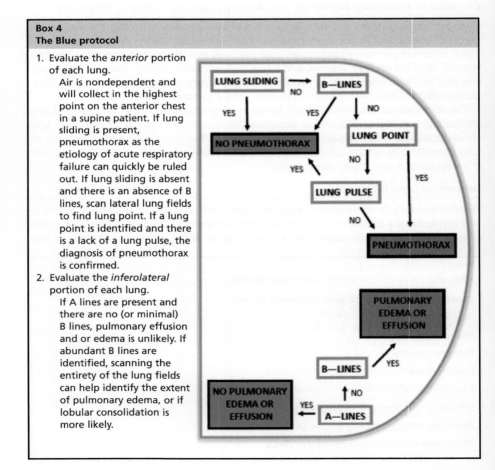

Box 5
Ultrasound probe transducers for lung ultrasound

Linear Probe
  The linear probe provides excellent imaging of the anterior pleura and is superior for the evaluation of pneumothorax.

Curvilinear Probe
  The curvilinear probe can detect consolidated lung at the level of the diaphragm and is superior for evaluation for effusion; however, due to its large footprint, image acquisition can be challenging to angulate between the ribs.

Phased Array Probe
  The phased array probe has a small footprint, enabling imaging between ribs, but sacrifices clarity.

---

sliding" seems as backward and forward movement of the pleura on ultrasound, reminiscent of *"ants marching."* Further evaluation of lung sliding can be performed in M mode on the ultrasound machine, which displays the movement of structures along a single axis of the ultrasound beam. Lung sliding in M mode is illustrated by the *"seashore sign."* Subcutaneous tissue above the pleural line generates horizontal straight lines and the movement of lung sliding appears as a sandy appearance below the pleural line (**Fig. 8**).[5]

Pathologic lung

After the appreciation of characteristics of the normal aerated lung, clinicians can identify and interpret ultrasonographic evidence of pathologic lung including pneumothorax, pulmonary edema/effusion, and consolidation.

Pneumothorax

- Although generally, A lines are indicative of the normal aerated lung tissue, A lines are also present with pneumothorax given that air introduced into the thorax generating the same artifact.
- There is an absence of lung sliding when a pneumothorax is present. This can be observed in M mode—given that the layers of pleura are not directly opposed,

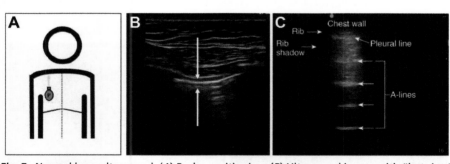

Fig. 7. Normal lung ultrasound. (*A*) Probe positioning. (*B*) Ultrasound image with "bat sign" and arrows pointing to the hyperechoic pleural line between 2 adjacent rib shadows with acoustic shadow. (*C*) Arrows pointing to A lines, an artifact of the aerated lung. (*Adapted from* Fein D, Abbasi MM. Lung and Pleural Ultrasound Technique. In: Soni NJ, Arntfield R, Kory P. Point-of- Care Ultrasound. Second edition. Philadelphia, PA: Elsevier, 2020. p. 53 to 62; with permission (Figure 8.4 A in original).)

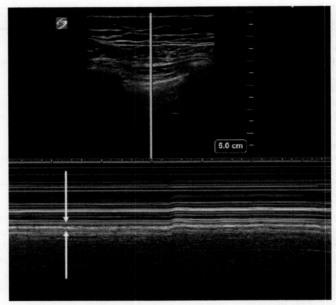

Fig. 8. Normal lung ultrasound - M mode. "Seashore sign" indicative of the presence of lung sliding; arrows pointing to the pleural line.

there will be a lack of "sand" and instead the *"barcode sign"* or *"stratosphere sign"* will be present (**Fig. 9**A).[5]

- Upon the identification of the absence of lung sliding, the ultrasound probe can be moved laterally across the chest to identify the *lung point*. The lung point is the point at which the 2 pleural layers rejoin one another (**Fig. 9**B).[5] On ultrasound, this is demonstrated by the return of lung sliding and the "seashore sign" in M mode. The identification of a lung point is pathognomonic for pneumothorax and confirms the diagnosis but can occasionally be difficult to identify.
- If no lung point is identified, a pneumothorax can be confirmed by the absence of a *lung pulse*. Lung pulse is the presence of T lines, or vertical lines extending from

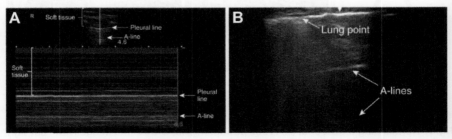

Fig. 9. Ultrasonographic evidence of pneumothorax. (*A*) "Barcode sign" in M mode indicative of pneumothorax. (*B*) Identification of a lung point confirms the diagnosis of pneumothorax. (*Images A-B adapted from* Ma I, Noble VE. Lung Ultrasound Interpretation. In: Soni NJ, Arntfield R, Kory P. Point-of-Care Ultrasound. Second edition. Philadelphia, PA: Elsevier, 2020. p. 63 to 75; with permission (Figure 9.5 and 9.6 in original).)

the pleural line to the bottom of the image in time with cardiac pulsation in M mode.[5]

Pulmonary edema, effusion, and/or consolidation

- The presence of *B lines* indicates fluid within the lung. B lines, or *"comet tails," "lung rockets,"* and *"Kerley B lines,"* are ultrasound artifacts that appear as long vertical hyperechoic lines from the pleural line down the full depth of the image (**Fig. 10**A). B lines result from the juxtaposition of alveolar air and septal thickening secondary to fluid or fibrosis.[5] One or 2 B lines between 2 adjacent ribs are normal; however, greater than or equal to 3 B lines between any 2 adjacent ribs are pathologic and indicates interstitial syndrome (eg, pulmonary edema, interstitial pneumonia/pneumonitis, pulmonary fibrosis).[14]
- The presence of *hepatization* or *"tissue-like sign"* indicates that the lung is highly fluid-filled or consolidated, representing the liver in echogenicity (**Fig. 10**B).[5]
- Pleural effusions are visualized as anechoic spaces between the parietal and visceral pleura at the base of the lung.[14]

Using lung ultrasound for guiding fluid resuscitation. Lung ultrasound and the presence or absence of B lines can help aid in fluid resuscitation and/or diuretic administration. The absence of B lines on lung ultrasound suggests that a fluid bolus (if clinically indicated) would likely not be detrimental to gas exchange. Practitioners can consider serial lung ultrasound examinations when giving fluid challenges; the appearance of B lines should be the stopping point to fluid resuscitation.[16] Conversely, serial examinations and the disappearance of B lines can illustrate a response to diuretic therapy.[17]

Using lung ultrasound in the preeclamptic parturient. Women with severe preeclampsia have more anterior B-lines, indicating increased extravascular lung water (EVLW) and filling pressures.[1] Ultrasound can be used to identify increased EVLW before overt clinical signs of pulmonary edema. Given that the number of B lines correlates with increasing severity of interstitial or alveolar involvement, this information could aid in proactive, rather than reactive interventions such as early fluid administration limitation and/or diuresis.

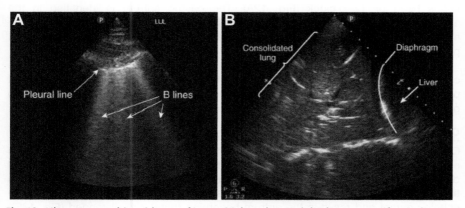

Fig. 10. Ultrasonographic evidence of interstitial syndrome. (*A*) B lines, an artifact indicating fluid within the lung. (*B*) Hepatization of lung indicating that the lung is highly fluid-filled or consolidated. (*Images A-B adapted from* Ma I, Noble VE. Lung Ultrasound Interpretation. In: Soni NJ, Arntfield R, Kory P. Point-of-Care Ultrasound. Second edition. Philadelphia, PA: Elsevier, 2020. p. 63 to 75; with permission (Figure 9.8 and 9.9 in original).)

The big picture

Lung ultrasound is the art of identifying artifacts, both normal and abnormal. Systematically approaching lung fields, as proposed by The Blue Protocol, can quickly rule out or identify etiologies of acute respiratory distress, facilitating expedited management. Lung ultrasound if used in succession can play a role in fluid management in the obstetric population, especially in the setting of preeclampsia and postpartum hemorrhage.

CLINICAL APPLICATION OF MULTIMODAL POCUS IN THE OBSTETRICAL PATIENT

Previous publications have detailed algorithms for assessing critically II obstetric patients with POCUS, such as ROSE (Rapid Obstetric Screening Echocardiography) which includes cardiac ultrasound with concurrent fetal heart rate assessment.[18] Additionally, the integrated use of cardiac and lung ultrasound, or "thoracic ultrasonography" (TUS), is superior to lung ultrasound alone in the diagnosis of the etiology of acute respiratory failure.[19]

We have created a multimodal approach to POCUS in the obstetric patient that combines information from both cardiac and lung ultrasound for a more comprehensive evaluation (**Fig. 11** and **Table 3**).[8,18,20]

GASTRIC ULTRASOUND

Obstetric patients are at baseline increased risk for pulmonary aspiration secondary to progesterone-mediated reduction in lower esophageal sphincter tone. Neuraxial opioids and labor also may contribute to aspiration risk secondary to delayed gastric emptying.

Gastric ultrasound is a useful tool to assess and individualize a parturient's aspiration risk for unscheduled procedures and/or unknown NPO statuses.

PERFORMING GASTRIC ULTRASOUND

Gastric ultrasound is performed in both supine and right lateral decubitus (RLD) positioning, using a curvilinear probe with the indicator pointed cephalad toward the patient's head or 12 o'clock (**Fig. 12A**). The gastric antrum is identified in the epigastric area, slightly to the right of the abdominal midline, using the liver, large abdominal vessels (aorta, inferior vena cava, superior mesenteric artery), and pancreas as internal landmarks (**Fig. 12B**).[21]

Similar to cardiac subcostal imaging, gastric ultrasound image acquisition can be challenging in obstetric patients. In addition to the steep angle between the xiphoid process and abdomen, there is the cephalad displacement of the stomach by the gravid uterus, as well as an increased depth of the antrum.[1]

Qualitative Evaluation

Qualitative gastric antrum evaluation consists of identifying whether the antrum is empty, contains clear fluids, or contains solid food. An empty antrum seems collapsed or flat, with an occasional *"bull's eye"* appearance owing to the varying echogenicity in tissue layers of the gastric wall (**Fig. 13A**). Clear fluids in the antrum appear as hypoechoic content and result in the antrum becoming round and distended (**Fig. 13B**). Solid food in a dilated antrum seems as a hyperechoic content with *"frosted glass"* appearance and ring down artifacts (**Fig. 13C**).[22]

Although the empty antrum and antrum with solid food clearly represent no or increased aspiration risk, respectively, the presence of clear fluid within the antrum

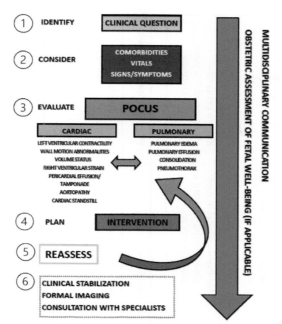

Fig. 11. Clinical application approach to cardiopulmonary POCUS in the Parturient. (1) Evaluation begins with a clinical question. Taking into context the patient's comorbidities, vitals, and signs/symptoms (2) a combined cardiac and pulmonary point-of-care ultrasound should be performed focusing on answering the clinical question at hand (3). Following evaluation and diagnosis, an intervention should be implemented (4) which requires follow-up and reassessment with POCUS (5). Upon patient stabilization, formal imaging and/or consultation with specialists can be obtained (6). Multidisciplinary communication throughout this process is vital. Obstetric assessment of the fetal-wellbeing should be frequently addressed (if applicable).

can be more challenging to assess aspiration risk with the qualitative evaluation. The Perlas grading system assigns a particular "grade" to gastric ultrasound evidence and its corresponding aspiration risk profile (**Box 6**).[7,23] This grading system is validated in pregnant patients[7] and has shown high interrater reliability.[24]

Quantitative Evaluation

Quantitative gastric ultrasound is performed by obtaining the antral cross-sectional area in the RLD position,[7] as antral cross-sectional area correlates with gastric fluid volume.[23] Two mathematical models have been suggested and validated,[7] with the Arzola *and colleagues* model validated in late pregnancy.[25] Based on quantitative models, gastric volumes up to 1.5 mL/kg are considered normal in fasted patients.[26] For parturients in their third trimester, an antral cross-sectional area in RLD greater than 9.6 cm^2 correlates with ingested volumes greater than 1.5 mL/kg with a sensitivity of 80% and specificity of 66.7%.[25]

The big picture

Ultimately, combined qualitative and quantitative ultrasound evaluation of the gastric antrum is best for clinical application and assessment of aspiration risk. There are proposed clinical decision-making algorithms[27,28] using this combined assessment

Table 3
Clinical application of POCUS in the obstetric patient.[a]

Symptoms	Hypotension	Dyspnea	Chest Pain	Arrest
Possible Etiologies	Postpartum hemorrhage sepsis peripartum cardiomyopathy hypovolemia	Asthma pulmonary edema embolism (pulmonary) pneumothorax aspiration	Severe hypertension aortic dissection myocardial infarction	Embolism (pulmonary, amniotic, air) Tension pneumothorax Pericardial tamponade Gross hypovolemia
Questions	What is the intravenous volume status? What is the left ventricular contractility?	What is the right ventricular size and contractility? Are there B lines?	Are there regional motion abnormalities? Is there a dilated aortic root?	Is there pericardial tamponade? Is there pulseless electrical activity?
Pocus Evaluation				
Parasternal Long Axis	LV function systolic anterior motion	RVOT size	Aortic root	MV RVOT size Aortic root
Parasternal Short Axis	LVEDV (filling) Global contractility	RV size interventricular septum positioning	Myocardial segments shortening wall motion abnormalities	LVEDV (filling) RV size Interventricular septum positioning
Apical 4-Chamber	Global contractility	RV size apex		Ventricular activity
Subcostal 4-Chamber		RV free wall function	Pericardial effusion	Ventricular activity Pericardial tamponade
Subcostal IVC long axis	IVC diameter			IVC
Lung	Absence of B lines	B lines Lung sliding Lung point Consolidation		Lung sliding Lung point

Abbreviations: IVC, inferior vena cava; RV, right ventricle; LVEDV, left ventricular end-diastolic volumes; RVOT, right ventricular outflow tract; MV, mitral valve
[a] Outlines a variety of clinical scenarios, signs and symptoms that may present in obstetric patients, as well as the clinical questions that need to be addressed and their potential answers provided by cardiopulmonary POCUS.

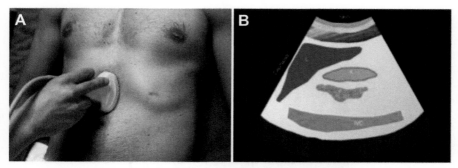

Fig. 12. Gastric ultrasound. (*A*) Patient positioning. (*B*) Anatomy of gastric antrum (A), liver (L), pancreas (P), and large vessels such as inferior vena cava (IVC) and aorta providing internal landmarks for this view. (*Adapted from* Talati C, Arzola C, Carvalho JC. The Use of Ultrasonography in Obstetric Anesthesia. *Anesthesiol Clin.* Mar 2017;35(1):35 to 58; with permission (see Figures. 5 and 6A in original).)

(**Fig. 14**). Gastric volumes greater than 1.5 mL/kg and/or the presence of solid contents in the gastric antrum suggest a high aspiration risk.[1]

NEURAXIAL ULTRASOUND

Neuraxial analgesia and anesthesia are the backbone of obstetric anesthesiology; however, the rate of difficult neuraxial blockade and abandoned neuraxial blockade has been shown to be 3.9% and 0.2%, respectively.[29] Functional neuraxial blockades can facilitate the avoidance of challenging emergent airway manipulation, which can be associated with increased maternal morbidity and mortality.

Ultrasound imaging for neuraxial placement can be used to identify the midline of the spine, locate the intervertebral level of choice, and measure the epidural space depth. Clinicians are correct in their assessment of intervertebral level approximately 30% of the time,[30] with mistaken identifications usually in the cephalad direction by 1 to 4 interspaces.[31] Neuraxial procedures should be performed below the conus level, which reaches the upper portion of L2 in 50% of women.[31] Ultrasound can also assist in estimated depth to the epidural space[32] potentially minimizing unintentional dural punctures and predict the need for extra-long spinal or epidural needles.[30]

Preprocedural ultrasound reduces the number of attempts (both punctures and re-directions) during neuraxial placement and decreases the risk of nonfunctional epidural catheters.[33] Additionally, neuraxial ultrasound reduces the risk of traumatic procedures, and thus may contribute to the safety of lumbar central neuraxial blocks[32,33] and reduce complications.[34]

PERFORMING NEURAXIAL ULTRASOUND

The goal of neuraxial ultrasound is the identification of the optimal puncture site by landmarking 1) the exact intervertebral level to avoid conus injury, 2) the midline of the spine, and 3) the depth and angle for proper needle insertion.

A curvilinear probe is used and optimal patient is positioning is the same as for neuraxial placement, seated in a bent forward position to enlarge the interspinous spaces (**Fig. 15**).

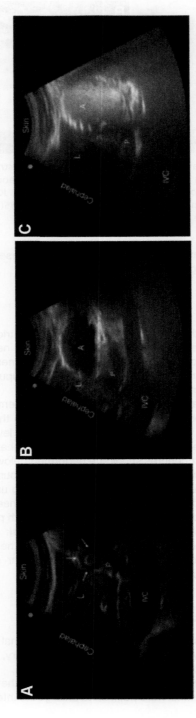

Fig. 13. Qualitative evaluation of gastric antrum. (A) Empty antrum with "bull's eye" appearance (*arrows*); liver (L), antrum (A), pancreas (P), and inferior vena cava (IVC). (B) Clear fluids in a dilated antrum. (C) Solid food in antrum with "frosted glass" appearance and ring down artifact. (*Adapted from* Talati C, Arzola C, Carvalho JC. The Use of Ultrasonography in Obstetric Anesthesia. *Anesthesiol Clin.* Mar 2017;35(1):35 to 58; with permission (see Figures 6B–D in original).)

Box 6

Perlas grading system for gastric ultrasound

Grade 0: empty antrum in both RLD[a] and supine positions indicating *lack of gastric contents*

Grade 1: fluid presenting in RLD only[b] indicating likely *low gastric volume (<100 mL)*

Grade 2: fluid in both RLD and supine positions indicating likely *high gastric volume (>250 mL)* and *increased aspiration risk*

[a]RLD = right lateral decubitus.

[b]The antrum enlarges with clear fluid content transitioning from the supine to RLD position as the fluid moves to more dependent areas.

Transverse Midline Approach

For the transverse midline approach, the probe is held horizontal, perpendicular to the long axis of spine (**Fig. 16**A). In this view, the hyperechoic spinous process is visualized immediately below the skin, which continues as a long triangular hypoechoic acoustic shadow and identifies midline (**Fig. 16**B). By sliding cephalad or caudad along the long axis of the spine between adjacent spinous processes, the lumbar interspace can be identified by the *"flying bat"* sign (**Fig. 16**C).[31,35] The angle of the transducer for which the lumbar interspace view is optimized can suggest the neuraxial procedure needle insertion angle. Within the lumbar interspace image, the first hyperechoic band at the midline closest to the transducer identifies the ligamentum flavum and the second hyperechoic band identifies the dura, producing the *"equal"* sign.[31,35] Thus, the

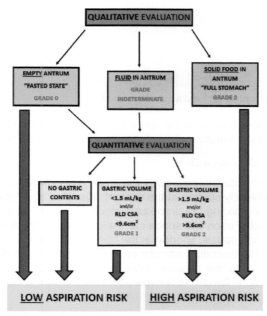

Fig. 14. Gastric POCUS clinical decision-making. Flow chart for the interpretation of findings and medical decision-making regarding aspiration risk based on combined qualitative and quantitative gastric POCUS findings. (RLD CSA = right lateral decubitus cross-sectional area).

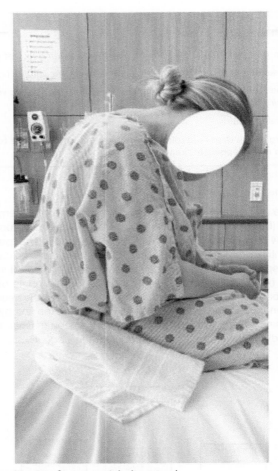

Fig. 15. Patient positioning for neuraxial ultrasound.

expected puncture depth to reach the epidural space from the skin to the inner surface of the ligamentum flavum–dura mater unit can be estimated with this view.

Paramedial Longitudinal Approach

For the paramedial longitudinal approach, the probe is held parallel along the long axis of the spine (**Fig. 17**A). By starting at the sacrum, identified as a hyperechoic wedge-shaped structure, and sliding the probe cephalad/cranially along the long axis of the spine, the exact level of each interspace can be identified.[31] The first lamina adjacent to the sacrum with an acoustic shadow is the L5 vertebra. This view reveals the *"saw tooth"* sign (**Fig. 17**B), illustrating articular processes as the teeth of the saw and the vertebral interspaces as the spaces between the teeth. By tilting the ultrasound medial, the ligamentum flavum as a hyperechoic band across adjacent lamina can be visualized (**Fig. 17**C).[31,35]

The big picture

Preprocedural neuraxial ultrasound identifies the optimal procedural puncture site from the coalescing of 2 marks made on skin—one coinciding with a midline (a vertical

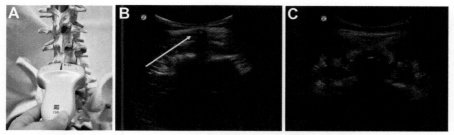

Fig. 16. Neuraxial ultrasound - transverse midline approach. (*A*) Probe positioning is horizontal or perpendicular to the long axis of the spine. (*B*) Hyperechoic spinous process (*arrow*) identifies the midline of spine. (*C*) Lumbar interspace identified by "flying bat" sign; "equal sign" sign identifies ligamentum flavum and dura (not seen in image).

line drawn from the middle of the probe during the transverse midline approach) and the other coinciding with the chosen interspace (a horizontal line drawn from the middle of the probe correlating with the middle of the interspace during the paramedial longitudinal approach) (**Fig. 18**).[35]

Preprocedural ultrasound has shown benefit for patients who were predicted to be difficult neuraxial placement and should be considered in patients with difficult spinal anatomy (eg, scoliosis, postsurgical), morbid obesity with poor quality surface landmarks, and soft interspinous ligament, and/or after the failure of standard insertion techniques. However, whereas shown to be beneficial in these subsets of patients, the advantage of preprocedural ultrasound is minimal in patients with easily discernible surface landmarks/palpable spinous processes.[34]

Neuraxial ultrasound takes time—it usually takes an average of 2 to 3 minutes for the ultrasound assessment of the spine.[35] However, the increased time to mark the insertion point with preprocedural ultrasound is offset by a shorter time to the identification of CSF and ultimate neuraxial placement.[34]

AIRWAY ULTRASOUND

Obstetric patients have a higher incidence of difficult airway in comparison to nonpregnant patients, with a failed airway rate of 2.6/1000 during general anesthetics

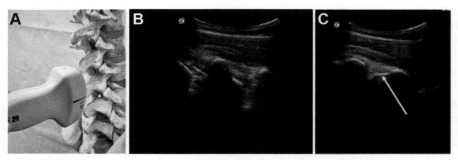

Fig. 17. Neuraxial ultrasound - paramedial longitudinal approach. (*A*) Probe positioning is vertical or along the long axis of the spine. (*B*) "Saw tooth" sign illustrating articular processes as the teeth of the saw and the vertebral interspaces as the spaces between the teeth. (*C*) Visualization of the ligamentum flavum as hyperechoic band across adjacent lamina (*arrow*).

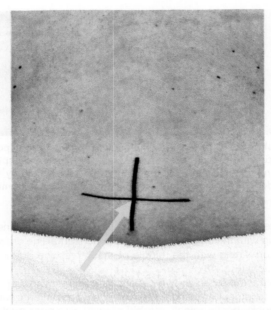

Fig. 18. Identification of the optimal puncture site. Preprocedural neuraxial ultrasound identifies the optimal procedural puncture site (*arrow*) from the coalescing of 2 marks made on skin—one coinciding with midline (a vertical *line* drawn from middle of the probe during the transverse midline approach) and the other coinciding with the chosen interspace (a horizontal *line* drawn from the middle of the probe correlating with the middle of the interspace during the paramedial longitudinal approach).

for obstetric procedures and 2.3/1000 for cesarean deliveries.[36] Physiologic changes during pregnancy including weight gain, enlarged breasts, and fluid retention resulting in oral mucosal soft tissue edema,[37] alter the oropharynx and can result in difficult intubation. There is a progressive worsening of Mallampati classification and a decrease in pharyngeal area[37] throughout labor.

Given the potential maternal morbidity and mortality associated with unanticipated difficult airway in the obstetric population, airway ultrasound has been examined for its utility as a tool for tracheal intubation confirmation, endobronchial intubation diagnosis, and cricothyroid membrane identification.

APPLICATIONS AND PERFORMING AIRWAY ULTRASOUND
Tracheal Intubation Confirmation

Airway ultrasound can provide rapid confirmation of successful endotracheal tube placement versus esophageal intubation.[1] Although capnographic confirmation of intubation is safe, fast, and easy, obstetric patients who are at high risk for aspiration may benefit from the early identification of esophageal intubation by airway ultrasound, given that increased gastric distention from subsequently assisted breaths while awaiting capnography could be detrimental and thus advantageously avoided.

For this verification, the ultrasound probe is placed transversely on the neck at the level of the suprasternal notch during intubation (**Fig. 19**A). Upon intubation, a

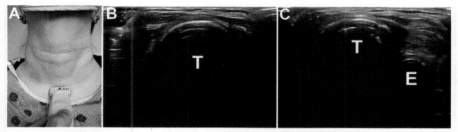

Fig. 19. Airway ultrasound - tracheal intubation confirmation. (*A*) Probe is placed transversely on the neck at the level of the suprasternal notch. (*B*) Tracheal (T) intubation; hyperechoic tube within trachea, observed dilation with endotracheal tube cuff inflation, and a single air–mucosa interface. (*C*) Esophageal (E) intubation; "double tract" sign due to 2 air–mucosa interfaces. (*Adapted from* Gottlieb M, Holladay D, Burns KM, Nakitende D, Bailitz J. Ultrasound for airway management: An evidence-based review for the emergency clinician. *Am J Emerg Med.* May 2020;38(5):1007 to 1013; with permission (see Figures 2 and 3 in original).)

hyperechoic tube will appear in the trachea (**Fig. 19**B) and tracheal dilation will be observed with endotracheal tube cuff inflation.[1] Esophageal intubation can be identified by the *"double tract"* sign (**Fig. 19**C). When the endotracheal tube is within the trachea, there is a single air–mucosa interface; however, with the endotracheal tube is within the esophagus, there will be 2 air–mucosa interfaces.[38]

Early endobronchial intubation recognition

Ultrasound has also shown to be more effective than auscultation for identifying tracheal versus bronchial endotracheal tube location,[39] and could potentially aid in the early recognition and prevention of trauma from endobronchial intubation.

Cricothyroid Membrane Identification

Cricothyroidotomy may be required in 1/60 "cannot ventilate, cannot intubate, cannot oxygenate" scenarios.[36] The most common complication of the procedure is the misidentification of the cricothyroid membrane, which can cause severe complications. In fact, there is only a 36% success rate in correct identification among

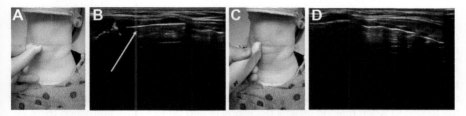

Fig. 20. Airway ultrasound - cricothyroid membrane identification. (*A*) Probe is placed transversely on the midline of the neck at the level of the cricoid cartilage. (*B*) Transverse approach; cricothyroid membrane is the hyperechoic line (*arrow*) between thyroid cartilage and cricoid cartilage. (*C, D*) Longitudinal approach; tracheal rings illustrated with "string of pearls" appearance. (*Adapted from* Gottlieb M, Holladay D, Burns KM, Nakitende D, Bailitz J. Ultrasound for airway management: An evidence-based review for the emergency clinician. *Am J Emerg Med.* May 2020;38(5):1007 to 1013; with permission (see Figures 7 and 8 in original).)

Box 7
POCUS limitations considerations

- Findings on POCUS evaluation should be taken into clinical context.

- Serial examinations may be more beneficial than a single observation.

- The practitioner should consider that the interpretation is flawed.

- Subtle abnormalities may be overlooked during the fast and directed assessment, thus the practitioner should not "lock in" or "lock out" diagnoses based on limited ultrasound data.

- Multiple views to assess the same clinical question should be used as applicable.

- As providers may be uncertain regarding any identified abnormalities, there should be a low threshold to obtain formal imaging and/or a second opinion to confirm findings.

---

anesthesiologists.[38] Airway ultrasound increases the rate of accurate cricothyroid membrane identification in comparison to palpation for cricothyroidotomy, especially in patients with poorly defined neck landmarks.[38]

Two approaches, the transverse approach and the longitudinal approach, can be performed to identify the cricothyroid membrane. A linear probe should be used in both approaches.[1,38]

Transverse approach
The ultrasound probe is placed transversely on the midline of the neck at the level of the cricoid cartilage (**Fig. 20**A). Slide the probe up and down the neck along the midline. The cricothyroid membrane is the hyperechoic line between the thyroid cartilage (cephalad) and cricoid cartilage (caudad) (**Fig. 20**B).[38]

Longitudinal approach
The ultrasound probe is placed at the level of the cricoid cartilage in the transverse orientation and then rotated 90° (**Fig. 20**C). The trachea visualized in this view will illustrate tracheal rings with a *"string of pearls"* appearance (**Fig. 20**D).[38]

The big picture
Maternal airway changes throughout pregnancy and labor can result in challenging airway manipulation. Airway ultrasound can assist in these scenarios to (1) confirm successful tracheal tube placement, (2) diagnose endobronchial intubation, and/or (3) accurately identify cricothyroid membrane for emergency airway access.

CONCLUSION
Pocus Limitations and Future Directions

Although POCUS is meant to be performed to answer a particular question, the narrow focus can potentially distract from the overall larger clinical picture. Given the concern that inaccurate diagnoses could lead to adverse outcomes, clinicians should consider the following when making clinical decisions based on POCUS information (**Box 7**).[4]

Barriers to the routine use of POCUS include the formation of training programs for practitioners to gain technical expertise, cost for equipment, and time. Formal education in ultrasound techniques is vital as minimal training may yield suboptimal imaging and unacceptable reproducibility on POCUS evaluation.[40]

Lastly, a divide remains between these beforementioned theoretic advantages of POCUS outlined in this article and actual demonstrated improvements in outcomes. Few high-quality clinical trials have been published on the impact of POCUS on overall morbidity and mortality. Upcoming research will need to link the application of POCUS in peripartum management to meaningful improvements in obstetric outcomes.[40]

SUMMARY

Ultrasound is a well-known tool for anesthesiologists for regional anesthesia and peripheral and/or central venous access. With the growing utility in the point-of-care evaluation of critically ill patients in the perioperative, intensive care, and peripartum settings; proficiency in POCUS is a vital skillset for the anesthesiologist. Particularly in the field of obstetric anesthesiology, utilization of cardiac, pulmonary, neuraxial, gastric, and airway ultrasound can aid in our clinical decision-making for common obstetric complications and ultimately aid in our role as critical care physicians in the multidisciplinary practice on labor and delivery.

CLINICS CARE POINTS

- Delayed recognition and management of the sick obstetric patient contribute to maternal morbidity and mortality.
- Owing to its noninvasiveness, ease of accessibility and use, and lack of radiation exposure, POCUS has a huge role in rapid diagnosis, clinical decision-making, and procedural assistance in the obstetric population.
- Combined cardiac and lung ultrasound can determine the presence of cardiopulmonary dysfunction, ascertain the etiology of acute respiratory failure, and assess overall volume status to help guide fluid administration and/or diuresis in obstetric patients.
- Gastric ultrasound, through combined qualitative and quantitative assessment, can identify stomach contents and/or volumes that may put obstetric patients at further increased risk for pulmonary aspiration.
- In a subset of the obstetric population (eg, morbidly obese, postsurgical, scoliotic patients), neuraxial ultrasound can increase efficacy, improve efficiency, and reduce complications of neuraxial procedures without significant prolongation of the total procedural time.
- Airway ultrasound can help confirm correct endotracheal tube placement and aid in locating the cricothyroid membrane for emergency front-of-neck airway access.
- Ultrasound findings should be taken into clinical context with the perspective that point-of-care evaluation can help answer clinical questions, but is not fully comprehensive; thus, a low threshold for formal imaging and second opinion should exist.

DISCLOSURE

The authors have nothing to disclose.

REFERENCES

1. Zieleskiewicz L, Bouvet L, Einav S, et al. Diagnostic point-of-care ultrasound: applications in obstetric anaesthetic management. Anaesthesia 2018;73(10): 1265–79.
2. Laursen CB, Sloth E, Lassen AT, et al. Point-of-care ultrasonography in patients admitted with respiratory symptoms: a single-blind, randomised controlled trial. Lancet Respir Med 2014;2(8):638–46.
3. Zieleskiewicz L, Lopez A, Hraiech S, et al. Bedside pocus during ward emergencies is associated with improved diagnosis and outcome: an observational, prospective, controlled study. Crit Care 2021;25(1):34.

4. Zimmerman JM. The nuts and bolts of performing focused cardiovascular ultrasound (FoCUS). Anesth Analg 2017;124(3):8.
5. Miller A. Practical approach to lung ultrasound. BJA Educ 2016;16(2):39–45.
6. Chalifoux LA, Sullivan JT. Applications of Focused Cardiac Ultrasound (FoCUS) in obstetrics. Curr anesthesiology Rep (Philadelphia) 2015;5(1):106–13.
7. Van de Putte P, Vernieuwe L, Bouchez S. Point-of-care ultrasound in pregnancy: gastric, airway, neuraxial, cardiorespiratory. Curr Opin Anaesthesiol 2020;33(3): 277–83.
8. Dennis A, Stenson A. The use of transthoracic echocardiography in postpartum hypotension. Anesth Analg 2012;115(5):1033–7.
9. Say L, Chou D, Gemmill A, et al. Global causes of maternal death: a WHO systematic analysis. Lancet Glob Health 2014;2(6):e323–33.
10. McNamara DM, Elkayam U, Alharethi R, et al. Clinical outcomes for peripartum cardiomyopathy in North America: results of the IPAC study (Investigations of Pregnancy-Associated Cardiomyopathy). J Am Coll Cardiol 2015;66(8):905–14.
11. Mhyre JM, Tsen LC, Einav S, et al. Cardiac arrest during hospitalization for delivery in the United States, 1998-2011. Anesthesiology 2014;120(4):810–8.
12. Vaught AJ, Kovell LC, Szymanski LM, et al. Acute cardiac effects of severe preeclampsia. J Am Coll Cardiol 2018;72(1):1–11.
13. Arbeid E, Demi A, Brogi E, et al. Lung ultrasound pattern is normal during the last gestational weeks: an observational pilot study. Gynecol Obstet Invest 2017; 82(4):398–403.
14. Volpicelli G, Elbarbary M, Blaivas M, et al. International evidence-based recommendations for point-of-care lung ultrasound. Intensive Care Med 2012;38(4): 577–91.
15. Lichtenstein DA, Meziere GA. Relevance of lung ultrasound in the diagnosis of acute respiratory failure: the BLUE protocol. Chest 2008;134(1):117–25.
16. Lichtenstein D. Fluid administration limited by lung sonography: the place of lung ultrasound in assessment of acute circulatory failure (the FALLS-protocol). Expert Rev Respir Med 2012;6(2):155–62.
17. Zieleskiewicz L, Lagier D, Contargyris C, et al. Lung ultrasound-guided management of acute breathlessness during pregnancy. Anaesthesia 2013;68(1): 97–101.
18. Dennis AT. Transthoracic echocardiography in obstetric anaesthesia and obstetric critical illness. Int J Obstet Anesth 2011;20(2):160–8.
19. Bataille B, Riu B, Ferre F, et al. Integrated use of bedside lung ultrasound and echocardiography in acute respiratory failure: a prospective observational study in ICU. Chest 2014;146(6):1586–93.
20. Griffiths SE, Waight G, Dennis AT. Focused transthoracic echocardiography in obstetrics. BJA Educ 2018;18(9):271–6.
21. Talati C, Arzola C, Carvalho JC. The use of ultrasonography in obstetric anesthesia. Anesthesiol Clin 2017;35(1):35–58.
22. Cubillos J, Tse C, Chan VW, et al. Bedside ultrasound assessment of gastric content: an observational study. Can J Anaesth 2012;59(4):416–23.
23. Van de Putte P, Perlas A. Ultrasound assessment of gastric content and volume. Br J Anaesth 2014;113(1):12–22.
24. Arzola C, Cubillos J, Perlas A, et al. Interrater reliability of qualitative ultrasound assessment of gastric content in the third trimester of pregnancy. Br J Anaesth 2014;113(6):1018–23.

25. Arzola C, Perlas A, Siddiqui NT, et al. Gastric ultrasound in the third trimester of pregnancy: a randomized controlled trial to develop a predictive model of volume assessment. Obstet Anesth Dig 2018;38(4):209–10.
26. Van de Putte P, Perlas A. The link between gastric volume and aspiration risk. In search of the Holy Grail? *Anaesthesia*. Mar 2018;73(3):274–9.
27. Roukhomovsky M, Zieleskiewicz L, Diaz A, et al. Ultrasound examination of the antrum to predict gastric content volume in the third trimester of pregnancy as assessed by MRI: A prospective cohort study. Eur J Anaesthesiol 2018;35(5):379–89.
28. Perlas A, Van de Putte P, Van Houwe P, et al. I-AIM framework for point-of-care gastric ultrasound. Br J Anaesth 2016;116(1):7–11.
29. Stendell L, Lundstrom LH, Wetterslev J, et al. Risk factors for and prediction of a difficult neuraxial block: a cohort study of 73,579 patients from the danish anaesthesia database. Reg Anesth Pain Med 2015;40(5):545–52.
30. Carvalho JC. Ultrasound-facilitated epidurals and spinals in obstetrics. Anesthesiology Clin 2008;26(1):145–58.
31. Sahin T, Balaban O. Lumbar ultrasonography for obstetric neuraxial blocks: sonoanatomy and literature review. Turk J Anaesthesiol Reanim 2018;46(4):257–67.
32. Perlas A, Chaparro LE, Chin KJ. Lumbar neuraxial ultrasound for spinal and epidural anesthesia: a systematic review and meta-analysis. Reg Anesth Pain Med 2016;41(2):251–60.
33. Shaikh F, Brzezinski J, Alexander S, et al. Ultrasound imaging for lumbar punctures and epidural catheterisations: systematic review and meta-analysis. BMJ 2013;346:f1720.
34. Young B, Onwochei D, Desai N. Conventional landmark palpation vs. preprocedural ultrasound for neuraxial analgesia and anaesthesia in obstetrics - a systematic review and meta-analysis with trial sequential analyses. Anaesthesia 2020;76(6):818–31.
35. Balki M. Locating the epidural space in obstetric patients-ultrasound a useful tool: continuing professional development. Can J Anaesth 2010;57(12):1111–26.
36. Kinsella SM, Winton AL, Mushambi MC, et al. Failed tracheal intubation during obstetric general anaesthesia: a literature review. Int J Obstet Anesth 2015;24(4):356–74.
37. Kodali BS, Chandrasekhar S, Bulich LN, et al. Airway changes during labor and delivery. Anesthesiology 2008;108(3):357–62.
38. Gottlieb M, Holladay D, Burns KM, et al. Ultrasound for airway management: an evidence-based review for the emergency clinician. Am J Emerg Med 2020;38(5):1007–13.
39. Ramsingh D, Frank E, Haughton R, et al. Auscultation versus point-of-care ultrasound to determine endotracheal versus bronchial intubation: a diagnostic accuracy study. Anesthesiology 2016;124(5):1012–20.
40. Sullivan JT. Adding diagnostic power to the physical exam: can employing focused cardiac ultrasound lead to improved obstetric outcomes? Int J Obstet Anesth 2018;34:3–4.

Ethics in the Labor and Delivery Unit

David G. Mann, MD, DBe[a], Caitlin D. Sutton, MD[b],*

KEYWORDS

- Ethics • Obstetric anesthesia • Informed consent • Shared decision-making

KEY POINTS

- A clinician's fiduciary obligations to their pregnant patients can be thought of as beneficence-based and autonomy-based obligations.
- The obstetric anesthesiologist has a fiduciary obligation to the pregnant woman because she is a patient. A fetus may also become a patient when (1) the pregnant woman presents it to the clinician as a patient, and (2) there is a clinical intervention that would provide greater good than harm to it.
- A patient with decision-making capacity has the ethical and legal right to provide informed consent or refusal for a procedure. Pregnancy does not negate that right.
- Clinicians should consider a shared decision-making approach for preference-sensitive choices.
- Ethical dilemmas surrounding the shared decision-making process may arise in the labor and delivery setting when the clinician has conflicting fiduciary obligations.

INTRODUCTION

On the surface, empowering patients to make ethically supportable decisions on the labor and delivery unit seems straightforward. Patients arrive expecting a joyful occasion, and clinicians and patients alike desire good outcomes. In reality, significant challenges exist: clinical situations can evolve quickly and dramatically, more than one patient may be impacted by a single decision, and patients can experience significant barriers to meaningful participation in the consent process. Each of these challenges contributes to the complexity of "doing the right thing." Addressing these challenges is necessary for the obstetric anesthesiologist to fulfill their fiduciary

[a] Department of Pediatric Anesthesiology, Perioperative, and Pain Medicine, Clinical Ethics, Texas Children's Hospital, Baylor College of Medicine, 6621 Fannin Street, Suite A3300, Houston, TX 77030, USA; [b] Department of Pediatric Anesthesiology, Perioperative, and Pain Medicine, Division of Maternal-Fetal Anesthesia, Texas Children's Hospital, Baylor College of Medicine, 6621 Fannin Street, Suite A3300, Houston, TX 77030, USA
* Corresponding author.
E-mail address: cdsutton@bcm.edu
Twitter: @caitlindsutton (C.D.S.)

Anesthesiology Clin 39 (2021) 839–849
https://doi.org/10.1016/j.anclin.2021.08.008   **anesthesiology.theclinics.com**
1932-2275/21/© 2021 Elsevier Inc. All rights reserved.

obligations to their patients. This article will use the ethical theory of principlism to provide a practical framework for the clinician striving to make ethically supportable decisions when ethical dilemmas arise.

MAKING ETHICALLY SUPPORTABLE DECISIONS

Declaring that a decision is "ethical" or "unethical" occurs commonly, yet these terms are often poorly understood. Ethics involves the use of a rational framework to identify actions that are the "right thing to do." The "rightness" of an act is determined using culturally acceptable justifications according to one of the numerous ethical theories. Decisions authorize actions, including the act of doing nothing. As acts in medicine are generally interventions, when there is justification, the "right" action is referred to as an appropriate intervention. A decision that authorizes an appropriate intervention based on culturally acceptable justifications is considered ethical. Thus, labeling a decision as ethically supportable means that there is some culturally acceptable justification to support performing the intervention.

ETHICAL THEORY: PRINCIPLISM

Principlism is probably the most common ethical theory applied in clinical medicine to provide the culturally acceptable justification for an appropriate intervention.[1] This theory identifies several ethical principles that apply consistently across many clinical situations, including the labor and delivery unit. The 4 most common principles are autonomy, beneficence, nonmaleficence, and justice. **Table 1** lists questions a clinician can use when considering whether a particular course of action is supported by these ethical principles.

Autonomy

The principle of autonomy upholds respect for individuals. It centers on the moral and legal right to self-rule that is unfettered by any type of coercion. Individuals are disrespected when their right to self-rule is removed through coercion, which is the act of exerting some influence to get an individual to behave in a manner that is not consistent with their choice. In the labor and delivery unit, the pregnant patient makes autonomy-based decisions by providing informed consent or informed refusal for any medical intervention(s) proposed by the clinician. Coercion may also originate from others. For example, a family member may exert pressure to convince a laboring woman to refuse an epidural for a reason that does not align with her own beliefs or values.

Table 1 Applying Ethical Principles	
Autonomy	Is the patient empowered to give consent for interventions that align with their expressed values, beliefs, and preferences?
Beneficence	Is the proposed intervention consistent with what the patient says is in their best interest?
Nonmaleficence	Despite the risks associated with any intervention, is it doing greater good than harm for this patient?
Justice	Is this patient being treated similarly to similarly situated patients? If not, what is the morally compelling explanation?

Beneficence and Nonmaleficence

The principle of beneficence is based on doing good or providing benefit. It is always balanced against the associated principle of nonmaleficence, which seeks to avoid causing unnecessary harm. The benefit to the pregnant patient through any intervention must be greater than the necessary harms she will experience to obtain the expected benefit. For example, a pregnant patient may have some discomfort during the placement of an epidural catheter; however, the expected benefits of a functioning catheter include labor analgesia and the ability to achieve effective and safe surgical anesthesia for a cesarean delivery if needed. These expected benefits far exceed the potential harm of discomfort during catheter placement.

Justice

One formulation for the principle of justice is that similarly situated persons are to be treated similarly unless there is a morally compelling reason for dissimilar treatment. Laboring patients would be considered a similarly situated group. Given that providing labor analgesia upon request is considered the standard of care, all laboring patients should receive a labor epidural upon request. However, there may be a morally compelling reason for some laboring women not to receive an epidural. One such reason could be resource allocation. For example, a single provider involved in an emergent cesarean delivery is unavailable at the time of another patient's request for neuraxial analgesia. Various theories of justice (eg, utilitarian, egalitarian, libertarian, etc.) are used to determine whether a reason is morally compelling. A full discourse on the various justice theories is beyond the scope of this article, but significant conflict may arise when two individuals are using differing theories of justice to determine a "morally compelling" reason.

WHAT ARE THE PHYSICIAN'S OBLIGATIONS TO A PATIENT?

Clinicians have a fiduciary obligation to their patients: the clinician should place the patient's health-related interests before their own. In terms of principlism, these obligations can be thought of as beneficence-based and autonomy-based obligations to the pregnant patient (**Box 1**). Offering appropriate interventions that are reliably expected to provide significantly more benefit than harm fulfills the clinician's beneficence-based obligations to the patient. Although some clinicians are reluctant to make explicit recommendations out of a well-intentioned concern for respecting patient autonomy, recommendations can (and often should) be made when an intervention, based on existing clinical evidence, is expected to advance the patient's health-related interests.

Supporting a patient in making decisions that advance her health-related interests fulfills the clinician's autonomy-based obligation to the patient. The clinician empowers her by providing the best possible clinical evidence for an intervention, interpreting the evidence when necessary, and offering counseling when appropriate. It is

---

Box 1
Physician's fiduciary obligations

- Maternal autonomy
- Maternal beneficence
- Fetal beneficence

important to remember that the patient has a unique understanding of her health-related interests that extends beyond the clinical evidence, and that it is the patient (not the clinician) who determines what is in her own best interest. Incorporating the patient's understanding of her own interests is a critical element of making ethically supportable decisions.

Empowering a pregnant patient to make ethically supportable decisions should be straightforward. In most cases, beneficence-based and autonomy-based obligations support the same action. The clinician offers appropriate interventions expected to provide significantly greater benefit than harm to all women in labor, makes recommendations where appropriate, and then respects the woman's choice to provide consent for or refusal of the proposed intervention to advance her health-related interests. Yet, for pregnant patients, it is not always so straightforward. Ethical dilemmas arise when autonomy-based and beneficence-based obligations support different or even opposing actions, and the presence of a fetus introduces additional layers of complexity. For example, a pregnant patient may make autonomy-based choices that seem inconsistent with her overall health-related interests, insisting that an intervention be performed to save her fetus at the cost of her own life or health. In such cases, both physicians and other providers can experience significant moral distress, making a clear understanding of how to proceed in an ethically supportable manner essential.

WHO IS A PATIENT?

The clinician's fiduciary obligations, both autonomy-based and beneficence-based, are to the pregnant woman because she is a patient. In the obstetric setting, the fetus represents another possible patient. It is essential for any clinician caring for a pregnant patient to understand when a fetus should be considered a patient, because if the fetus is a patient, then the clinician has beneficence-based obligations to it as well. There are no autonomy-based obligations because the fetal central nervous system is not yet sufficiently developed to legitimately claim any awareness of its own health-related interests. Further complicating the situation, this relative vulnerability serves to increase the importance of the clinician's fiduciary beneficence-based obligations to the fetal patient.

In an approach that does not require the impossible task of determining when precisely a fetus possesses the independent moral status of personhood, Chervenak and colleagues claim the fetus becomes a patient when (1) the pregnant woman presents it to the clinician as a patient, and (2) there is a clinical intervention that would provide greater good than harm to it.[2] As a viable fetus can survive the neonatal period to become a child with independent moral status, the clinician has beneficence-based obligations to the viable fetal patient. This makes directive counseling (eg, "It would be appropriate to do this for its benefit to both you and your fetus.") about proposed interventions ethically supportable. The previable fetus may also be a patient, but *only* as a function of the pregnant woman's autonomous choice, because by definition, it cannot survive the neonatal period to become a child. Therefore, the clinician's beneficence-based obligations may change based on the pregnant woman's choice to withhold, confer, or rescind the previable fetus' status as a patient. For the previable fetal patient, only nondirective counseling (eg, "This intervention may benefit your fetus without imposing undue burden on you, if you choose to provide consent for it.") would be ethically supportable. The clinician must always balance beneficence-based obligations to the fetal *patient* with both the beneficence-based and autonomy-based obligations to the pregnant patient.

INFORMED CONSENT ON THE LABOR AND DELIVERY UNIT

Each of these fundamental requirements (autonomy and beneficence, the clinician's fiduciary obligations, and identifying who should be considered a patient) is important when a decision about performing an intervention is required. Understanding these basics allows the clinician to confidently and effectively approach the process of informed consent. Before considering some complexities unique to the labor and delivery unit, one must determine if the patient is able to participate in a valid consent process.

Determining Decision-Making Capacity

A patient must have decision-making capacity to provide informed consent or refusal. In contrast to competency, which is a legal designation, decision-making capacity is a medico-ethical determination. A person with decision-making capacity possesses the emotional, psychological, and intellectual ability to weigh data in relation to their personal values, principles, and life goals. Some elements for assessing decision-making capacity are outlined in **Box 2**.

Some ethicists incorporate whether a patient's value set is stable into the assessment of decision-making capacity.[3] The right to change one's mind is irrefutable, but occasionally a patient's capacity may be called into question when a longstanding, clearly communicated stance changes. Such position shifts are not uncommon if a situation changes or if more information is received. On the labor and delivery unit, questions about the stability of a value set may arise when a patient requests a labor analgesia option that is different from what is reflected in a clearly written birth plan. **Box 3** uses principlism to consider an approach to such a situation.

Capacity in the Laboring Patient

Many challenges to the informed consent process are ubiquitous in the labor and delivery setting. Despite multiple studies demonstrating that patients would prefer that the consent process for labor analgesia occur before the onset of labor,[4,5] it is not uncommon for a patient's first encounter with an anesthesiologist to be after admission to the labor and delivery unit. By this point, patients often have defined expectations for their birth experience which may be influenced by inaccurate or inadequate information.[6] They may be in significant pain, or they may have received medications impacting their cognition to varying degrees, such as opioids, magnesium, or nitrous oxide. Furthermore, patients' preferences for risk communication can vary significantly. Many studies[4,5,7] have attempted to identify which risks patients want to know, but the mixed results underscore the importance of tailoring any discussion of risks to the individual patient. Contrary to common teaching, studies in laboring women have demonstrated that opioid administration, pain, or anxiety level do not

---

Box 2
Four elements to evaluate decision-making capacity[11]

1. Does the patient understand the information relevant to her situation?

2. Does the patient appreciate the possible outcomes and their likelihood? Does she understand how these outcomes may impact her life?

3. Has the patient communicated a choice?

4. Does the patient use reasoning to reach a conclusion that aligns with her stated values and goals?

Box 3
Case 1: A patient with a Change of Heart

A 35-year-old G1P0 presents to the labor and delivery unit for induction at 41 weeks' gestation with an extremely detailed, typed birth plan. The document explains the patient's desires for her delivery in detail and includes clear language about how she does not want an epidural under any circumstance. During your routine preanesthesia consultation, she again expresses her desire for an unmedicated childbirth. After a prolonged induction, her nurse calls to inform you that she is requesting a labor epidural.

Beneficence:

- Placing a labor epidural is expected to relieve the patient's pain.
- A functioning labor epidural increases the likelihood of safe conversion to neuraxial anesthesia in case emergency cesarean delivery is required.

Nonmaleficence:

- Ensuring the patient has no medical contraindications will minimize the risk of harm associated with labor epidural placement.
- Supporting the patient emotionally may decrease feelings of distress or disappointment associated with her change in plans.

Autonomy:

- The requested labor epidural aligns with the patient's autonomous choice.

Justice:

- The standard of care supports the administration of labor epidurals for similarly situated patients (ie, healthy laboring patients requesting an epidural).

Possible approach:

- Recall that the patient now has more information about the labor process, and a change in preferences does not indicate a lack of decision-making capacity.
- Ensure that the patient is making an uncoerced request for the labor epidural.
- Promote a supportive and encouraging environment by advocating for the patient if judgmental comments are made.

---

diminish a patient's self-reported ability to understand the information shared during the consent process.[4,5] Still, clinicians should strive to perform preanesthetic consultations as early as possible during the labor process to optimize the likelihood of achieving effective and timely communication, as well as align with the stated preferences of most patients. **Box 4** describes an approach to questions about the impact of these variables on decision-making capacity in labor.

SHARED DECISION-MAKING ON THE LABOR AND DELIVERY UNIT

Although informed consent should be obtained before any procedure, certain interventions warrant an even more considered approach in which patients are actively supported through a multistep approach referred to as shared decision-making. Elwyn and colleagues have developed a 3-step model for shared decision-making including choice talk, option talk, and decision talk.[8] Choice talk is a preparatory step in which patients are made aware that reasonable options exist. This step is important because some patients are not aware that they can participate in their health care decision-making, and others are not aware of the uncertainty that exists in the practice of medicine. Option talk includes an evaluation of a patient's existing knowledge, a

---

Box 4
Case 2: A patient who declines to hear risks

A 22-year-old G1P0 arrives to your labor and delivery unit with a cervical dilation of 9 cm. She reports 10/10 pain and is requesting an epidural for labor analgesia. When you arrive to the bedside to obtain informed consent, she states that she does not want to hear the risks of the procedure.

Beneficence:

- An effective consent process can help set expectations and relieve anxiety.
- An efficient consent process, aligned with her specific refusal to hear risks, facilitates rapid relief of her pain.

Nonmaleficence:

- Forcing a patient to listen to risks that they understand exist but specifically decline to hear, is unnecessary, delays pain relief, and may interfere with the therapeutic relationship.[12]

Autonomy:

- Ideally patients will participate actively in the discussion, but respect for autonomy supports allowing the patient to determine their role in the consent process.[8]
- The patient's autonomous choice to not participate or to delegate their role in the consent process should be respected.
- This is in contrast to *assuming* that a patient would not want to be involved in the consent process; patients must clearly understand that risks associated with the procedure exist.

Justice:

- Patients in pain are a similarly situated group, and no other circumstances exist in which it would be acceptable to deny treatment of severe pain amenable to safe intervention[13]

Possible approach:

- Allow patients to determine their role in the consent process. An active, autonomous decision to not hear risks should be accepted (and documented).
- Allow patients to determine the amount of information and level of detail that they want to receive during the informed consent process. Patients should not be coerced into discussing risks if they decline to do so.
- Ensure patients are aware that risks exist, and that you are willing to discuss them at any time.
- Consider treatment with a low dose of opioids to facilitate pain relief if the patient would like to discuss risks but is unable to participate because of pain.
- Preventive ethics: Strive to complete the preanesthetic consultation early in labor to facilitate a robust consent process when possible.

---

discussion of the alternatives with the associated benefits and risks that are expected with each, and may use decision support tools such as decision aids when possible. Recognizing that patients who are better informed often choose differently from those who do not underscores the importance of this step.[9] Decision talk involves eliciting patient preferences, decision-making, and confirming mutual understanding. This final step is important, as the evidence demonstrates that clinicians perform poorly when guessing what patients would want, and that power dynamics inhibit many patients from speaking up to express their preferences.[9]

Given the high number of decisions made in every clinical encounter (one study[10] identified an average of 14 decisions per encounter in the hospital setting), it would

---

Box 5
Case 3: A patient who refuses cesarean delivery

A 31-year-old G2P1 at 30 weeks' gestation presents to your OB anesthesia high-risk clinic with a history of post-traumatic stress disorder after a prior emergency cesarean under general anesthesia. The obstetrician's note states that she has refused cesarean delivery "under any circumstances." When you call the obstetrician to discuss this further, he says that she is unlikely to need a cesarean delivery and that he is sure she will change her mind "if the time comes."

Beneficence:

- Pregnant patient: Best interests are defined by the patient rather than the clinician, and include dimensions beyond physiologic health outcomes.[14] For some indications (eg, placenta previa), cesarean delivery is expected to improve maternal morbidity and mortality.

- Fetal patient: Benefits of indicated cesarean delivery include improved neonatal morbidity and mortality.

Nonmaleficence:

- Pregnant patient: Possible risks associated with cesarean delivery, in general, include injury, bleeding, infection, increased likelihood of placental pathology or uterine rupture with future pregnancies, and so forth.[15] Harms associated with coerced cesarean delivery also include psychological distress, trauma, impaired maternal-infant bonding, and loss of trust/ therapeutic relationship with the clinician. Risks associated with refusal of cesarean delivery vary depending on the indication for cesarean.

- Fetal patient: Possible risks associated with cesarean include possible injury, neonatal respiratory distress, or immunologic disorders.[16] Risks associated with refusal of cesarean delivery include fetal hypoxic-ischemic encephalopathy or demise.

Autonomy:

- Pregnant patient: Patients with decision-making capacity have the right to give informed refusal for any intervention.

Justice:

- Pregnancy is not considered to be a morally compelling reason to violate the right of a patient to provide informed refusal for an intervention.

Possible approach:

- Multidisciplinary planning, as well as early and ongoing discussion, can improve the effectiveness of communication and may facilitate a shared decision-making process.

- Open-ended questions can help identify barriers and areas of misunderstanding that may be overcome (eg, anxiety that could be managed with cognitive-behavioral interventions or anxiolytics).

- When obligations to maternal autonomy conflict with beneficence-based obligations to the viable fetal patient, persuasive counseling is often acceptable and may be warranted.

---

be impossible to use this shared decision-making model for every decision. Pragmatically, clinicians should consider a shared decision-making approach for preference-sensitive choices. Preference-sensitive choices occur when more than one reasonable option exists and when the likely consequences of each choice differ enough to justify the time and effort that is required to help the patient understand the impact of these differences.[8] For example, in most cases, a shared decision-making approach to the choice between a spinal versus a combined spinal-epidural for cesarean delivery is not necessary because her experience would be essentially equivalent regardless of the specific technique chosen. If, however, during the informed consent

---

Box 6
Case 4: A patient who asks for a risky procedure

A 26-year-old G1P0 at 25 and 6/7 weeks' gestation is scheduled to undergo prenatal repair of a fetal neural tube defect. The day before her scheduled procedure, she is diagnosed with COVID-19. You inform her that her surgery will be canceled, and her baby will need to undergo postnatal repair. She becomes distraught and tells you that she is not worried about the risks associated with anesthesia for herself, and that she will "sign anything" to be able to undergo prenatal repair.

Beneficence:

- Pregnant patient: A patient *may* define her best interests as including the emotional and psychological benefit that is associated with improved outcomes related to the prenatal repair of a fetal neural tube defect.

- Fetal patient: Prenatal repair of neural tube defects is expected to be associated with decreased incidence of shunting and improved motor and developmental outcomes.[17]

Nonmaleficence:

- Pregnant patient: Proceeding with surgery and general anesthesia in the setting of lower respiratory infection can increase the likelihood of maternal morbidity and mortality. Fetal surgery, in general, is associated with pain and surgical risks that the pregnant patient would not incur if postnatal repair were pursued.

- Fetal patient: Increased maternal morbidity and mortality is associated with worse fetal outcomes. Fetal surgery in general is associated with an increased risk of prematurity.

Autonomy:

- Pregnant patient: A patient has the right to request a medical intervention but cannot compel a clinician to perform an intervention deemed to be medically inappropriate.

Justice:

- The standard of care supports cancellation of a procedure if a patient has a symptomatic lower respiratory infection and an appropriate alternative is available (eg, postnatal repair).

Possible approach:

- The use of the shared decision-making model does not compel a clinician to perform a medically inappropriate intervention, but it can help improve communication and decrease the distress surrounding cancellation of a desired procedure.

- If another physician or center is willing to provide an intervention, it is appropriate to refer the patient for evaluation.

---

process regarding neuraxial anesthesia, a patient expresses a specific value-laden preference (she has a specific concern about the ability to extend the duration of anesthesia based on a prior experience) that may result in a different choice between a spinal or combined spinal-epidural anesthetic, a shared decision-making approach would be appropriate.

Ethical dilemmas surrounding the shared decision-making process may arise in the labor and delivery setting when the clinician has conflicting fiduciary obligations. For example, a pregnant patient may provide informed refusal for a procedure that is expected to benefit herself and/or her fetus. **Box 5** uses principlism to consider an approach to determining whether a patient can refuse an indicated procedure. Alternatively, a patient may request an intervention that prioritizes the health of her fetus over significant risks to herself. **Box 6** describes an approach to determining whether a patient can compel a clinician to perform such an intervention.

SUMMARY

Obstetric anesthesiologists can use the tenets of principlism to address the challenges of complex decision-making on the labor and delivery unit. This approach begins with recognizing and upholding the fiduciary obligations that every physician has to their patient. For the pregnant patient, these obligations are both autonomy-based and beneficence-based. Additional beneficence-based obligations arise in cases where the fetus is also a patient. Ethical dilemmas result from conflict between any of these obligations. A shared decision-making model that incorporates the foundational principles of ethics can be used to resolve these conflicts, leaving clinicians and patients confident that an ethical decision-making process has resulted in an ethically supportable decision.

DISCLOSURE

The authors have nothing to disclose.

REFERENCES

1. Beauchamp TL. Methods and principles in biomedical ethics. J Med Ethics 2003; 29(5):269–74.
2. Chervenak FA, McCullough LB. The fetus as a patient: an essential concept for the ethics of perinatal medicine. Am J Perinatol 2003;20(8):399–404.
3. Lo B. Assessing decision-making capacity. L Med Health Care Fall 1990;18(3): 193–201.
4. Jackson A, Henry R, Avery N, et al. Informed consent for labour epidurals: what labouring women want to know. Can J Anaesth 2000;47(11):1068–73.
5. Pattee C, Ballantyne M, Milne B. Epidural analgesia for labour and delivery: informed consent issues. Can J Anaesth 1997;44(9):918–23.
6. Murphy J, Vaughn J, Gelber K, et al. Readability, content, quality and accuracy assessment of internet-based patient education materials relating to labor analgesia. Int J Obstet Anesth 2019;39:82–7.
7. Bethune L, Harper N, Lucas DN, et al. Complications of obstetric regional analgesia: how much information is enough? Int J Obstet Anesth 2004;13(1):30–4.
8. Elwyn G, Frosch D, Thomson R, et al. Shared decision making: a model for clinical practice. J Gen Intern Med 2012;27(10):1361–7.
9. Mulley AG, Trimble C, Elwyn G. Stop the silent misdiagnosis: patients' preferences matter. BMJ 2012;345:e6572.
10. Ofstad EH, Frich JC, Schei E, et al. Clinical decisions presented to patients in hospital encounters: a cross-sectional study using a novel taxonomy. BMJ Open 2018;8(1):e018042.
11. Appelbaum PS, Grisso T. Assessing patients' capacities to consent to treatment. N Engl J Med 1988;319(25):1635–8.
12. Meisel A, Kuczewski M. Legal and ethical myths about informed consent. Arch Intern Med 1996;156(22):2521–6.
13. American College of O, Gynecologists' Committee on Practice B-O. ACOG practice bulletin no. 209: obstetric analgesia and anesthesia. Obstet Gynecol 2019; 133(3):e208–25.
14. Malek J. What really is in a child' s best interest? Toward a more precise picture of the interests of children. J Clin Ethics 2009;20(2):175–82.

15. Timor-Tritsch IE, Monteagudo A. Unforeseen consequences of the increasing rate of cesarean deliveries: early placenta accreta and cesarean scar pregnancy. A review. Am J Obstet Gynecol 2012;207(1):14–29.
16. Stjernholm YV, Petersson K, Eneroth E. Changed indications for cesarean sections. Acta Obstet Gynecol Scand 2010;89(1):49–53.
17. Farmer DL, Thom EA, Brock JW, et al. The management of myelomeningocele study: full cohort 30-month pediatric outcomes. Am J Obstet Gynecol 2018; 218(2):256.e1-13.

Neurocognitive Effects of Fetal Exposure to Anesthesia

Olutoyin A. Olutoye, MD, MSc[a],*, Candace Style, MD, MS[b],
Alicia Menchaca, MD[b]

KEYWORDS

- Fetal surgery • Neuroapoptosis • Nonobstetrical surgery • Animal models
- Fetal neurodevelopment

KEY POINTS

- Although many studies attempt to define anesthetic and surgical effects on fetal neurodevelopment, much remains to be discovered.
- Maternal surgical procedures, which promote maternal health, should be prioritized over fetal neurodevelopmental concerns, given lack of sufficient data and worsened outcomes with progressive maternal disease.
- Animal models used for assessing fetal anesthetic effects are not perfectly matched to human gestation and development, and deserve critical consideration when interpreting research results.
- Future work should expand on modern anesthetic combinations to elucidate mechanistic effects of dual anesthetics, which may balance toxicities.

INTRODUCTION

Surgery during pregnancy is a topic of much debate with clinical practice often governed by gestalt and past practice. In the last 20 years or so, investigators have sought to establish evidenced-based practice of if, when, and how surgery should take place during pregnancy, keeping in mind the ever-fragile balance of risk and benefit to both the mother and the growing fetus. Briefly, this section will give an overview of surgeries commonly performed on the mother and fetus, when these interventions take place during gestation, as well as the available information to date on the effect of anesthesia on the developing fetal brain.

[a] Department of Anesthesiology, Perioperative and Pain Medicine, Texas Children's Hospital, Baylor College of Medicine, 6621 Fannin Street, Suite A-3300, Houston, TX 77030, USA;
[b] Abigail Wexner Research Institute, Center for Regenerative Medicine, Nationwide Children's Hospital, 575 Children's Crossroad, Columbus, OH 43205, USA
* Corresponding author.
E-mail address: oaolutoy@texaschildrens.org

Anesthesiology Clin 39 (2021) 851–869
https://doi.org/10.1016/j.anclin.2021.08.015
1932-2275/21/© 2021 Elsevier Inc. All rights reserved.

MATERNAL SURGERY
Appendectomy

The most common surgery performed in pregnant women for nonobstetrical indications is appendectomy.[1] Over the years, there has been much debate regarding the safest method of performing this operation in pregnancy (open vs laparoscopic) and questions still remain. A 2020 review of meta-analyses determined the quality of published meta-analyses to be poor and results inconclusive.[2] In addition, the question has been raised as to whether conservative management with antibiotics is a feasible option. A recent small retrospective study by Liu and colleagues[3] compared outcomes among pregnant women with uncomplicated appendicitis who underwent surgery versus those who received antibiotic therapy only. The findings revealed that appendicitis recurred during pregnancy in one patient and in two following delivery in the antibiotic group, but there were no differences between the groups in fetal outcomes including gestational age at birth, mode of delivery, birth weight, and APGAR scores. Although consensus may not be reached regarding the best mode of therapy, there is consensus that once a diagnosis of appendicitis is made, it must be treated urgently regardless of the trimester of pregnancy in which it occurs. This is of utmost importance to avoid both fetal and maternal complications, which can include fetal demise or maternal mortality.

Cholecystectomy

Cholecystectomy is a common nonobstetrical operation performed in a pregnant woman with an incidence of 1 to 8/10,000 pregnancies.[4] Indications for cholecystectomy in pregnancy are typically infectious or inflammatory processes that require urgent intervention including acute cholecystitis, cholangitis, or gallstone pancreatitis. If left untreated, these pathologies can lead to pregnancy complications including fetal demise. The question of when this operation should be performed in pregnancy has generally been left to clinical preference with the thought that anesthesia and the stress of surgery in the first trimester may be teratogenic or lead to fetal demise. The third trimester, however, poses specific technical challenges for laparoscopic surgery and may be complicated by preterm labor. The second trimester is therefore normally preferred for cholecystectomy. A recent study by Cheng and colleagues,[5] however, sought to answer this question of timing by looking at the outcomes of pregnancies when the operation was performed in the first or third trimester compared to the second. They found there was no difference in complication rates during the first trimester compared to the second for either the mother or the fetus but comparing the third trimester to the second there was a higher rate of preterm delivery and overall maternal and fetal complications. Their findings may suggest that this operation can be safely performed in the first trimester although the effects of anesthesia on the fetus were not accounted for, and the third trimester should be avoided if possible.

Oncologic Surgery

Malignancies during pregnancy cover a broad range of diagnoses that are beyond the scope of this review. Briefly, one of the more common malignancies, breast cancer, can occur at any age or stage of life, including pregnancy, and is worth mentioning. Most often invasive breast cancer is treated at the time of diagnosis with surgery alone as first-line therapy, with few exceptions, given that most adjuvant therapies typically used in conjunction with surgery are teratogenic to the fetus.

FETAL INTERVENTIONS OR SURGERY

Several life-threatening, or high morbidity conditions in the fetus are amenable to surgical intervention in utero. To halt the disease progression and subsequent fetal demise, these procedures are commonly performed midgestation at varying periods of brain development in the fetus.

Lower Urinary Tract Obstruction

Lower urinary tract obstruction is a fetal anomaly that affects the outflow tract of the bladder and can be caused by posterior urethral valves, urethral stenosis, or urethral atresia. It is typically diagnosed midgestation by fetal anatomic survey ultrasound. Although there is no consensus on which fetuses should receive in utero intervention, a commonly used algorithm is to determine if oligohydramnios or anhydramnios is present. If either is present, kidney function is assessed with vesicocentesis and analysis of urinary markers predictive of kidney damage such as electrolytes and β-2 microglobulin. To date, these markers have not been found to be reliable indicators of postnatal renal function.[6] Nevertheless, if urine analysis is favorable and the bladder refills with urine after serial vesicocenteses, demonstrating the kidneys are still functional, then the mother is offered fetal intervention to relieve the fetal urinary obstruction typically in the second trimester. Less commonly, fetal intervention can occur in the first trimester, but it may also be offered in the third trimester if oligohydramnios or anhydramnios develop later in gestation.

Sacrococcygeal Teratoma

Sacrococcygeal teratoma is the most common fetal tumor characterized by a multilineage growth arising from the coccyx. The decision on when and how to intervene in utero is one in which multiple predictive tools have been used to better predict which fetuses are likely to succumb to the condition in utero and therefore benefit from fetal intervention. Those models include a tumor-to-fetal ratio of greater than 0.12 before 24 weeks' gestation,[7] solid tumor volume index,[8] and tumor growth rate[9] to name a few. Ultimately, the goal is to avoid lethal high-output cardiac failure in utero, as this tumor can act as a large arteriovenous fistula. Most commonly, fetal intervention for this anomaly takes place in the second trimester. Rarely, intervention may be performed in the third trimester, at the time of delivery via resection during ex utero intrapartum therapy (EXIT-to-resection).

Twin Anomalies

Twin reversed arterial perfusion (TRAP) sequence is a phenomenon that occurs in monochorionic twin gestation in which one fetus fails to fully form a functioning heart, leading to an acardiac twin and the pump twin that supports both fetuses. Often the acardiac twin is not fully formed, and in all cases is not viable outside the womb. There is no consensus as to when fetal intervention should occur to stop or reduce blood flow to the acardiac twin so the pregnancy may continue as a singleton gestation, and there is an ongoing clinical trial seeking to answer that very question (NCT02621645). Currently, most interventions take place between 16 and 18 weeks; however, there is evidence for and against earlier intervention in the literature.[10]

Twin-Twin Transfusion Syndrome (TTTS) is another fetal complication that can occur in monochorionic diamniotic twins. It occurs when placental blood flow is unequally distributed between the twins with one twin receiving less blood and the other twin receiving more. At times, the extra blood is too much for the recipient fetus to handle, leading to high output cardiac failure. Other complications include poor development in the donor fetus, neurologic sequelae, polyhydramnios, and/or fetal or perinatal demise of one or both fetuses. In light of this, interventions have been developed, which largely include fetoscopic laser therapy to coagulate the abnormal placental anastomoses between the fetuses. The standard intervention based on a randomized clinical trial published in the *New England Journal of Medicine* in 2004 is fetoscopic laser ablation before 26 weeks' gestation.[11] Interventions can take place after 26 weeks, but a recent meta-analysis looking at outcomes of expectant management, laser ablation, amniocentesis, or delivery when TTTS occurs later in gestation could not make definitive conclusions because of the poor quality of included studies.[12]

Congenital Lung Malformations

Congenital pulmonary airway malformations (CPAMs) make up at least 30% of all diagnosed congenital lung malformations.[13] These lesions are located within the lung parenchyma, share blood supply with the lung, and exhibit hamartomatous growth of terminal respiratory structures.[14] When CPAMs require in utero intervention, it is most often for hydrops or cardiac compromise. A review looking at fetal outcomes following fetal intervention for congenital lung malformations found that the average gestational age at which intervention was performed was 27.2 weeks in the absence of hydrops and 24.9 weeks when hydrops was present.[14]

In contrast to CPAMs, bronchopulmonary sequestration lesions are separate from the pulmonary parenchyma, and as such do not share blood supply but instead have their own arterial supply from branches of the aorta. They can further be classified as intralobar if located within the pulmonary pleura, or extralobar if they have their own visceral pleura.[14] In-utero intervention when required, occurs on average at 27.4 weeks of gestation.[14] With the more liberal use of fetal echocardiography to assess cardiac function and prenatal steroids to decrease the growth of the lung malformations, midgestation resection of fetal lung malformations is now rarely performed. Fetuses with persistently large masses may undergo resection at the time of delivery via an ex-utero intrapartum treatment (EXIT)-to-resection strategy (which is outside the scope of this article).

Myelomeningocele

Myelomeningocele is a neural tube defect that occurs during embryogenesis leading to exposure of the spinal cord and meninges to amniotic fluid as it protrudes outside of the spinal canal.[15] Progressive damage of the exposed spinal cord results in lower extremity, bladder, and anorectal dysfunction. A randomized control trial published in the *New England Journal of Medicine* showed that fetal surgery for myelomeningocele was associated with improved postnatal motor function compared to postnatal repair. This finding among other benefits led to the early termination of the trial.[16] In this trial, fetal surgery was performed between 19 and 25.9 weeks of gestation, although the question has been raised as to whether intervention should take place earlier in gestation for this repair as recent studies have shown that neural damage can occur even before 16 weeks of gestation.[15]

These are a few examples of the many reasons why a gravid patient, or the fetus she is carrying, may need to undergo surgery during pregnancy. In all these situations, the operation is never elective, and the well-being of both patients is taken into consideration before the final decision is made to intervene. Many studies have looked at fetal outcomes in terms of survival and postnatal morbidity following surgery during pregnancy. However, a question that remains to be fully answered is, what effect do surgery and anesthesia have on the developing fetal brain? Several studies have been performed examining the effect of anesthesia on the developing brain. Until recently, however, only a few of these studies involved concomitant surgery on the fetus as occurs with in-utero fetal surgery.

The following sections present an overview of brain development and the literature attempting to answer the question of the effect of anesthesia alone, and anesthesia plus surgery, on the developing brain in different animal models. Several studies examining the effect of anesthesia on the developing fetal brain have been conducted in rodents, nonhuman primates (NHPs), and rabbits. The ovine animal model is the prototype model for the establishment of fetal surgical procedures.[17] As such, most in-utero interventions have initially been performed in the pregnant sheep to test for feasibility and long-term outcomes before performance of these procedures in humans.

Overview of Brain Development

Fetal brain development in humans follows a series of highly coordinated steps that interpolates both structural and functional changes mediated by genetic cues, maternal hormones, and environmental stimuli. Structurally, central nervous system (CNS) development begins early in embryogenesis (~ day 25 of gestation) with the formation of the notochord.[18] This initiates neurulation, in which the ectoderm layer overlying the notochord forms the neural plate, which subsequently invaginates along the central axis to form the neural groove and lateral folds. Caudal and cranial fusion of these folds results in the neural tube, which separates from the ectoderm and becomes the structural basis for the brain and spinal cord.[19] Anatomically, by week 10 of gestation, the basics of the neural system are established and continue to develop driven primarily by external sensory input.[20–22] By midgestation, neurogenesis and dramatic changes at the cellular level initiate the production of signaling molecules for communication between nerve cells at a temporary layer of γ-aminobutyric acid (GABA)-ergic and glutamatergic neurons located between the cerebral cortex and white matter in various regional zones.[23] These immature neurons subsequently migrate to their terminal destinations. Both neurogenesis and neuronal migration are thought to peak in the second trimester, but also continue postnatally up to 2.5 years of age.[24]

During this time of rapid in-utero brain maturation, synaptogenesis (excitatory synapse formation), a pivotal aspect of functional neurodevelopment, begins midgestation and extends into the third trimester[25] Synapses are the neurobiological substrate of most cell-to-cell communication and rely on the activation of calcium channels to establish synaptic connections with analogous neurons in-utero. During synaptogenesis, these calcium channels are regulated indirectly by GABA and an N-methyl D-aspartate (NMDA) subtype of glutamate receptors leading to coordinated biochemical and morphologic changes of both presynaptic and postsynaptic features.[26] Compatibility of the biochemical connection and correct timing are essential for synapse maturation and any interference during this stage can be detrimental to the developing brain. Simultaneously, glia, astrocytes, oligodendrocytes, and Schwann cells—the support cells of the CNS that are integral for function, proliferate, migrate, and initiate axonal myelination.[27]

Amidst the myriad signaling sources, proper neurodevelopment is incomplete without developmental neuronal apoptosis which occurs during both prenatal and postnatal development. This process of programmed cell death is tightly regulated and any noxious agent or alteration in environmental stimuli that perturbs the balance can result in structural and/or functional neurologic damage.[28–30] Given that even minor perturbations can have significant and long-lasting consequences well into adulthood, nuances of the developing fetal brain and the effect of anesthetics must be rigorously studied.

Animal Models Studying Anesthesia and the Developing Brain

Research in the pregnant human to identify and discriminate any causative mechanisms of injury and to develop neuroprotective therapies pose ethical restrictions and therefore requires the use of animal models. No animal model of brain development exactly mimics that of humans, but the key stages of cortical development are surprisingly conserved among mammalian phylogeny.[25] Selecting the proper model of fetal brain injury is a crucial first step in ensuring that critical periods of development are assessed, particularly when evaluating the effects of drug and anesthesia exposure beyond teratogenicity.[31] When choosing a model to study in-utero anesthetic effects, the following criteria should be evaluated: the proportion of in-utero or prenatal brain development in the selected species; the ability to deliver the insult or stimuli in-utero at a congruent stage of development; feasibility of monitoring the outcome in-utero, ideally with testing of neurofunctional outcomes postnatally; and similarity in the volume of white to gray matter.[32] Below we review different animal models and the evaluation of fetal CNS development.

Rodents (Mice, Rats)

Perhaps the most widely used animals in anesthetic research, rodents have a practical advantage, given their low cost and ease of maintenance. They tend to have large litters and can easily be genetically manipulated to study numerous disease models over a short period as the typical gestation in rodents is 20 to 22 days compared with a human gestation of 266 to 280 days.[33] Although feasible to use to study the developing brain, several key differences are important to keep in mind when interpreting the results of rodent studies. In rodents, structural development occurs much later in gestation. Neural tube formation occurs at midgestation (day 10.5–11 in rats and 9–9.5 in mice) as opposed to day 24 (week 3) out of 280 in humans.[19,33] Similarly, hippocampal formation takes place perinatally, whereas the hippocampus is formed by the third trimester in humans.[20,34] Gyrification via cortical folding is notably absent in rodents, although the significance of this as it relates to brain development is largely debated.[35] Aside from structural architecture, the timing of regional cell differentiation also differs in rodents and humans. Although the processes are indeed parallel, they occur along different time scales. This is particularly true for synaptogenesis, which happens postnatally in rodents but begins late in the second trimester for humans. Although synaptogenesis, which has been considered the peak of fetal brain development, has been identified as a key component in the neurotoxicity of drugs,[29,33,36] most studies performed on rodents regarding neurotoxicity come from animal studies that are conducted postnatally, making it difficult to ascertain the true effects of pharmacologic agents delivered in-utero.

Rodents (Guinea Pigs)

Also, in the genus *Rodentia,* but unlike the rats and mice, guinea pigs have litters of only 3 to 4 offspring with triple the gestational time frame (67 days).[37,38] As an animal model, there are similarities with humans of the placental barrier and maternal hormonal production, making guinea pigs a popular choice in obstetric research. Guinea pig models have gained traction in studying the placental effects on perinatal brain development.[39–42] Like humans, much of guinea pig neurodevelopment occurs prenatally, with peak brain growth around 50 days gestation (75%), or 5 times longer than their rodent counterparts.[38] Their larger size also allows for easier maternal monitoring although their stature is not quite large enough to allow for direct monitoring of fetal well-being.[43] Similar to rats and mice, this model has recently been used to demonstrate an increase in neuroapoptosis after in-utero exposure to anesthetics.[43]

Nonhuman Primates (Monkeys)

NHPs are often considered for research of fetal brain development, given their close phylogenetic relationship to humans in physiology, reproduction, neuroanatomy, and cognition. Old World monkeys, particularly the macaque monkey, rhesus monkey, and baboons, have longer gestation periods (164–187 days), similar multivillious placental blood flow, and in-utero brain development, including peak growth, gyrification, and myelination, that have been mapped and equilibrated to human gestation.[44] The proximity to humans is seemingly ideal to study the effects of anesthetics on neurodevelopment; however, the use of higher-order primates in research has long been debated.[45] Before utilization, it is important to note that NHPs have a significant cost and require full-time care. The facility and staff must be specialized and highly skilled to work with the specific species. In addition, the advantages of the model must be weighed against ethical concerns especially regarding the possible affliction of pain.

Sheep

Limitations in the preclinical use of the rodent model have yielded a resurgence in the use of the large animal ovine model for studying the biological basis of injury to the developing brain. The placental barrier of sheep is distinct from humans, they give birth to 1 to 2 lambs that are neurodevelopmentally mature,[38] and weigh approximately the same as a term newborn at birth. Sheep are generally easy to handle, and pregnant sheep tolerate invasive procedures well, making for a translatable model for fetal physiology. While the sheep is considered a prenatal developer as opposed to humans who are postnatal developers, there are benefits to evaluating the ovine brain. Neuroblast formation occurs at a similar time proportionally to human brain development. In sheep, neuroblast formation occurs midgestation, around day 70 to 90 of a 145-day total gestation and in humans this cell formation occurs around 10 to 18 weeks, making it easy to choose the proper vulnerable timing for the study of effects of drugs midgestation.[46,47] This model has been proven to be suitable for the study of fetal lamb brains following anesthetic exposure after undergoing tracheal occlusion for congenital diaphragmatic hernia as baseline neuroapoptosis was readily detectable by immunohistochemistry.[48]

Whatever the animal model selected for investigation, the relative duration of anesthetic exposure to the fetal gestation must be taken into consideration. A 2-hour fetal anesthetic exposure in mice, rabbits, guinea pigs, or sheep comprises significantly different proportions of their gestational period (20, 35, 67, and 145 days, respectively) and imparts a more potent exposure than a 2-h fetal exposure in a human fetus (280 days gestation). These considerations may explain the disparate findings with fetal anesthetic exposure in animal models and the human experience.

Anesthetic Agents Implicated in Neurotoxicity to the Developing Brain

Inhalational anesthetics, such as isoflurane, [49,50]desflurane,[51] sevoflurane,[52,53] and nitrous oxide,[54] as well as intravenous agents propofol,[55–57] ketamine,[58] and midazolam,[59] have all been implicated in anesthetic-induced neurotoxicity. The neurotoxic effects are mediated by action on either GABA[60] or N-methyl-D-aspartate receptors.[61] Research suggests the increased neuroapoptotic activity secondary to GABA receptor agonism (from inhalational agents, propofol and midazolam) and NMDA antagonists (such as ketamine and nitrous oxide) can have detrimental long-term consequences in developing fetuses and young children.[62] Some of these agents are used in nonobstetrical invasive interventions during pregnancy as placental transfer yields some fetal anesthesia thereby reducing the known damaging effects of fetal distress.[63,64] Initial studies in the rat model blocked NMDA glutamate receptors on 7-day-old rat pups and noted dose-dependent but widespread apoptotic neurodegeneration prompting concerns of neurotoxicity with pediatric and fetal anesthesia use.[61] The macaque model has also been used to examine the effects of ketamine on the fetal and neonatal brain. Pregnant macaques and neonates were administered ketamine for 5 hours on gestational day 120 and postnatal day 6, respectively. The fetal and neonatal brains had a significantly higher apoptotic cell death count compared with the controls. However, the fetal brain exposed to ketamine had neuronal cell death that was 2.2 times higher compared with the neonatal brain exposed to ketamine.[65] Fortunately, ketamine is rarely used in pregnancy. Studies in rats focused on the use of inhaled anesthetics also yielded similar apoptotic results.

Evaluating the in-utero effects of GABA agonists, Palanisamy and colleagues[66] administered 1.4% isoflurane to gravid rats on gestational day 14 over 6 hours. Only adult male offspring were evaluated to avoid potential confounding effects of the estrus stage on female cognitive behavior. There were no deficits in object recognition memory, spontaneous locomotor activity, or spontaneous alterations, but a significant increase in errors of omission was made during radial arm maze testing and open arm entries during elevated plus maze testing compared with the controls. This evidence was suggestive of isoflurane having a neurodegenerative effect on spatial memory acquisition which could promote the development of anxiety-related behaviors.[66] In a study conducted by Zheng and colleagues,[67] pregnant mice also evaluated at gestational day 14 were exposed to 2.5% sevoflurane for 2 hours. Ex-vivo primary mouse neurons were also exposed to 4.1% sevoflurane for 6 hours. A marked increase in IL-6 levels, a reduction of synapse marker PSD-95, and caspase-3 activation, all markers of apoptosis, were detected in the primary mouse neurons. In addition, offspring tested in a Morris water maze at 31 days of age were found to have a deficit in learning and memory, manifested as increased escape latency from the water maze.[67] How these findings in rodents compare to equivalent exposure durations in the human fetus is unclear.

The implications of the aforementioned studies prompted the United States Food and Drug Administration (FDA) to issue a warning in late 2016 regarding the repeated or lengthy use of volatile anesthetics and intravenous sedation agents in children younger than 3 years or in pregnant women in the third trimester, because of a concern for possible impaired development of children's brains.[68,69] The body of literature in existence at the time this warning was released was composed primarily of studies with anesthetic exposure only and did not address the component of surgical stimulation to the fetus that occurs during fetal intervention.[69] Nonobstetrical procedures in pregnancy and in-utero fetal surgery usually occur in the second trimester with lower doses of general anesthesia than that described in a significant number of the anesthesia neurotoxicity studies. Addressing this and the known limitations of rodent and NHP models, effects of isoflurane on the developing brain were also evaluated using fetal sheep. We exposed pregnant ewes at midgestation (day 70 of 145) to either isoflurane 2% for 1 hour, 4% for 3 hours, or repeated exposure to 2% isoflurane for 1 hour every other day for 3 cycles to mimic various anesthetic exposures that may occur with fetal intervention. No significant neuroapoptosis was observed in either of the single exposure groups, but repeated isoflurane exposure resulted in increased neuroapoptosis of the frontal cortex sparing the hippocampus, cerebellum, and the basal ganglia.[70] Furthermore, also using the sheep model of tracheal occlusion, we had noted that isoflurane administered in conjunction with dexmedetomidine, a selective α-2 adrenoreceptor agonist, over the same duration attenuated neuroapoptosis of the hippocampus compared to isoflurane-only fetuses.[48]

Table 1 shows recent studies examining anesthesia-induced neurotoxicity in which concomitant surgical manipulation was implemented and lists the observed neuropathology in the developing brain.

Neuroprotection of the Fetal Brain and Dual Anesthetic Use in the Animal Model

The proposed mechanism of neurotoxicity with GABA agonists and NMDA antagonists is linked to derangement of synaptogenesis via blockade of GABA and glutamate receptors.[60,61] Dexmedetomidine has no interaction with the aforementioned receptors and actually reduces doses of volatile anesthetics while providing anxiolysis, hypnosis, and analgesia in the clinical setting. Bypassing both GABAergic and glutaminergic systems makes dexmedetomidine, an α-2 agonist, a top agent in the study of neuroprotection of the fetal brain. Similar to findings we observed in the ovine model,[48] protective effects of dexmedetomidine were also noted in a fetal rat model where pregnant rats at gestational day 14 received 1.5% isoflurane for 4 hours and were injected with dexmedetomidine 15 minutes before and after inhalation in incremental doses. Of all dosing intervals, 20 μg/kg of dexmedetomidine effectively blunted neuroapoptosis caused by isoflurane and inhibited downregulation of brain-derived neurotrophic factor expression. Animals in this group also performed similarly to controls in spatial and learning memory exhibiting minimal neurocognitive defect in water maze testing.[71]

Xenon, a noble gas, is an ideal anesthetic agent that has cytoprotective properties and has been shown to ameliorate anesthetic-induced neurotoxicity both in vitro and in animal models.[72–75] However, cost and scarcity limit its widespread clinical use.[76] Other agents such as lithium[77,78] and melatonin[79] have also been studied in preclinical models and have been shown to offer some neuroprotection as well.[77]

Intravenous anesthetics and GABA agonists, such as propofol and midazolam, have been associated with neurotoxicity,[43,57] although there is little evidence to demonstrate the same pronounced effects as their inhalational counterparts. Propofol is a popular anesthetic induction and maintenance agent that quickly crosses the placenta and is rapidly metabolized by the fetus. Creeley and colleagues[57] investigated the safety of propofol on the fetal and neonatal brain using the macaque model in late gestation and postnatally. Fetuses and neonates were exposed to propofol for 5 hours at gestational day 120 and at postnatal day 6, respectively. Both the fetal and neonatal groups experienced increases in neuron and oligodendrocyte cell death. In the fetal brain, cell death was concentrated in the subcortical and caudal regions, whereas cell death was mostly seen in the neocortical regions of the neonatal brain. Interestingly, this group also noted that while propofol and isoflurane affected similar regions of the brain, propofol resulted in less apoptotic cell death compared with isoflurane exposure alone.[57]

Further evidence of propofol mitigating neurodegeneration caused by isoflurane was noted by Nie and colleagues.[80] Using a mouse model to study the effects of isoflurane-propofol administration on neurotoxicity in the fetal and neonatal brain, pregnant mice were split into groups of control, isoflurane, propofol, and isoflurane + propofol. Anesthesia was administered at gestation day 15 and fetal brains were then examined for levels of interleukin-6 (IL-6) and poly-ADP polymerase (PARP) fragment. Neonatal hippocampal tissues from postnatal day 31 pups were used to measure postsynaptic density-95 (PSD-95) and synaptophysin levels. Isoflurane alone significantly increased levels of IL-6 and PARP fragment in fetuses, significantly decreasing PSD-95 and synaptophysin levels, and a deficit in cognitive function was noted in neonates. However, propofol administered in conjunction with isoflurane

Table 1
Summary of studies involving effects of anesthesia and surgery on the developing brain

Study	Authors	Species	Anesthetic	Anesthetic Time	Surgery	Endpoint	Outcome	Conclusion
Histologic evaluation of fetal brains following maternal pneumo-peritoneum	Garcia-Oria et al, 2001[87]	Guinea pigs	1% Isoflurane	40 min	Maternal CO_2 insufflation Maternal open laparotomy	Fetal central nervous system injury	No evidence of brain injury in any of the groups (anesthesia only, pneumo-peritoneum, laparotomy). Cerebral cortex, hippocampus, basal ganglia, brain stem, and cerebellum examined	Maternal Pneumoperitoneum at 5 mm Hg for 40 min does not produce fetal brain injury
Maternal surgery during pregnancy has a transient adverse effect on the developing fetal rabbit brain	Van der Veeken et al, 2019[88]	Rabbit	Sevoflurane at 1 MAC (3.8 vol%)	2 h	Maternal 5 cm median laparotomy, minimal organ manipulation + partial exposure of uterus	Motor and sensory neurologic testing	POD1: Surgery pups had significantly lower motor, sensory, and neurobehavioral scores and lower brain:body weight ratio than sham group	Surgery had a measurable impact on neonatal neurologic function and brain morphology Pups had a slower motor neurodevelopment, but by 7 wk the effect became almost undetectable.

Desflurane and Surgery Exposure During Pregnancy Decreased Synaptic Integrity and Induced Functional Deficits in Juvenile Offspring	Zou et al, 2020[89]	Mice	10% Desflurane	3 h	Maternal sciatic nerve hemitransection surgery	Cognition and memory function of juvenile offspring	7 wk postop: Significantly lower neuron density in hippocampus, lower proliferation rates and synaptophysin expression No difference in neuron density or synaptophysin, improved neurobehavioral impairment Surgery group had cognitive impairment, significantly lower hippocampal levels of postsynaptic density (PSD)-95 levels in the hippocampus compared to control (sham)	Anesthetic exposure together with surgery during pregnancy may induce detrimental effects in juvenile offspring of mice via the induction of cell death and disruption of synaptic integrity

(continued on next page)

Table 1
(continued)

Study	Authors	Species	Anesthetic	Anesthetic Time	Surgery	Endpoint	Outcome	Conclusion
Effects of Maternal Abdominal Surgery on Fetal Brain Development in the Rabbit Model	Bleeser et al, 2021[90]	Rabbit	1 MAC of sevoflurane in 30% oxygen	2 h	Maternal laparoscopic appendectomy	Neuron density in frontal cortex, neuro-behavioral assessment	Neuron densities were significantly lower in the surgery group in the caudate nucleus ($P = .0180$), no other regions No differences in neuro-behavioral assessment	Abdominal surgery in pregnant rabbits at a gestational age corresponding to the end of human second trimester results in limited neurohistological changes but not in neurobehavioral impairments. High intrauterine mortality limits translation to clinical scenario, where fetal mortality is close to zero.
Fetal Surgery Decreases Anesthesia Induced Neuro-apoptosis in the Mid-Gestational Fetal Ovine Brain	Olutoye et al, 2019[91]	Sheep	2% Isoflurane 4% Isoflurane Low dose (LD) = 2% + 1 h High dose (HD) = 4% + 3 h	1 h and 3 h	Surgery (S) = fetal femoral cutdown	Fetal brain neuro-apoptosis	Neuroapoptosis in **dentate gyrus** was significantly less in the HD + S group vs the HD, or control Neuroapoptosis in the pyramidal layer of the	Fetal surgery decreases isoflurane-induced neuroapoptosis in the dentate gyrus and the pyramidal layer of mid-gestational fetal sheep. Long-term effects of these observations on memory and learning deserve further exploration.

Study	Animal	Drugs	Time	Outcome measure	Results	Conclusion
					hippocampus was significantly less in the HD + S vs HD or control	
Van der Veeken et al, 2021[92]	Rabbit	Sevoflurane at 1 MAC (3.8 vol%) *plus* Fetal drugs: Fentanyl 0.2 mcg, Cisatracurium 10 mcg & Atropine 0.2 mcg	1 h	Maternal median laparotomy · Neuro-behavioral assessment & neuron density	No difference in motor or sensory scores in pups who received medication and the sham pups Comparable neuron densities in both groups of pups; higher synaptic density in medicated pups but no translation to any measurable functional impact	Fetal injected medication (atropine-fentanyl-curare), does not result in measurable short term neurocognitive effects Fetally injected drugs for immobilization and analgesia do not modify fetal brain development in a rabbit model.

Abbreviation: MAC, minimum alveolar concentration.

resulted in a significant reduction of the neurotoxic effects seen in both fetal and neonatal mice exposed only to isoflurane. In addition, the cognitive impairment seen in postnatal day 31 pups exposed to isoflurane was attenuated with the addition of propofol.[80]

Midazolam, a benzodiazepine, has been implicated in anesthetic-induced neurotoxicity,[43] but has also been shown to ameliorate brain injury in some instances. For example, the neurodegenerative effects of ketamine were decreased by midazolam in a study by Li and colleagues.[81] In this study, using the rat model, pregnant rats at G19 were exposed to either ketamine alone, ketamine in combination with midazolam or midazolam alone with results verified in vitro. Ketamine alone increased reactive oxidative species which can trigger apoptosis by upregulating autophagy, decreased total antioxidant capacity, and increased levels of malondialdehyde, a naturally occurring marker of oxidative stress. These harmful effects were all decreased by midazolam.[81] Additional studies on clinically relevant and available drugs that exhibit neuroprotective effects are required.

As preclinical studies continue to help us better understand the role of coincidental surgery and/or supplemental fetal anesthesia on anesthesia-induced neurotoxicity in fetal animals, we should exercise caution in interpretation. All these studies provide intriguing preclinical information that would need to be validated in longitudinal observational studies in pregnant women, particularly the studies demonstrating dual anesthetic use and mitigation of neurotoxicity, once ethical challenges can be circumvented with good study design. It is important to note that similar concerns have been raised about the effects of anesthesia on the brain development of infants and young children. However, prospective studies in young children following anesthetic exposures of short duration have so far not confirmed preclinical observations.[82–84]

In summary, anesthetic agents acting via the GABA and NMDA pathways cause perturbations in fetal brain development that may be deleterious. Some of these neurotoxic effects can be easily mediated by combination therapy of implicated agents (eg, propofol, isoflurane) or the addition of α-2 adrenoreceptor agonists such as dexmedetomidine. Coincidental or concomitant surgery may be somewhat protective compared with unchallenged anesthetic exposure. Given the wide differences in proportional gestational exposure to anesthetics in the animal models, the true clinical impact on newborns following in-utero anesthetic exposure is unclear and would require longitudinal studies. Nevertheless, the possible risks to the fetus should be considered alongside the potential benefit of the procedure and anesthetic to the mother and/or fetus. This should be discussed as part of the informed consent. Ultimately, brain function is not impacted only by what happens during fetal development but also by exposure or insults to the brain during other significant stages of brain development such as from birth to age 5 years and adolescence.[85,86]

CLINICS CARE POINTS

- Maternal and surgical societies support surgical procedures and interventions as appropriate in any trimester of pregnancy.
- When counseling a pregnant patient undergoing maternal or fetal anesthesia and surgery, it is important to note that preclinical animal model-based research findings have not been entirely replicated in humans.
- Consider dual anesthetic agents for general anesthesia, including use of dexmedetomidine, as these agents appear to have favorable neuroapoptotic outcomes in animal models.

REFERENCES

1. Kort B, Katz VL, Watson WJ. The effect of nonobstetric operation during pregnancy. Surg Gynecol Obstet 1993;177(4):371–6.
2. Augustin G, Boric M, Barcot O, et al. Discordant outcomes of laparoscopic versus open appendectomy for suspected appendicitis during pregnancy in published meta-analyses: An overview of systematic reviews. Surg Endosc 2020;34(10):4245–56.
3. Liu J, Ahmad M, Wu J, et al. Antibiotic is a safe and feasible option for uncomplicated appendicitis in pregnancy - A retrospective cohort study. Asian J Endosc Surg 2021;14(2):207–12.
4. Kuy S, Roman SA, Desai R, et al. Outcomes following cholecystectomy in pregnant and nonpregnant women. Surgery 2009;146(2):358–66.
5. Cheng V, Matsushima K, Ashbrook M, et al. Association between trimester and outcomes after cholecystectomy during pregnancy. J Am Coll Surg 2021; 233(1):29–37.e1.
6. Morris RK, Quinlan-Jones E, Kilby MD, et al. Systematic review of accuracy of fetal urine analysis to predict poor postnatal renal function in cases of congenital urinary tract obstruction. Prenat Diagn 2007;27(10):900–11.
7. Akinkuotu AC, Coleman A, Shue E, et al. Predictors of poor prognosis in prenatally diagnosed sacrococcygeal teratoma: A multiinstitutional review. J Pediatr Surg 2015;50(5):771–4.
8. Coleman A, Kline-Fath B, Keswani S, et al. Prenatal solid tumor volume index: Novel prenatal predictor of adverse outcome in sacrococcygeal teratoma. J Surg Res 2013;184(1):330–6.
9. Coleman A, Shaaban A, Keswani S, et al. Sacrococcygeal teratoma growth rate predicts adverse outcomes. J Pediatr Surg 2014;49(6):985–9.
10. Vitucci A, Fichera A, Fratelli N, et al. Twin reversed arterial perfusion sequence: Current treatment options. Int J Womens Health 2020;12:435–43.
11. Senat MV, Deprest J, Boulvain M, et al. Endoscopic laser surgery versus serial amnioreduction for severe twin-to-twin transfusion syndrome. N Engl J Med 2004;351(2):136–44.
12. Sileo FG, D'antonio F, Benlioglu C, et al. Perinatal outcomes of twin pregnancies complicated by late twin-twin transfusion syndrome: A systematic review and meta-analysis. Acta Obstet Gynecol Scand 2021;100(5):832–42.
13. Zobel M, Gologorsky R, Lee H, et al. Congenital lung lesions. Semin Pediatr Surg 2019;28(4):150821.
14. Witlox RS, Lopriore E, Oepkes D, et al. Neonatal outcome after prenatal interventions for congenital lung lesions. Early Hum Dev 2011;87(9):611–8.
15. Ben Miled S, Loeuillet L, Van Huyen Duong, et al. Severe and progressive neuronal loss in myelomeningocele begins before 16 weeks of pregnancy. Am J Obstet Gynecol 2020;223(2):256.e1–9.
16. Adzick NS, Thom EA, Spong CY, et al. A randomized trial of prenatal versus postnatal repair of myelomeningocele. N Engl J Med 2011;364(11):993–1004.
17. Nathanielz PW. Animal models in fetal medicine. North-Holland, Amsterdam: Elsevier; 1980.
18. Huang H, Vasung L. Gaining insight of fetal brain development with diffusion MRI and histology. Int J Dev Neurosci 2014;32:11–22.
19. Rice D, Barone S. Critical periods of vulnerability for the developing nervous system: Evidence from humans and animal models. Environ Health Perspect 2000; 108(Suppl 3):511–33.

20. Altman J. Morphological and behavioral markers of environmentally induced retardation of brain development: An animal model. Environ Health Perspect 1987;74:153–68.

21. Gierthmuehlen M, Wang X, Gkogkidis A, et al. Mapping of sheep sensory cortex with a novel microelectrocorticography grid. J Comp Neurol 2014;522(16): 3590–608.

22. Studholme C. Mapping fetal brain development in utero using magnetic resonance imaging: The big bang of brain mapping. Annu Rev Biomed Eng 2011; 13:345–68.

23. Bayer SA, Altman J, Russo RJ, et al. Timetables of neurogenesis in the human brain based on experimentally determined patterns in the rat. Neurotoxicology 1993;14(1):83–144.

24. Clancy B, Darlington RB, Finlay BL. Translating developmental time across mammalian species. Neuroscience 2001;105(1):7–17.

25. Clancy B, Finlay BL, Darlington RB, et al. Extrapolating brain development from experimental species to humans. Neurotoxicology 2007;28(5):931–7.

26. Crossley KJ, Nitsos I, Walker DW, et al. Steroid-sensitive GABAA receptors in the fetal sheep brain. Neuropharmacology 2003;45(4):461–72.

27. Baud O, Saint-Faust M. Neuroinflammation in the developing brain: Risk factors, involvement of microglial cells, and implication for early anesthesia. Anesth Analg 2019;128(4):718–25.

28. Andropoulos DB. Effect of anesthesia on the developing brain: Infant and fetus. Fetal Diagn Ther 2017. https://doi.org/10.1159/000475928.

29. Bree B, Gourdin M, De Kock M. Anesthesia and cerebral apoptosis. Acta Anaesthesiol Belg 2008;59(3):127–37.

30. Colon E, Bittner EA, Kussman B, et al. Anesthesia, brain changes, and behavior: Insights from neural systems biology. Prog Neurobiol 2017;153:121–60.

31. Palanisamy A. Maternal anesthesia and fetal neurodevelopment. Int J Obstet Anesth 2012;21(2):152–62.

32. Rees S, Harding R, Walker D. The biological basis of injury and neuroprotection in the fetal and neonatal brain. Int J Dev Neurosci 2011;29(6):551–63.

33. Semple BD, Blomgren K, Gimlin K, et al. Brain development in rodents and humans: Identifying benchmarks of maturation and vulnerability to injury across species. Prog Neurobiol 2013;106-107:1–16.

34. Rees S, Inder T. Fetal and neonatal origins of altered brain development. Early Hum Dev 2005;81(9):753–61.

35. Dubois J, Benders M, Borradori-Tolsa C, et al. Primary cortical folding in the human newborn: An early marker of later functional development. Brain 2008;131(Pt 8):2028–41.

36. Jevtovic-Todorovic V. Developmental synaptogenesis and general anesthesia: A kiss of death? Curr Pharm Des 2012;18(38):6225–31.

37. Dobbing JSJ. Growth and development of the brain and spinal cord of the guinea pig. Brain Res 1970;17(1):115–23.

38. Dobbing J, Sands J. Comparative aspects of the brain growth spurt. Early Hum Dev 1979;3(1):79–83.

39. Nelson PS, Gilbert RD, Longo LD. Fetal growth and placental diffusing capacity in guinea pigs following long-term maternal exercise. J Dev Physiol 1983;5(1):1–10.

40. Sun SY, Zhang W, Han X, et al. Cell proliferation and apoptosis in the fetal and neonatal ovary of guinea pigs. Genet Mol Res 2014;13(1):1570–8.

41. Thompson LP, Turan S, Aberdeen GW. Sex differences and the effects of intra-uterine hypoxia on growth and in vivo heart function of fetal guinea pigs. Am J Physiol Regul Integr Comp Physiol 2020;319(3):R243–54.

42. Williams D, Dunn S, Richardson A, et al. Time course of fetal tissue invasion by listeria monocytogenes following an oral inoculation in pregnant guinea pigs. J Food Prot 2011;74(2):248–53.

43. Rizzi S, Carter LB, Ori C, et al. Clinical anesthesia causes permanent damage to the fetal guinea pig brain. Brain Pathol 2008;18(2):198–210.

44. Liu Z, Wang X, Newman N, et al. Anatomical and diffusion MRI brain atlases of the fetal rhesus macaque brain at 85, 110 and 135 days gestation. Neuroimage 2020;206:116310.

45. Grigsby PL. Animal models to study placental development and function throughout normal and dysfunctional human pregnancy. Semin Reprod Med 2016;34(1):11–6.

46. Dobbing J, Sands J. Quantitative growth and development of human brain. Arch Dis Child 1973;48(10):757–67.

47. McIntosh GH, Baghurst KI, Potter BJ, et al. Foetal brain development in the sheep. Neuropathol Appl Neurobiol 1979;5(2):103–14.

48. Olutoye OA, Lazar DA, Akinkuotu AC, et al. Potential of the ovine brain as a model for anesthesia-induced neuroapoptosis. Pediatr Surg Int 2015;31(9):865–9.

49. Kong FJ, Tang YW, Lou AF, et al. Effects of isoflurane exposure during pregnancy on postnatal memory and learning in offspring rats. Mol Biol Rep 2012;39(4):4849–55.

50. Kong FJ, Ma LL, Hu WW, et al. Fetal exposure to high isoflurane concentration induces postnatal memory and learning deficits in rats. Biochem Pharmacol 2012;84(4):558–63.

51. Kodama M, Satoh Y, Otsubo Y, et al. Neonatal desflurane exposure induces more robust neuroapoptosis than do isoflurane and sevoflurane and impairs working memory. Anesthesiology 2011;115(5):979–91.

52. Wu B, Yu Z, You S, et al. Physiological disturbance may contribute to neurode-generation induced by isoflurane or sevoflurane in 14 day old rats. PLoS One 2014;9(1):e84622.

53. Hirotsu A, Iwata Y, Tatsumi K, et al. Maternal exposure to volatile anesthetics in-duces IL-6 in fetal brains and affects neuronal development. Eur J Pharmacol 2019;863:172682.

54. Zhen Y, Dong Y, Wu X, et al. Nitrous oxide plus isoflurane induces apoptosis and increases beta-amyloid protein levels. Anesthesiology 2009;111(4):741–52.

55. Xiong M, Li J, Alhashem HM, et al. Propofol exposure in pregnant rats induces neurotoxicity and persistent learning deficit in the offspring. Brain Sci 2014;4(2):356–75.

56. Xiong M, Zhang L, Li J, et al. Propofol-induced neurotoxicity in the fetal animal brain and developments in modifying these effects-an updated review of propofol fetal exposure in laboratory animal studies. Brain Sci 2016;6(2). https://doi.org/10.3390/brainsci6020011.

57. Creeley C, Dikranian K, Dissen G, et al. Propofol-induced apoptosis of neurones and oligodendrocytes in fetal and neonatal rhesus macaque brain. Br J Anaesth 2013;110(Suppl 1):29.

58. Wang C, Sadovova N, Hotchkiss C, et al. Blockade of N-methyl-D-aspartate re-ceptors by ketamine produces loss of postnatal day 3 monkey frontal cortical neurons in culture. Toxicol Sci 2006;91(1):192–201.

59. Young C, Jevtovic-Todorovic V, Qin YQ, et al. Potential of ketamine and midazolam, individually or in combination, to induce apoptotic neurodegeneration in the infant mouse brain. Br J Pharmacol 2005;146(2):189–97.

60. Zhao YL, Xiang Q, Shi QY, et al. GABAergic excitotoxicity injury of the immature hippocampal pyramidal neurons' exposure to isoflurane. Anesth Analg 2011; 113(5):1152–60.

61. Ikonomidou C, Bosch F, Miksa M, et al. Blockade of NMDA receptors and apoptotic neurodegeneration in the developing brain. Science 1999; 283(5398):70–4.

62. Jevtovic-Todorovic V, Hartman RE, Izumi Y, et al. Early exposure to common anesthetic agents causes widespread neurodegeneration in the developing rat brain and persistent learning deficits. J Neurosci 2003;23(3):876–82.

63. Bonnet MP, Bruyere M, Moufouki M, et al. Anaesthesia, a cause of fetal distress? Ann Fr Anesth Reanim 2007;26(7–8):694–8.

64. Schepanski S, Buss C, Hanganu-Opatz IL, et al. Prenatal immune and endocrine modulators of offspring's brain development and cognitive functions later in life. Front Immunol 2018;9:2186.

65. Brambrink AM, Evers AS, Avidan MS, et al. Ketamine-induced neuroapoptosis in the fetal and neonatal rhesus macaque brain. Anesthesiology 2012;116(2):372–84.

66. Palanisamy A, Baxter MG, Keel PK, et al. Rats exposed to isoflurane in utero during early gestation are behaviorally abnormal as adults. Anesthesiology 2011; 114(3):521–8.

67. Zheng H, Dong Y, Xu Z, et al. Sevoflurane anesthesia in pregnant mice induces neurotoxicity in fetal and offspring mice. Anesthesiology 2013;118(3):516–26.

68. United States Food and Drug Administration. FDA drug safety communication: FDA review results in new warnings about using general anesthetics and sedation drugs in young children and pregnant women. . Updated 2017. Accessed July 06, 2017. Available at: https://www.fda.gov/drugs/drug-safety-and-availability/fda-drug-safety-communication-fda-review-results-new-warnings-about-using-general-anesthetics-and.

69. Olutoye OA, Baker BW, Belfort MA, et al. Food and drug administration warning on anesthesia and brain development: Implications for obstetric and fetal surgery. Am J Obstet Gynecol 2018;218(1):98–102.

70. Olutoye OA, Sheikh F, Zamora IJ, et al. Repeated isoflurane exposure and neuroapoptosis in the midgestation fetal sheep brain. Am J Obstet Gynecol 2016; 214(4):542.e1–8.

71. Su ZY, Ye Q, Liu XB, et al. Dexmedetomidine mitigates isoflurane-induced neurodegeneration in fetal rats during the second trimester of pregnancy. Neural Regen Res 2017;12(8):1329–37.

72. Maze M, Laitio T. Neuroprotective properties of xenon. Mol Neurobiol 2020;57(1): 118–24.

73. Campos-Pires R, Onggradito H, Ujvari E, et al. Xenon treatment after severe traumatic brain injury improves locomotor outcome, reduces acute neuronal loss and enhances early beneficial neuroinflammation: A randomized, blinded, controlled animal study. Crit Care 2020;24(1):667–9.

74. Gill H, Pickering AE. The effects of xenon on sevoflurane anesthesia-induced acidosis and brain cell apoptosis in immature rats. Paediatr Anaesth 2021; 31(3):372–4.

75. Liu F, Liu S, Patterson TA, et al. Protective effects of xenon on propofol-induced neurotoxicity in human neural stem cell-derived models. Mol Neurobiol 2020; 57(1):200–7.

76. Robel R, Caroccio P, Maze M. Methods for defining the neuroprotective properties of xenon. Methods Enzymol 2018;602:273–88.
77. Straiko MM, Young C, Cattano D, et al. Lithium protects against anesthesia-induced developmental neuroapoptosis. Anesthesiology 2009;110(4):862–8.
78. Young C, Straiko MM, Johnson SA, et al. Ethanol causes and lithium prevents neuroapoptosis and suppression of pERK in the infant mouse brain. Neurobiol Dis 2008;31(3):355–60.
79. Yon JH, Carter LB, Reiter RJ, et al. Melatonin reduces the severity of anesthesia-induced apoptotic neurodegeneration in the developing rat brain. Neurobiol Dis 2006;21(3):522–30.
80. Nie Y, Li S, Yan T, et al. Propofol attenuates isoflurane-induced neurotoxicity and cognitive impairment in fetal and offspring mice. Anesth Analg 2020;131(5): 1616–25.
81. Li Y, Li X, Zhao J, et al. Midazolam attenuates autophagy and apoptosis caused by ketamine by decreasing reactive oxygen species in the hippocampus of fetal rats. Neuroscience 2018;388:460–71.
82. Davidson AJ, Disma N, de Graaff JC, et al. Neurodevelopmental outcome at 2 years of age after general anaesthesia and awake-regional anaesthesia in infancy (GAS): An international multicentre, randomised controlled trial. Lancet 2016;387(10015):239–50.
83. McCann ME, de Graaff JC, Dorris L, et al. Neurodevelopmental outcome at 5 years of age after general anaesthesia or awake-regional anaesthesia in infancy (GAS): An international, multicentre, randomised, controlled equivalence trial. Lancet 2019;393(10172):664–77.
84. Sun LS, Li G, Miller TL, et al. Association between a single general anesthesia exposure before age 36 months and neurocognitive outcomes in later childhood. JAMA 2016;315(21):2312–20.
85. Mayberry RI, Lock E, Kazmi H. Linguistic ability and early language exposure. Nature 2002;417(6884):38.
86. Ko WR, Liaw YP, Huang JY, et al. Exposure to general anesthesia in early life and the risk of attention deficit/hyperactivity disorder development: A nationwide, retrospective matched-cohort study. Paediatr Anaesth 2014;24(7):741–8.
87. Garcia-Oria M, Ali A, Reynolds JD, et al. Histologic evaluation of fetal brains following maternal pneumoperitoneum. Surg Endosc 2001;15(11):1294–8.
88. Van der Veeken L, Van der Merwe J, Devroe S, et al. Maternal surgery during pregnancy has a transient adverse effect on the developing fetal rabbit brain. Am J Obstet Gynecol 2019;221(4):355.e1–19.
89. Zou S, Wei ZZ, Yue Y, et al. Desflurane and Surgery Exposure During Pregnancy Decrease Synaptic Integrity and Induce Functional Deficits in Juvenile Offspring Mice. Neurochem Res 2020;45(2):418–27.
90. Bleeser T, Van Der Veeken L, Devroe S, et al. Effects of Maternal Abdominal Surgery on Fetal Brain Development in the Rabbit Model. Fetal Diagn Ther 2021; 48(3):189–200.
91. Olutoye OA, Cruz SM, Akinkuotu AC, et al. Fetal Surgery Decreases Anesthesia-Induced Neuroapoptosis in the Mid-Gestational Fetal Ovine Brain. Fetal Diagn Ther 2019;46(2):111–8.
92. Van der Veeken L, Inversetti A, Galgano A, et al. Fetally-injected drugs for immobilization and analgesia do not modify fetal brain development in a rabbit model. Prenat Diagn 2021;41(9):1164–70.

UNITED STATES POSTAL SERVICE®
Statement of Ownership, Management, and Circulation (All Periodicals Publications Except Requester Publications)

1. Publication Title	2. Publication Number	3. Filing Date
ANESTHESIOLOGY CLINICS	000 – 275	9/18/2021

4. Issue Frequency	5. Number of Issues Published Annually	6. Annual Subscription Price
MAR, JUN, SEP, DEC	4	$368.00

7. Complete Mailing Address of Known Office of Publication (Not printer) (Street, city, county, state, and ZIP+4®)

ELSEVIER INC.
230 Park Avenue, Suite 800
New York, NY 10169

Contact Person
Malathi Samayan

Telephone (Include area code)
91-44-4299-4507

8. Complete Mailing Address of Headquarters or General Business Office of Publisher (Not printer)

ELSEVIER INC.
230 Park Avenue, Suite 800
New York, NY 10169

9. Full Names and Complete Mailing Addresses of Publisher, Editor, and Managing Editor (Do not leave blank)

Publisher (Name and complete mailing address)

DOLORES MELONI, ELSEVIER INC.
1600 JOHN F KENNEDY BLVD. SUITE 1800
PHILADELPHIA, PA 19103-2899

Editor (Name and complete mailing address)

JOANNA COLLETT, ELSEVIER INC.
1600 JOHN F KENNEDY BLVD. SUITE 1800
PHILADELPHIA, PA 19103-2899

Managing Editor (Name and complete mailing address)

PATRICK MANLEY, ELSEVIER INC.
1600 JOHN F KENNEDY BLVD. SUITE 1800
PHILADELPHIA, PA 19103-2899

10. Owner (Do not leave blank. If the publication is owned by a corporation, give the name and address of the corporation immediately followed by the names and addresses of all stockholders owning or holding 1 percent or more of the total amount of stock. If not owned by a corporation, give the names and addresses of the individual owners. If owned by a partnership or other unincorporated firm, give its name and address as well as those of each individual owner. If the publication is published by a nonprofit organization, give its name and address.)

Full Name	Complete Mailing Address
WHOLLY OWNED SUBSIDIARY OF REED/ELSEVIER, US HOLDINGS	1600 JOHN F KENNEDY BLVD. SUITE 1800 PHILADELPHIA, PA 19103-2899

11. Known Bondholders, Mortgagees, and Other Security Holders Owning or Holding 1 Percent or More of Total Amount of Bonds, Mortgages, or Other Securities. If none, check box ▸ ☐ None

Full Name	Complete Mailing Address
N/A	

12. Tax Status (For completion by nonprofit organizations authorized to mail at nonprofit rates) (Check one)
The purpose, function, and nonprofit status of this organization and the exempt status for federal income tax purposes:
☒ Has Not Changed During Preceding 12 Months
☐ Has Changed During Preceding 12 Months (Publisher must submit explanation of change with this statement)

PS Form **3526**, July 2014 [Page 1 of 4 (see instructions page 4)]   PSN: 7530-01-000-9631   PRIVACY NOTICE: See our privacy policy on www.usps.com

---

13. Publication Title		14. Issue Date for Circulation Data Below
Anesthesiology Clinics		JUNE 2021

15. Extent and Nature of Circulation		Average No. Copies Each Issue During Preceding 12 Months	No. Copies of Single Issue Published Nearest to Filing Date
a. Total Number of Copies (Net press run)		220	176
b. Paid Circulation (By Mail and Outside the Mail)	(1) Mailed Outside-County Paid Subscriptions Stated on PS Form 3541 (Include paid distribution above nominal rate, advertiser's proof copies, and exchange copies)	79	68
	(2) Mailed In-County Paid Subscriptions Stated on PS Form 3541 (Include paid distribution above nominal rate, advertiser's proof copies, and exchange copies)	0	0
	(3) Paid Distribution Outside the Mails Including Sales Through Dealers and Carriers, Street Vendors, Counter Sales, and Other Paid Distribution Outside USPS®	94	73
	(4) Paid Distribution by Other Classes of Mail Through the USPS (e.g., First-Class Mail®)	0	0
c. Total Paid Distribution (Sum of 15b (1), (2), (3), and (4))	▸	173	141
d. Free or Nominal Rate Distribution (By Mail and Outside the Mail)	(1) Free or Nominal Rate Outside-County Copies included on PS Form 3541	29	18
	(2) Free or Nominal Rate In-County Copies Included on PS Form 3541	0	0
	(3) Free or Nominal Rate Copies Mailed at Other Classes Through the USPS (e.g., First-Class Mail)	0	0
	(4) Free or Nominal Rate Distribution Outside the Mail (Carriers or other means)	0	0
e. Total Free or Nominal Rate Distribution (Sum of 15d (1), (2), (3) and (4))	▸	29	18
f. Total Distribution (Sum of 15c and 15e)	▸	202	159
g. Copies not Distributed (See Instructions to Publishers #4 (page 83))	▸	18	17
h. Total (Sum of 15f and g)	▸	220	176
i. Percent Paid (15c divided by 15f times 100)	▸	85.64%	88.67%

* If you are claiming electronic copies, go to line 16 on page 3. If you are not claiming electronic copies, skip to line 17 on page 3.

16. Electronic Copy Circulation		Average No. Copies Each Issue During Preceding 12 Months	No. Copies of Single Issue Published Nearest to Filing Date
a. Paid Electronic Copies	▸		
b. Total Paid Print Copies (Line 15c) + Paid Electronic Copies (Line 16a)	▸		
c. Total Print Distribution (Line 15f) + Paid Electronic Copies (Line 16a)	▸		
d. Percent Paid (Both Print & Electronic Copies) (16b divided by 16c × 100)	▸		

☒ I certify that 50% of all my distributed copies (electronic and print) are paid above a nominal price.

17. Publication of Statement of Ownership

☒ If the publication is a general publication, publication of this statement is required. Will be printed
in the DECEMBER 2021 issue of this publication.

☐ Publication not required.

18. Signature and Title of Editor, Publisher, Business Manager, or Owner	Date
Malathi Samayan - Distribution Controller *Malathi Samayan*	9/18/2021

I certify that all information furnished on this form is true and complete. I understand that anyone who furnishes false or misleading information on this form or who omits material or information requested on the form may be subject to criminal sanctions (including fines and imprisonment) and/or civil sanctions (including civil penalties).

PS Form **3526**, July 2014 (Page 2 of 4)   PRIVACY NOTICE: See our privacy policy on www.usps.com

Moving?

Make sure your subscription moves with you!

To notify us of your new address, find your **Clinics Account Number** (located on your mailing label above your name), and contact customer service at:

Email: journalscustomerservice-usa@elsevier.com

800-654-2452 (subscribers in the U.S. & Canada)
314-447-8871 (subscribers outside of the U.S. & Canada)

Fax number: 314-447-8029

Elsevier Health Sciences Division
Subscription Customer Service
3251 Riverport Lane
Maryland Heights, MO 63043

Printed and bound by CPI Group (UK) Ltd, Croydon, CR0 4YY
08/05/2025
01864704-0001